Medicinal Plants and Natural Compounds in Health and Disease: Progresses, Challenges, Opportunities

Medicinal Plants and Natural Compounds in Health and Disease: Progresses, Challenges, Opportunities

Editors

Marilena Gilca
Adelina Vlad

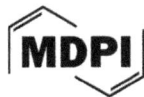

Basel • Beijing • Wuhan • Barcelona • Belgrade • Novi Sad • Cluj • Manchester

Marilena Gilca
Biochemistry Department
Carol Davila University of
Medicine and Pharmacy
Bucharest
Romania

Adelina Vlad
Physiology Department
Carol Davila University of
Medicine and Pharmacy
Bucharest
Romania

Editorial Office
MDPI AG
Grosspeteranlage 5
4052 Basel, Switzerland

This is a reprint of the Special Issue, published open access by the journal *International Journal of Molecular Sciences* (ISSN 1422-0067), freely accessible at: www.mdpi.com/journal/ijms/special_issues/X71A174148.

For citation purposes, cite each article independently as indicated on the article page online and using the guide below:

Lastname, A.A.; Lastname, B.B. Article Title. *Journal Name* **Year**, *Volume Number*, Page Range.

ISBN 978-3-7258-1652-1 (Hbk)
ISBN 978-3-7258-1651-4 (PDF)
https://doi.org/10.3390/books978-3-7258-1651-4

© 2024 by the authors. Articles in this book are Open Access and distributed under the Creative Commons Attribution (CC BY) license. The book as a whole is distributed by MDPI under the terms and conditions of the Creative Commons Attribution-NonCommercial-NoDerivs (CC BY-NC-ND) license (https://creativecommons.org/licenses/by-nc-nd/4.0/).

Contents

About the Editors vii

Laura Toma, Mariana Deleanu, Gabriela Maria Sanda, Teodora Barbălată, Loredan Ştefan Niculescu and Anca Volumnia Sima et al.
Bioactive Compounds Formulated in Phytosomes Administered as Complementary Therapy for Metabolic Disorders
Reprinted from: *Int. J. Mol. Sci.* **2024**, 25, 4162, doi:10.3390/ijms25084162 1

Yebin Kim, Seonghyeon Nam, Jongbin Lim and Miran Jang
Autumn Olive (*Elaeagnus umbellata* Thunb.) Berries Improve Lipid Metabolism and Delay Aging in Middle-Aged *Caenorhabditis elegans*
Reprinted from: *Int. J. Mol. Sci.* **2024**, 25, 3418, doi:10.3390/ijms25063418 41

Chang Wang, Yitian Yang, Jinyan Chen, Xueyan Dai, Chenghong Xing and Caiying Zhang et al.
Berberine Protects against High-Energy and Low-Protein Diet-Induced Hepatic Steatosis: Modulation of Gut Microbiota and Bile Acid Metabolism in Laying Hens
Reprinted from: *Int. J. Mol. Sci.* **2023**, 24, 17304, doi:10.3390/ijms242417304 55

Syed Sayeed Ahmad, Khurshid Ahmad, Ye Chan Hwang, Eun Ju Lee and Inho Choi
Therapeutic Applications of Ginseng Natural Compounds for Health Management
Reprinted from: *Int. J. Mol. Sci.* **2023**, 24, 17290, doi:10.3390/ijms242417290 71

Jialuan Wang, Fengyi Zhao, Wenlong Wu, Lianfei Lyu, Weilin Li and Chunhong Zhang
Ellagic Acid from Hull Blackberries: Extraction, Purification, and Potential Anticancer Activity
Reprinted from: *Int. J. Mol. Sci.* **2023**, 24, 15228, doi:10.3390/ijms242015228 86

Aseel Ali Hasan, Elena Kalinina, Julia Nuzhina, Yulia Volodina, Alexander Shtil and Victor Tatarskiy
Potentiation of Cisplatin Cytotoxicity in Resistant Ovarian Cancer SKOV3/Cisplatin Cells by Quercetin Pre-Treatment
Reprinted from: *Int. J. Mol. Sci.* **2023**, 24, 10960, doi:10.3390/ijms241310960 104

Tsz Ki Wang, Shaoting Xu, Yuanjian Fan, Jing Wu, Zilin Wang and Yue Chen et al.
The Synergistic Effect of Proanthocyanidin and HDAC Inhibitor Inhibit Breast Cancer Cell Growth and Promote Apoptosis
Reprinted from: *Int. J. Mol. Sci.* **2023**, 24, 10476, doi:10.3390/ijms241310476 121

Teodora-Cristiana Grădinaru, Marilena Gilca, Adelina Vlad and Dorin Dragoș
Relevance of Phytochemical Taste for Anti-Cancer Activity: A Statistical Inquiry
Reprinted from: *Int. J. Mol. Sci.* **2023**, 24, 16227, doi:10.3390/ijms242216227 134

Xiaoyue Li, Zewen Liu, Ting Gao, Wei Liu, Keli Yang and Rui Guo et al.
Tea Polyphenols Protects Tracheal Epithelial Tight Junctions in Lung during *Actinobacillus pleuropneumoniae* Infection via Suppressing TLR-4/MAPK/PKC-MLCK Signaling
Reprinted from: *Int. J. Mol. Sci.* **2023**, 24, 11842, doi:10.3390/ijms241411842 156

Lei Chen, Tong Yu, Yiman Zhai, Hongguang Nie, Xin Li and Yan Ding
Luteolin Enhances Transepithelial Sodium Transport in the Lung Alveolar Model: Integrating Network Pharmacology and Mechanism Study
Reprinted from: *Int. J. Mol. Sci.* **2023**, 24, 10122, doi:10.3390/ijms241210122 173

Qilin Huang, Wei Li, Xiaohan Jing, Chen Liu, Saad Ahmad and Lina Huang et al.
Naringin's Alleviation of the Inflammatory Response Caused by *Actinobacillus pleuropneumoniae* by Downregulating the NF-B/NLRP3 Signalling Pathway
Reprinted from: *Int. J. Mol. Sci.* **2024**, 25, 1027, doi:10.3390/ijms25021027 . . . . **192**

Laura Floroian and Mihaela Badea
In Vivo Biocompatibility Study on Functional Nanostructures Containing Bioactive Glass and Plant Extracts for Implantology
Reprinted from: *Int. J. Mol. Sci.* **2024**, 25, 4249, doi:10.3390/ijms25084249 . . . . **207**

About the Editors

Marilena Gilca

Marilena Gilca is Professor at the "Carol Davila" University of Medicine and Pharmacy, Faculty of Medicine, Biochemistry Department, 050474 Bucharest, Romania. Her research interests include oxidative stress, antioxidants, medicinal plants, and ethnopharmacology. Orcid ID: 0000-0002-8073-1596.

Adelina Vlad

Adelina Vlad is an Associate Professor at the "Carol Davila" University of Medicine and Pharmacy, Faculty of Medicine, Physiology Department, 050474 Bucharest, Romania. Her research interests include atherosclerosis, coronary artery disease, scavenger receptors, anesthetic preconditioning, endothelial progenitor cells, non-coding RNA, nutraceuticals, and phytocompounds. Orcid ID: 0000-0002-2282-6802.

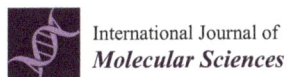
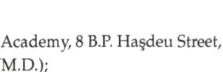

Review

Bioactive Compounds Formulated in Phytosomes Administered as Complementary Therapy for Metabolic Disorders

Laura Toma, Mariana Deleanu, Gabriela Maria Sanda, Teodora Barbălată, Loredan Ştefan Niculescu ®, Anca Volumnia Sima and Camelia Sorina Stancu *

Institute of Cellular Biology and Pathology "Nicolae Simionescu" of the Romanian Academy, 8 B.P. Haşdeu Street, 050568 Bucharest, Romania; laura.toma@icbp.ro (L.T.); mariana.deleanu@icbp.ro (M.D.); gabriela.sanda@icbp.ro (G.M.S.); teodora.barbalata@icbp.ro (T.B.); loredan.niculescu@icbp.ro (L.Ş.N.); anca.sima@icbp.ro (A.V.S.)
* Correspondence: camelia.stancu@icbp.ro

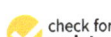

Citation: Toma, L.; Deleanu, M.; Sanda, G.M.; Barbălată, T.; Niculescu, L.Ş.; Sima, A.V.; Stancu, C.S. Bioactive Compounds Formulated in Phytosomes Administered as Complementary Therapy for Metabolic Disorders. *Int. J. Mol. Sci.* **2024**, *25*, 4162. https://doi.org/10.3390/ijms25084162

Academic Editor: David Arráez-Román

Received: 10 March 2024
Revised: 2 April 2024
Accepted: 5 April 2024
Published: 9 April 2024

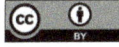

Copyright: © 2024 by the authors. Licensee MDPI, Basel, Switzerland. This article is an open access article distributed under the terms and conditions of the Creative Commons Attribution (CC BY) license (https:// creativecommons.org/licenses/by/ 4.0/).

Abstract: Metabolic disorders (MDs), including dyslipidemia, non-alcoholic fatty liver disease, diabetes mellitus, obesity and cardiovascular diseases are a significant threat to human health, despite the many therapies developed for their treatment. Different classes of bioactive compounds, such as polyphenols, flavonoids, alkaloids, and triterpenes have shown therapeutic potential in ameliorating various disorders. Most of these compounds present low bioavailability when administered orally, being rapidly metabolized in the digestive tract and liver which makes their metabolites less effective. Moreover, some of the bioactive compounds cannot fully exert their beneficial properties due to the low solubility and complex chemical structure which impede the passive diffusion through the intestinal cell membranes. To overcome these limitations, an innovative delivery system of phytosomes was developed. This review aims to highlight the scientific evidence proving the enhanced therapeutic benefits of the bioactive compounds formulated in phytosomes compared to the free compounds. The existing knowledge concerning the phytosomes' preparation, their characterization and bioavailability as well as the commercially available phytosomes with therapeutic potential to alleviate MDs are concisely depicted. This review brings arguments to encourage the use of phytosome formulation to diminish risk factors inducing MDs, or to treat the already installed diseases as complementary therapy to allopathic medication.

Keywords: bioactive compounds; cardiovascular diseases; diabetes mellitus; dyslipidemia; hepatic disorders; inflammatory stress; metabolic disorders; metabolic syndrome; oxidative stress; phytosomes

1. Introduction

Metabolic disorders (MDs) are the main cause of life-threatening diseases such as diabetes mellitus (DM), cardiovascular diseases (CVDs) and liver pathologies, affecting people worldwide, despite the various therapies developed for their treatment [1–6]. Connections between these pathologies were established, and the underlying mechanisms interconnecting them are intricated and involve the activation of different molecular pathways [7–9]. Extensive experimental and clinical evidence identified oxidative stress and inflammatory stress as common denominators and important players in the inception and progression of MDs [7,8,10]. Risk factors such as hyperglycemia, increased levels of advanced glycation end-products and of free fatty acids, decreased levels of high-density lipoprotein cholesterol (HDL-C) that appear in dyslipidemia, obesity, DM or non-alcoholic fatty liver disease (NAFLD) determine the activation of pro-oxidative nicotinamide adenine dinucleotide phosphate (NADPH) oxidase (NADPHox), the uncoupling of endothelial nitric oxide synthase (eNOS) or the dysfunction of mitochondria. Thus, the increased production of oxygen reactive species (ROS) is determined. In parallel, the downregulation of the antioxidant defense system including superoxide dismutase (SOD), catalase (CAT) and the enzymes involved in the metabolism of glutathione (GSH) is induced, resulting in a diminished detoxification of ROS [8,10]. The increased oxidative stress further acts as a trigger for the inflammatory stress, determining the increase in tumor necrosis factor alpha (TNF α), C-reactive protein (CRP), nucleotide-binding oligomerization domain (NOD)-like receptor protein 3 (NLRP3) inflammasome, nuclear factor kappa B (NF-kB), mitogen-activated protein kinases (MAPK), Janus kinases (JNKs), interleukins (ILs), etc., further exacerbating the pathological processes [8]. In addition, the excessive levels of ROS contribute to the oxidation of low-density lipoproteins (LDLs) and HDLs, endothelial cell dysfunction or apoptosis, vascular remodeling and atheroma formation [11], contributing to the development of cardiovascular diseases (CVDs), one of the major complications of NAFLD, obesity or diabetes.

Many therapies designed to treat MDs have failed completely or partially (cholesteryl ester transfer protein inhibitors, troglitazone, vitamins), or were too expensive to be applied to the entire population at CVD risk (apolipoprotein A-I Milano). Other treatments have been successful, but they induce considerable side effects (statins, sulfonylureas, calcium channel blockers, renin–angiotensin system inhibitors) [12–14]. Therefore, the exploration for new products to prevent or treat MDs is of high and continued interest. In the last decade, scientific researchers turned their attention to phytochemicals as effective, safe and low-cost natural bioactive compounds for MD treatment [15–18]. Phytochemicals such as polyphenols, alkaloids and terpenoids have good antioxidative activity and anti-inflammatory effects, due to their ability to bind free radicals with their functional groups. The main signaling pathways by which numerous natural bioactive compounds exert anti-oxidant and anti-inflammatory actions involve the modulation of transcription factors, the inhibition of NLRP3 inflammasome and NF-κB, activation of nuclear factor erythroid 2-related factor 2 (Nrf2) and protein kinase B (PKB/Akt), and the consequent stimulation of eNOS, of antioxidant enzymes and the inhibition of NADPHox [19–21] (Figure 1). In addition, notable lipid-regulatory effects have been described for some phytochemicals; they inhibit the lipid absorption in the small intestine, stimulating the excess cholesterol excretion via the gallbladder or small intestine, and impeding de novo lipid synthesis in the liver. The molecular mechanisms responsible for the lipid-lowering effects of some natural compounds involve the activation of essential transcription regulators, such as sirtuin 1 (SIRT-1), liver X receptors (LXRs) and the peroxisome proliferator-activated receptors (PPARs) [19,22–24] (Figure 1).

In addition, it is widely accepted that drugs derived from plant extracts are safer than their synthetic equivalents [25]. It has been proven that natural compounds administered as combined total extracts exert additive effects compared to their individual counterparts' administration [26]. Despite all these benefits acknowledged for phytochemicals, there are no substantial clinical studies to prove the clear advantages of the therapies with phytochemicals in CVDs, DM or hepatic disorders [18,27,28]. An explanation for the lack of consistent data from clinical studies could be the limited solubility and low stability of the natural bioactive compounds in circulation [18,28]. The polyphenols are compounds with very high antioxidant and anti-inflammatory potential, but their bioavailability is very limited, due to their rapid enzymatic modification in vivo that blocks the hydroxyl groups which exert their antioxidant effect [19]. Another category of compounds that cannot fully exert their beneficial properties are phytochemicals which cannot pass through the intestinal membranes by passive diffusion, due to their large chemical structure [29]. For an ideal bioavailability, the phytochemical molecules should be able to exhibit a hydrophilic–lipophilic balance [30]. Therefore, the delivery system must be developed to increase the solubility and stability of the bioactive compounds from extracts. To overcome these limitations, researchers developed new advanced drug delivery systems for phytochemicals. There are many types of nanosystems that have been created for therapeutic purposes and classified in inorganic nanoparticles (silica nanoparticles, magnetic nanoparticles, carbon nanotubes, polymeric nanoparticles, polymerosomes) and organic nanoparticles, the latter including liposomes (50–450 nm), phytosomes (50–10,000 nm), ethosomes (50–400 nm/2000–5600 nm), transferosomes (<300 nm), nanostructured lipid carriers (50–500 nm), cubosomes (100–500 nm), solid lipid nanoparticles (10–1000 nm), hexosomes, nanoparticles (10 to 1000 nm), niosomes (100–2000 nm), nanocrystals (<1000 nm), nanomicelles (10–100 nm), nanoemulsions (100–600 nm, 10–1000 nm), nanofibers (50–1000 nm) and microspheres (6–735 µm) [30–35].

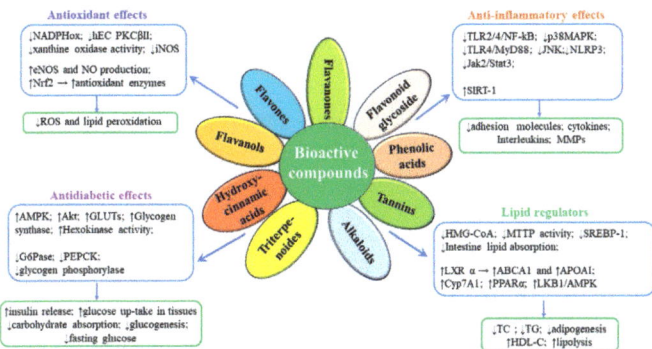

Figure 1. Schematic representation of the signaling pathways by which phytochemicals exert their therapeutic actions in MD. ABCA1, ATP-binding cassette A1; AMPK, AMP-activated protein kinase; ApoA1, Apolipoprotein A-I; CYP7A1, cholesterol 7alpha-hydroxylase; eNOS, endothelial nitric oxide synthase; ERK, extracellular signal-regulated kinase; GLUTs, glucose transporters; G6Pase, Glucose-6-phosphatase; HDL-C, high-density lipoproteins cholesterol; hECs, human endothelial cells; HMG-CoA, hydroxymethylglutaryl coenzyme A; iNOS, inducible nitric oxide synthase; Jak2/Stat3, Janus kinase 2/Signal transducer and activator of transcription 3; LKB1, Liver kinase B1; JNK, c-Jun N-terminal kinases; LXRs, liver X receptors; MAPK, mitogen-activated protein kinases; MD, metabolic disorders; NADPHox, nicotinamide adenine dinucleotide phosphate (NADPH) oxidase; MMPs, Matrix metalloproteinases; MTTP, Microsomal triglyceride transfer protein; MyD88, NF-κB, nuclear factor kappa B; NLRP3, nucleotide-binding oligomerization domain (NOD)-like receptor protein 3; NO, nitric oxide; Nrf2, nuclear factor erythroid 2-related factor 2; p38MAPK, p38 mitogen-activated protein kinases; PEPCK, phosphoenolpyruvate carboxykinase; PKB/Akt, Protein kinase B; PKCβII, protein kinase CβII; PPARα, peroxisome proliferator-activated receptor α; ROS, reactive oxygen species; SIRT1, sirtuin 1; SREBP, Sterol regulatory element-binding protein; TC, total cholesterol; TGs, triglycerides; TLR2/4, Toll-like receptor 2/4; upwards arrow (↑) represents increases; downwards arrow (↓) represents decreases.

Among these, the phyto-phospholipid complexes, named phytosomes, are self-assembling vesicular structures in aqueous environments, forming a unique and stable arrangement due to the electrostatic interactions and hydrogen bonds formed between the polar head of phospholipid (ammonium and negative phosphate groups) and the functional groups of phytochemicals having an active hydrogen atom (-COOH, -OH, -NH$_2$) (Figure 2).

There are important physico-chemical differences between phytosomes and liposomes, giving important advantages to the former: (i) the size of phytosomes is smaller than that of liposomes; (ii) the phytosomes are more stable due to the hydrogen bonds formed between phospholipids and the carried active compounds, whereas no chemical bonds are formed in liposomes; (iii) the molar ratio of phospholipids and natural compounds is 1:1 or 2:1 in phytosomes, which confers a very low susceptibility to oxidation, while in liposomes there are hundreds or even thousands of oxidation-prone phospholipids surrounding the water-soluble compounds [36].

The phytosomes help to minimize the loss of bioactive compounds along the digestive tract by limiting their degradation by the digestive enzymes and microbiota, improving their retention in the small intestine and increasing their absorption. Thus, the phytosomes' formulation increases the bioavailability of phytochemicals, strengthening their efficacy, and allowing for an in vivo non-invasive delivery (oral or topic administration) [18,36].

The phytosomes containing phytochemicals may be helpful for patients who are intolerant to allopathic drugs or those who are not able to attain targeted parameters at the maximally tolerated dose of the allopathic drug.

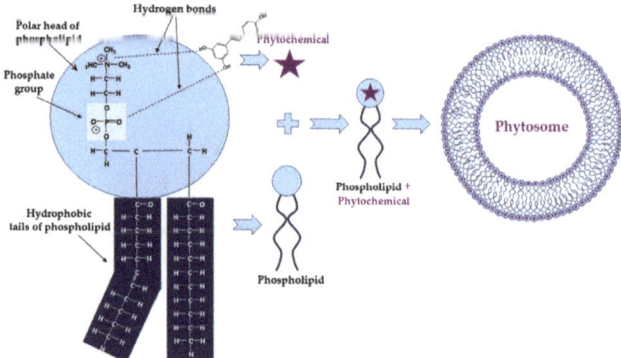

Figure 2. Schematic representation of the chemical bonds established during phytosome formation and their structure. The phytochemical (e.g., resveratrol) and the polar head of the phospholipid form hydrogen bonds which are represented by dashed lines.

The rationale of the present review is to highlight the scientific proof for the improved benefic action of phytochemicals formulated in phytosomes compared to their free form in order to stimulate the use of these phyto-phospholipid complexes as remedies for MD, administered as complementary therapies to allopathic drugs. We briefly present specific methods for the preparation and characterization of phytosomes, followed by scientific evidence of their increased stability and bioavailability compared to unformulated phytochemicals. We depict the data about the use of phytosomes with bioactive compounds or plant extracts to safely alleviate oxidative and inflammatory stress, dyslipidemia, hyperglycemia and insulin resistance, the main risk factors in MD evolution.

The strategy to identify the pre-clinical and clinical studies that investigated the therapeutic potential of bioactive compounds formulated in phytosomes involved searching for publications on PubMed, Scopus and Web of Science from 2000 to 2024, with restriction to English language. The main keyword used was "phytosomes", and the secondary keywords were "metabolic disorders", "oxidative stress", "inflammatory stress/inflammation", "dyslipidemia", "diabetes", "metabolic syndrome", "hepatic disorders/NAFLD" and "cardiovascular diseases". The resulting total number of papers was 941, out of which we excluded the duplicates and retained only the articles with the full text available (excluded proceeding papers and conference abstracts). Thus, the final number of papers that met the selection criteria was 132. Using the same exclusion criteria, the number of papers that addressed the methods of phytosome preparation and characterization, and the techniques for measuring the bioavailability of active compounds from phytosomes, was 57.

2. Preparation and Characterization of Phytosomes with Bioactive Compounds

2.1. Preparation of Phytosomes with Bioactive Compounds

Phytosomes are prepared by complexing the natural bioactive compounds with phospholipids in a suitable solvent. The phospholipids are glycerophospholipids such as phosphatidylcholine (PC), phosphatidylethanolamine, phosphatidylserine, phosphatidic acid, phosphatidylinositol and phosphatidylglycerol. Among these phospholipids, PC is the most frequently used to prepare phyto-phospholipid complexes because it exhibits amphipathic properties which ensure moderate solubility in water and lipid environments [36]. In addition, PC shows low toxicity and robust biocompatibility because it is an essential component of the cell membrane. Different solvents have been used for phyto-phospholipid complex formulation. Aprotic solvents, such as methylene chloride, chloroform, tetrahydrofuran, dimethylsulfoxide, ethyl acetate or acetone have been used to prepare phytosomes, but they have been largely replaced by protic solvents like ethanol, because it is a food grade solvent, leaves less residues and causes minimal damage [37,38]. Regarding the stoichiometric ratio of bioactive compounds and phospholipids, the phyto-phospholipid complexes are employed by reacting the ingredients in a molar ratio ranging from 0.5 to 2.0 [39]. The stoichiometric ratio of 1:1 was considered optimal in many studies to prepare phyto-phospholipid complexes [30], but this ratio should be adjusted every time a new combination of phytochemicals and phospholipids is tested. The solvent, stoichiometric ratio of active ingredients, reaction temperature and reaction duration are the primary variables that influence the formation of phyto-phospholipid complexes [40]. Phytosomes can be prepared by three main techniques: solvent evaporation/thin film hydration, anti-solvent precipitation and freeze–drying [18]. A widely used technique for preparing phyto-phospholipid complexes is the solvent evaporation/thin-layer hydration method, according to which the PC and standardized extracts or bioactive compounds are combined in a round bottom flask and dissolved in a proper solvent by heating at an ideal constant temperature for a predetermined time duration. The complexes prepared in this way can be finally obtained by evaporating the solvent under vacuum. The resulting dry film can be sieved and stored in a desiccator or can be hydrated with the optimum volume of water, followed by controlled sonication in order to obtain a certain size for the phytosome particles. Then, the phyto-phospholipid complexes can be freeze–dried for long-term preservation, and later formulated in capsules (Figure 3) [38,41,42].

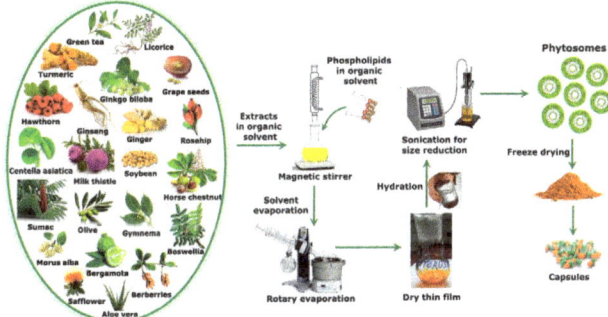

Figure 3. The main steps for phytosome preparation by solvent evaporation/thin-film method.

The anti-solvent precipitation technique is the second most used method for the preparation of phytosomes. According to this technique, the phyto-phospholipid complexes obtained as in the previously described method are finally precipitated by using a suitable solvent, such as n-hexan [43,44]. By using the freeze–drying method, the bioactive compound solubilized in the suitable solvent is mixed with the phospholipid alcoholic solution, allowed to react in predetermined conditions followed by lyophilization in order to obtain the phytosomes [42].

2.2. Characterization of Phytosomes with Bioactive Compounds

Several techniques were employed to establish the phytosomes' size, composition, morphology and other physical characteristics. Some of the physical properties of phytosomes can be explored by more than one technique. The main parameters for characterization of phytosomes are: (i) size and shape; (ii) surface charge; (iii) chemical composition and structure; (iv) stability; (v) encapsulation efficiency (EE%) and (vi) release behavior. The size and morphology of particles are important indicators of the phytosomes' quality. Different techniques can be used for phytosome size characterization, such as dynamic light scattering (DLS) [18,38,45–47], transmission electron microscopy (TEM) [18,38,47–50], scanning electron microscopy (SEM) [18,47–49,51,52], atomic force microscopy (AFM) [53] and size-exclusion chromatography (SEC) [54]. The measurement of size distribution and polydispersity of phytosomes gives information about their physical stability; it can be evaluated by DLS, an easy, very fast and precise method [18,38,45–47]. Zeta potential represents the complete charge generated by medium, defines the surface charge of phytosomes in emulsions and reflects the stability of the phytosomes in the medium. This parameter can be negative, positive or neutral, depending on the composition of the phytosomes. A zeta potential greater than +30 mV or less than −30 mV is known to correspond to a stable emulsion of phytosomes [51,52,55,56]. The electrostatic properties of phytosomes can be measured using Zeta Sizer [51,52,55,56]. The chemical composition and interaction between phospholipid and phytochemicals are evaluated by high-performance liquid chromatography (HPLC) [38,46,52] and liquid chromatography coupled to mass-spectrometry (LC-MS) [51]. To characterize the solid-state matter in the complex form, the thermal analysis is widely used. In differential scanning calorimetry (DSC), the determination of changes in solid-state properties, in accordance with the temperature change, provide important information about the phytosomes' stability, degradation and melting (Table 1). Phyto-phospholipid complexation and molecular interactions in solution are studied by employing spectroscopic techniques like proton (^{1}H) nuclear magnetic resonance (NMR), carbon-13 (^{13}C) NMR, phosphorus-31(^{31}P) NMR, and Fourier transform infrared (IR) spectroscopy (FTIR). Formation of the hydrogen bonds is associated with specific signals like changes in chemical shift and line broadening in NMR spectra and with appearance of new bands in IR spectra [38]. Studies of the phytosomes' stability are performed to explore the phytochemical changes in phytosomes during storage, and can be measured over several months by determining average size, zeta potential, size distribution and drug content with the same techniques. Determination of the encapsulation efficiency (EE%) begins with the removal of free, unencapsulated phytochemicals from the phytosomes emulsion by different methods, such as ultracentrifugation [18,38,46,52,57,58], the Sephadex gel column or dialysis method (specific cut-off) for several hours against buffer solution [18,45]. The formula for EE% calculation is as follows:

EE (%) = [(Initial amount of phytochemical − amount of free phytochemical from filtrate)/initial amount phytochemical] × 100

Table 1. General methods for the characterization of phytosomes containing bioactive compounds.

Parameter	Techniques	References
Average size and shape	• Dynamic light scattering (DLS) • Scanning electron microscopy (SEM) • Transmission electron microscopy (TEM) • Cryo-TEM and freeze-fracture-TEM • Fluorescence microscopy • Atomic force microscopy (AFM) • Field flow fractionation • Size-exclusion chromatography	[18,38,45–47] [18,48,49,51,52] [18,47–50,52] [59] [52,60] [53] [54] [54]
Surface charge	• DLS	[51,52,55,56]
Chemical composition and structure	• Gas chromatography-mass spectrometry (GC-MS) • High-performance liquid chromatography (HPLC) • Fourier-transform infrared spectroscopy (FTIR) • ^{1}H NMR (Nuclear Magnetic Resonance spectroscopy) • ^{13}C NMR (Nuclear Magnetic Resonance spectroscopy) • ^{31}P NMR (Nuclear Magnetic Resonance spectroscopy) • Differential scanning calorimetry (DSC) • Powder X-ray diffraction (PXRD)	[61] [38,46,52] [47,49,51,52,61,62] [63–65] [65] [38] [47,49,51,52,62] [47,49,52]
Stability	• ^{31}P (Nuclear Magnetic Resonance spectroscopy) • Electron microscopy methods • DSC • DLS • UV–Vis	[38] [48,59] [62] [46,55,56] [18,47,58]

Table 1. Cont.

Parameter	Techniques	References
Encapsulation efficiency (EE%) and release behavior	• Mini-column centrifugation • HPLC • UV–Vis • Dialysis • Enzymatic assays • Gel electrophoresis • Liquid chromatography mass spectrometry	[18,38,52,57,58] [38,46,49,52] [58] [38,46,49,52] [18] [18] [51]

The amounts of free (unloaded) phytochemicals in filtrate could be measured spectrophotometrically (UV–Vis) [47,58] or by HPLC, ultra-performance liquid chromatography (UPLC) or LC-MS methods [38,46,49,52]. The release of phytochemicals from phytosomes can be abrupt or sustained. In vitro drug release is explored by introducing the phytosomal solution into a dialysis membrane which is dipped into a container containing release medium at a constant stirring speed and temperature. The phytochemical released in the medium is quantified by spectrophotometry or HPLC, LC-MS methods. The established and accepted methods for the characterization of phytosomes with bioactive compounds are summarized in Table 1.

3. Evaluation of the Bioavailability of Active Compounds Formulated in Phytosomes

The phyto-phospholipid complexes being amphiphilic allows for a better dissolution in the gastrointestinal fluid and very good absorption through the lipophilic membranes or intestinal cells. Moreover, Wang H. et al. [66] indicated that the phospholipid molecules have the potential to act as chaperones for the drugs, transporting them through the biological membranes and improving their bioavailability. They also improve the drugs' stability by encapsulating them into the formed nanocarriers and protecting the drug molecules from the aggressive environment in the gastrointestinal tract. Thus, the phyto-phospholipid complexes can be transported via the microfold (M)-cell of the intestinal mucosa [28]. Many studies have been dedicated to the development and in vitro characterization of phytosomes, but in vivo studies need to be conducted to prove their effectiveness and to determine their oral bioavailability that is expressed as the rate and extent of the bioactive compound absorption which can reach into the bloodstream. The experiments for measuring the bioavailability of a bioactive compound can be achieved in animal models or humans. After in vivo administration of the phytosomes and unformulated extracts, the amount of drug entering into the systemic circulation is measured at different time points and plotted to acquire the maximum drug concentration (Cmax), peak time (Tmax) and area under the curve (AUC). These are the kinetic parameters that can be used to characterize the properties of phytosomes in terms of bioavailability [67]. The relative bioavailability of a bioactive compound can be calculated by dividing the value measured for AUC of the compound in the phytosome by the AUC value of the unformulated compound. The main parameters to be measured in order to establish the level of bioavailability of the bioactive compounds formulated in phytosomes compared to unformulated compounds are summarized in Table 2. An important advantage of the phytosomes is that they can be administered through non-invasive routes. Thus, most of the products based on phytosomes are designed for oral administration (see Table 3), but there are also phytosomes created for nasal [68] or topic administration [69].

The commercially available products based on bioactive compounds or plant extracts formulated into phytosomes and suitable for prevention or treatment of MD are reviewed in Table 3.

Table 2. Parameters to be measured in order to establish the level of bioavailability for various bioactive compounds formulated in phytosomes.

Subject	Dose of Bioactive Compound	Cmax ± SD Unformulated Bioactive Compound	AUC ± SD Unformulated Bioactive Compound	Tmax ± SD (h) Unformulated Bioactive Compound	Cmax ± SD Bioactive Compound in Phytosome	AUC ± SD Bioactive Compound in Phytosome	Tmax ± SD Bioactive Compound in Phytosome	References
Sprague Dawley rats	Curcumin 340 mg/kg	6.5 ± 4.5 (nM)	4.8 (μg*min/mL)	30 (min)	33.4 ± 7.1 (nM)	26.7 (μg*min/mL)	15 (min)	[70]
Rats	Berberine 50 mg/kg	66.01 ± 15.03 (ng/mL)	384.45 ± 108.62 (ng*h/mL)	0.5 (h)	219.67 ± 6.02 (ng/mL)	1169.19 ± 93.75 (ng*h/mL)	2 (h)	[52]
Rats	Apigenin 100 mg/kg	0.14 ± 0.15 (μg/mL)	0.84 ± 0.42 (μg*h/mL)	2.0 ± 0.23 (h)	0.20 ± 0.25 (μg/mL)	1.31 ± 0.46 (μg*h/mL)	4.0 ± 0.34 (h)	[43]
Sprague Dawley rats	Baicalein 75 mg/kg	1.61 ± 0.37 (μg/mL)	664.68 ± 75.50 (μg*min/mL)	170.00 ± 65.73 (min)	8.68 ± 1.35 (μg/mL)	1748.20 ± 280.80 (μg*min/mL)	33.33 ± 8.67 (min)	[71]
Rats	Ursolic acid 20 mg/kg	8 ± 0.21 (μg/mL)	13.15 ± 0.34 (μg*h/mL)	1.5 ± 1.23 (h)	9 ± 2.17 (μg/mL)	60.33 ± 2.19 (μg*h/mL)	2 ± 0.43 (h)	[72]
Male Albino rats	Resveratrol 25 mg	0.24 ± 0.12 (μg/mL)	24.31 ± 4.31 (μg*min/mL)	30 (min)	2.27 ± 0.51 (μg/mL)	257.15 ± 40.26 (μg*min/mL)	60 (min)	[73]
Human	Curcuminoids 376 mg	5.2 ± 0.2 (ng/mL)	39.6 ± 1.5 (ng*h/mL)	9.5 ± 0.2 (h)	8.7 ± 0.4 (ng/mL)	65.3 ± 2.3 (ng*h/mL)	1.7 ± 0.4 (h)	[74]
Human	Curcuminoids 376 mg	0.9 ± 0.1 (ng/mL)	10.4 ± 1.3 (ng*h/mL)	4 (h)	18.0 ± 6.4 (ng/mL)	86.9 ± 12.1 (ng*h/mL)	1 (h)	[67]
Human	Coenzyme Q10 30 mg	0.10 ± 0.05 (μg/mL)	1.43 ± 1.96 (μg*h/mL)	16.83 ± 19.73 (h)	0.13 ± 0.08 (μg/mL)	3.92 ± 3.56 (μg*h/mL)	24 ± 18.68 (h)	[75]
Human	Quercetin 500 mg	10.93 ± 2.22 (ng/mL)	4774.93 ± 1190.61 (ng*min/mL)	290 ± 31.19 (min)	223.10 ± 16.32 (ng/mL)	96,163.87 ± 9291.31 (ng*min/mL)	202.50 ± 35.97 (min)	[76]
Human	Curcumin 207 mg	2.03 ± 1.79 (nM)	19.06 ± 17.47 (nM*h)	6.92 ± 5.96 (h)	16.61 ± 10.10 (nM)	147.9 ± 67.84 (nM*h)	6.92 ± 8.34 (h)	[77]
Human	Berberine 188 mg	69.95 ± 14.54 (pg/mL)	1057 ± 117 (pg*h/mL)	4.55 ± 0.29 (h)	375.57 ± 41.56 (pg/mL)	4146 ± 431 (pg*h/mL)	4.50 ± 0.30 (h)	[78]

AUC; Area under the curve (0-t); C_{max}; Maximum concentration of the drug in plasma; T_{max}; Time of maximum drug concentration measured in the plasma.

Table 3. Commercial products based on phytochemicals formulated in phytosomes and their beneficial effects in MDs.

No.	Commercial Product; Doses and Administration Protocol	Company	Phytochemicals	Beneficial Effects; Mechanisms of Action	References
1	Berberine–phospholipid complex-based phytosomes (100 mg/kg orally administered to db/db mice 4 weeks)	-	Berberine	Anti-diabetic (decreased glucose levels in plasma and TG in the liver)	[52]
2	Casperome® phytosome (250 mg/day orally administered to subjects with musculoskeletal conditions, 1–4 weeks)	Indena	*Boswellia serrata*–Resin	Anti-inflammatory (lower the pain score, decrease CRP levels)	[79]
3	Curcumin phytosome (1 g × 2/day, corresponding to 200 mg curcumin, orally to humans with acute muscle injury, 4 days)	Indena	*Curcuma longa* L.–Rhizome	Anti-inflammatory (decreased IL-8)	[80]
4	Greenselect® / Green Tea Phytosome (2 × 150 mg/day Greenselect and 30 mg piperine orally administered to obese women, 3 months)	Indena	*Camellia sinensis* L.–Leaf	Bodyweight regulator (reduction in weight and fat mass, improvement of lipidic profile growth hormone, insulin-like growth factor-1, insulin and cortisol)	[81,82]
5	Monoselect Camellia (MonCam) 1 tablet eq to 300 mg/day of Greenselect phytosomes for 24 weeks	PharmExtracta (Pontenure, Italy)	*Camellia sinensis*	Improver of lipidic profile, antioxidant (reduced fasting glucose, increased HDL, decreased TG, reduced plasma free radicals)	[83]
6	Hawthorn Phytosome (100 mg, orally)	Indena	Flavonoids of *Crataegus* species	Blood pressure regulator, cardioprotective	[84,85]
7	Leucoselect® / Grape Seed Phytosome (300 mg grape procyanidin extracts eq, to healthy smoking adults, 4 weeks)	Indena	*Vitis vinifera* L.–Seed	Antioxidant, cardioprotective (reduced lipid peroxidation in LDL, increased the lag phase of LDL oxidation)	[86]
8.	Ginseng Phytosome (100 or 200 mg per day for eight weeks orally administered to diabetic patients)	Natural Factors (Monroe, WA, USA)	*Panax Ginseng*	Antidiabetic effects (decreased fasting blood glucose, reduced hemoglobin A_{1C} values for 200 mg dose)	[18,87]
9	Naringenin Phytosome (Approx 3 mg Naringenin eq, intratracheary administered to rats with acute lung injury, 4 h)	-	*Citrus aurantium*	Anti-inflammatory, antioxidant (increased SOD2 mRNA, decreased COX2 and ICAM-1 gene expression, decreased p-p38MAPK in the lungs)	[88]
10	Quercefit™ Phytosome (1–2 tabs/day administered to human subjects with both asthma and rhinitis, for 30 days)	Indena	Quercetin	Antioxidant (reduction of plasma-free radicals)	[89]
11	Siliphos® (120 mg, orally administered)	Indena	Silybin of *Silybum marianum*	Antioxidant, hepatoprotective	[85,90]
12	Green Tea Phytosome 1 capsule 2–3 times/day orally administered to obese subjects for 90 days)	Natural Factors	Green tea polyphenols	Antioxidant, bodyweight regulator (thermogenic effect, improvements in weight and body mass index)	[91]
13	Ubiqsome™ Phytosome (150–300 mg corresponding to 30–60 mg CoQ10, administered orally to healthy humans for two periods of two weeks)	Indena	Co-enzyme Q10	Antioxidant; a good absorbance of CoQ10	[75]
14	Vazguard™ Phytosome (1000 mg/L of bergamot phytosome subjected to simulated gastric digestion and further incubated to fecal slurries from healthy women)	Indena	Bergamot extract	Regulator of plasma glucose and lipid levels, bodyweight regulator (modulator of gut microbiota: Firmicutes, Proteobacteria, Bacteroidetes, Actinobacteria)	[92]
15	Vazguard™/Naringin Phytosome (oral administration to type 2 diabetic patients)	Indena	Bergamot extract	Antioxidant, cardioprotective (improvement in lipid profile, reduction in small, dense LDLs and decreased glucose levels in plasma)	[93]

4. Pathologies Addressed by Natural Bioactive Compounds Formulated in Phytosomes

4.1. Oxidative and Inflammatory Stress

It is generally accepted that oxidative and inflammatory stress are responsible for the initiation and progression of numerous diseases, including MD, and many therapies have been attempted, but without remarkable results [27]. In the last quarter century, numerous phytochemical formulations in phytosomes have been prepared and demonstrated to have antioxidant and anti-inflammatory effects. Here, we display those with potential impact on MDs. The first indication that a chemical bond is formed between phospholipids and natural bioactive compounds in phytosomes came from the group of Bombardelli E. in 1989 [94]. After this moment, an increasing number of laboratories have approached and developed this biotechnology.

4.1.1. Preclinical Studies

The extracts of *Ginkgo biloba* leaves have been found to possess multiple beneficial properties, the main active constituents being flavone glycosides, such as kaempferol, quercetin and isorhamnetin [95]. The Ginkgoselect Phytosome® (Indena SpA, Milan, Italy) prepared by mixing a stoichiometric amount of soy phospholipids and *Ginkgo biloba* leaf extract has been tested for antioxidant properties in Wistar rats with rifampicin-induced hepatotoxicity (500 mg/kg, for 30 days). Simultaneously administered, Ginkgoselect Phytosome® at 25 mg/kg and 50 mg/kg significantly lowered the plasma levels of lipid peroxides, and elevated the amounts of GSH, SOD, CAT, glutathione peroxidase (GPx) and glutathione reductase (GR) in liver homogenates, in a dose-dependent manner. No significant differences between the groups treated with phytosomes or silymarin (100 mg/kg, positive control) were observed [96].

The bioactive compound most frequently formulated in phytosomes and tested is curcumin, the primary polyphenol found in turmeric (*Curcuma longa*) [18]. The antioxidant activity of curcumin is due to its ability to scavenge radicals generated in oxidation processes, and its anti-inflammatory effects are based on the down-regulation of cyclooxygenase-2, MAPK and JNK, and the prevention of TNFα and ILs production [97,98]. Curcumin formulated in nanophytosome (at a dose of 15 mg/kg for seven days) improved the antioxidant effects in a mouse model of inflammation [99]. Acute inflammation in the mice was induced by the administration of carrageenan (1%) into the subplantar region of the paw. The pre-treatment with curcumin formulated in nanophytosomes induced a significant increased enzymatic activity of CAT, SOD, GR and GPx, compared to unformulated curcumin [99]. This study brings evidence that the phytosomal formulation of curcumin improves its therapeutic potential.

Ginger (*Zingiber officinale*) rhizomes are used as food and drink spices and in traditional medicine for their antioxidant, anti-inflammatory, hypolipidemic, antidiabetic and anticoagulant effects [100–104]. The most abundant bioactive compounds of the ginger extract are gingerols and shogaols, able to trigger multiple signaling pathways to exert their therapeutic effects, but having low bioavailability due to their low solubility [105]. Therefore, high doses of ginger extracts are used with the intent to increase its benefits. Some side effects have been described in these conditions, such as digestive tract irritation, bleeding or cardiac arrhythmias [106]. The rosehip fruits (*Rosa canina*) have been used in traditional medicine to reduce pain or as hypolipemic and hypoglycemic treatment, being characterized as having antioxidant, anti-inflammatory, anti-obesity, hepatoprotective, nephroprotective and cardioprotective properties [107,108]. The major bioactive constituents of rosehips, flavonoids, anthocyanins and phenolic compounds are lipophilic and present low bioavailability. Thus, Deleanu M. et al. [38] developed a new formulation of phytosomes with bioactive compounds from ginger and rosehips extracts, and demonstrated that those with the mass ratio ginger extract:rosehip extract:phosphatidylcholine—0.5:0.5:1 had the most effective antioxidant and anti-inflammatory effects in cultured human enterocytes. Moreover, they showed that the phytosome formulation had doubled the plasma concentration of bioactive compounds, compared to unformulated extracts, by increasing their absorption from the digestive tract and accumulation in the liver and kidneys of C57Bl/6J mice. In addition, Deleanu et al. [38] evidenced that the antioxidant and anti-inflammatory effects of the extracts were significantly improved by the phytosome formulation. These properties have been demonstrated in mice with lipopolysaccharide (LPS)-induced systemic inflammation as the increased plasma level of SOD2 and paraoxonase 1 (PON1), and decreased protein expression of TNFα and IL-1 beta (IL-1β) in the liver and small intestine. All these data confirm the enhanced therapeutic properties of ginger and rosehip extracts formulated in phytosomes.

Gallic acid is a well-known flavonoid and the main bioactive compound of sumac (*Rhus coriaria* L.), having antioxidant, anti-inflammatory and antitumoral activity [109,110]. Despite these beneficial activities, the therapeutic potential of gallic acid is limited due to its low absorption, poor bioavailability and rapid elimination [111,112]. The group of Abbasalipour H. et al. [113] formulated gallic acid and sumac extract in phytosomes and tested their antioxidant properties at doses of 20 mg/kg daily in a rat model of valproic acid-induced oxidative stress in the nervous system. Both types of phytosomes showed superior antioxidant effects measured as increased plasma activity of GPx, GR, SOD, CAT and GSH level, compared to unformulated gallic acid or sumac extract [113]. The mechanism involves the Nrf2 signaling pathway that regulates the expression of various antioxidant enzymes and is activated as a defense mechanism against oxidative stress [114]. Gallic acid and sumac extract formulated in phytosomes, compared to the unformulated extract, manifested better solubility and bioavailability, induced the doubling of Nrf2 gene expression and blocked the binding of Nrf2 to Kelch-like ECH-associated protein 1 (Keap1), leading to the activation of downstream antioxidative enzymes [113]. These results show that the phytosomal formulation of plant extracts or of their active constituents can improve their beneficial effects.

Berberine is a benzylisoquinoline alkaloid found in many plants, particularly in barberry (*Berberis vulgaris* L. and *Berberis aristata* DC.), and has antihypertensive, hypoglycemic and hepatoprotective effects [115–117]. It has high water solubility, but its bioavailability is low when orally administered due to its high molecular weight and self-aggregation tendency that impede its passage through the intestinal wall. Thus, the absolute bioavailability of berberine is low, and high doses are necessary for administration in clinical studies, which unfortunately causes adverse gastrointestinal effects [52,118]. To increase berberine bioavailability and efficacy, the group of Güngör-Ak A. et al. [29] used the Quality by Design method for the formulation design and selection of the optimum formula to prepare berberine–phospholipid complexes using the reverse phase evaporation method. The resulting berberine phytosomes have a small particle size and narrow particle size distribution. The antipyretic activity was detected in rats only at high dose (209 mg/kg versus 104.5 mg/kg), and for longer periods of time (from 6–10 days to 8–14 days) compared to unformulated berberine. The analgesic and anti-inflammatory effects of berberine in phytosomes have been shown for the high dose only (209 mg/kg), which reduced the hind paw edema induced by carrageenan and serotonin, the subcutaneous air-pouch Freund's complete adjuvant-induced inflammation, and inhibited the acetic acid-induced capillary permeability in mice [29].

The wild leek (*Allium ampeloprasum*) is known for its nutritional and therapeutic properties as antiplatelet, antidiabetic and anti-atherosclerotic effect [119]. Very recently, the group of Shoeibi A. et al. [120] formulated in phytosomes a fraction enriched in polyphenols extracted from leek and tested their antioxidant properties in BALB/c mice with colon carcinoma. Administered at a dose of 50 mg total phenolic compounds/kg for 28 days, the phytosomes increased the gene expression of GPx and SOD in the liver, and reduced the lipid peroxides measured as malondialdehyde (MDA) levels, compared to the group receiving unformulated leek extract [120].

The *Gymnema inodorum* leaf extract contains bioactive compounds, such as phenolic acids, flavonoids, triterpenoids and pregnane glycosides, which have been shown to have antioxidant and anti-inflammatory properties and are beneficial for diabetic control, but have low bioavailability [121,122]. Very recently, Nuchuchua O. et al. [26] developed phytosomes with *G. inodorum* extract to overcome this limitation. The formulation of *G. inodorum* phytochemicals in phytosomes significantly changed the particles' surface charge from neutral (blank phytosome) to negative (−35 mV to −45 mV), allowing for the bioactive compounds to be embedded in the phospholipid membrane. Nanoparticles at sizes lower than 200 nm show direct diffusion via the intestinal mucosal sites. Phytosomes with *G. inodorum* extract exhibited increased anti-inflammatory activity in LPS-stimulated RAW 264.7 macrophages, by lowering the production of nitric oxide (NO) induced by pro-inflammatory conditions, compared to unformulated *G. inodorum* extract [26]. All these data confirm the enhanced antioxidant and anti-inflammatory effects of plant extracts following the phytosomal formulation.

Tripterine, also known as celastrol, is a phytochemical derived from the plant of *Trypterygium wilfordii* and belongs to the family of quinone methides [123]. Tripterine exhibits anti-inflammatory effects by modulating proinflammatory cytokines, such as IL-18 and IL-1β, and inhibiting the effects of LPS or interferon gamma (IFNγ) in macrophages [124]. Due to its low bioavailability and certain toxicity at high doses, tripterine has limited clinical applications; thus, phytosome formulation was used as a method to increase tripterine absorption and sustained release. In addition, selenium supplementation of phytosomes for the improvement of SOD was also used to increase the beneficial effects of tripterine [125–127]. Pyroptosis is an inflammasome-mediated programmed cell death dependent on caspase-1, and it may be a major cause of multiple organ dysfunction [128]. Thus, in the attempt to develop new drugs to treat inflammatory diseases, Liu S. et al. formulated tripterine into phytosomes and functionalized them with selenium (Se@Tri-PTs) to attenuate the cytotoxic effect of phytochemical and potentiate its anti-inflammatory effect [124]. Formulation in phytosomes increased the tripterine solubility by ~500-fold and their uptake by murine J774A.1 macrophage, while the cytotoxicity decreased. Se@Tri-PTs inhibited the activation of NRLP3 inflammasome and pyroptosis by reducing the cleavage of gasdermin D and release of IL-1β in a dose-dependent manner (in a rage of 50–200 ng/mL) [124]. Thus, tripterine becomes safer and effective following formulation in phytosomes.

For hesperidin, a flavanoid within the flavanone subclass, numerous biological effects have been described, such as anti-inflammatory, heart and blood vessels protection, anti-diabetic and neuroprotective [19,129,130]. Due to its poor water solubility, which is further diminished by the acidic environment, the reported bioavailability is low (<25%) and the transmembrane permeability is reduced following oral administration. The group of Kalita B. and Patwary B.N. [131] formulated phospholipid complexes with hesperidin and demonstrated their enhanced solubility in a basic buffer system and a very balanced partition coefficient, suggesting a good membrane permeation efficiency. In addition, the complexes showed a concentration-dependent increase in the anti-oxidant activity, similar to ascorbic acid [131].

4.1.2. Clinical Studies

In the late nineties, Nuttall S.L. et al. [132] prepared an extract from grape seeds formulated in phytosomes (Leucoselect™ Phytosome®, Indena SpA, Milan, Italy), starting from the observation that, in countries with increased consumption of red wine, the incidence of coronary artery disease is lower compared to other countries. Grape seed proanthocyanidins have been reported to inhibit lipid peroxidation, capillary fragility and platelet aggregation, and regulate the activity of phospholipase A2, cyclooxygenase and lipoxygenase [133,134]. Nuttall S.L. et al. [132] administered an equivalent of 300 mg of grape procyanidins to 20 young healthy volunteers and induced a doubling of the serum total antioxidant activity for over 3 h from ingestion. This observation marked a change in perception according to which antioxidant consumption is part of a healthy diet for the concept of therapeutic strategy in diseases which are known to be aggravated by oxidative stress.

Studies have shown that, when administered orally, curcumin has a very short half-life (10 min) due to its rapid metabolization, low absorption in the gastro-intestinal tract and rapid excretion [135–139]. In order to boost curcumin activity, its complexation with phospholipids to form phytosomes seems to be the most promising technology, due to the demonstrated improvement in its intestinal absorption and metabolic stability [139]. Recently, it has been shown that a six months treatment with curcumin formulated in phytosomes (Meriva®, Indena SpA, Milan, Italy, 500 mg tablet × 2/day, equivalent of 100 mg curcuminoids/tablet) significantly reduced plasma pro-inflammatory mediators, such as monocyte chemoattractant protein-1 (MCP-1/CCL-2), IFNγ and IL-4, as well as lipid peroxidation products (thiobarbituric acid reactive substances, TBARS) in chronic kidney disease patients [140]. Gut microbiota has been also influenced by Meriva® treatment, the *Escherichia-Shigella* being significantly lowered, while *Lachnoclostridium* and *Lactobacillaceae* spp. being considerably increased, the latter being known as playing an important role in the maintenance of the gut barrier function. It is important to mention that no adverse effects have been observed in the treatment group, confirming the good tolerance of curcumin phytosomes even on long-term administration [140].

4.2. Dyslipidemia

Dyslipidemia, defined as increased plasma concentrations of total cholesterol (TC), low-density lipoproteins cholesterol (LDL-C), triglycerides (TGs), low plasma concentrations of HDL-C or a combination of these, is a well-known major risk factor for CVD [141]. Dyslipidemia can trigger the accumulation of lipids in the arterial wall, which results in the development of the atherosclerotic plaque, the underlying cause of CVD [142]. Many types of drugs have been developed in order to decrease circulating levels of cholesterol. Among these, statins are one of the most widely used. They target endogen cholesterol synthesis, by inhibiting hydroxymethylglutaryl coenzyme A (HMG-CoA) reductase, the rate-limiting enzyme in the cholesterol biosynthesis pathway. Another class of drugs used for this purpose are Niemann-Pick C1-Like 1 (NPC1L1) inhibitors, such as ezetimibe, which inhibits the absorption of cholesterol in the intestine [143]. A novel class of lipid-lowering drugs that has emerged are monoclonal antibodies, such as evolocumab, an inhibitor for proprotein convertase subtilisin/kexin type 9 (PSCK9), a known ligand of LDL receptor (LDLR) [144]. One common aspect for all these drugs are their side effects, such as dizziness, nausea, muscle weakness or headaches [145]. This is why the complementary therapies to all these drugs are the bioactive compounds that present lipid-lowering properties with minimal side effects. Therefore, their formulation in phytosomes may be a valid complementary therapy to allopathic lipid-lowering drugs.

4.2.1. Preclinical Studies

The curry tree (*Murraya koenigii*) is a rich source of alkaloids, coumarins and phytochemicals such as girinimbin, iso-mahanimbin and koenimbine, which are known to have antioxidant, antidiabetic and lipid-lowering properties, but have low bioavailability due to their limited absorption through biological membranes [146]. Therefore, the group of Rani A. et al. [51] prepared phytosomes containing *M. koenigii* extract to improve its bioavailability and assessed the hypolipidemic effects in vivo, using streptozotocin (STZ)-induced diabetic Wistar rats. The animals were treated for 21 days with phytosomes (100 mg/kg and 200 mg/kg) or unformulated *M. koenigii* extract (200 mg/kg and 400 mg/kg). Animals displayed significantly reduced levels of serum TC, TG, LDL-C and very low-density lipoproteins cholesterol (VLDL-C), and increased levels of HDL-C compared to the untreated group. The phytosomes-treated group showed a tendency for lower concentrations of TC, TG, LDL-C and VLDL-C and for higher concentrations of HDL-C compared to the group treated with unformulated extract, but these differences were not statistically significant [51].

Crataegus aronia is recognized to have lipid-lowering and antidiabetic properties [147,148]. The ethanolic leaf extract was found to be strongly enriched in phenols, flavonoids, alkaloids and tannins. Altiti A.J. et al. [50] formulated the *Crataegus aronia* leaf ethanolic extract in phytosomes and evaluated their potential to improve the lipidic profile of STZ-induced diabetic Wistar albino rats, by comparing the effects to those of unformulated extract at similar concentrations (150 and 250 mg/kg). Both the phytosomes and the extract displayed lipid-lowering properties, by reducing the serum levels of TC, TG and LDL-C and by increasing the levels of HDL-C at 21 days after the administration, but there was no statistically significant difference between the two groups in this respect [50]. These results show that, in some cases, the phytosomal formulation may not improve the therapeutic effects of the bioactive compounds.

Caffeic acid is a very active hydroxycinnamic acid, being found in fruits, vegetables, coffee and wine [149]. It possesses many health benefits, among which is the lipid regulatory effect, but caffeic acid displays poor water solubility and poor oral absorption [150]. To improve these aspects, Mangrulkar S. et al. [151] formulated caffeic acid in phytosomes by encapsulating the bioactive compound in Phospholipon® 90H (Lipoid, Ludwigshafen, Germany). They evaluated the lipid regulatory potential of the phytosomes on Sprague Dawley rats fed a high fat diet for 8 weeks. The results show that formulated caffeic acid significantly lowered the levels of TC, TG, LDL-C, VLDL-C and increased the level of HDL-C, proving superior lipid regulatory action compared to the pure caffeic acid, at the same concentration of 40 mg/kg [151].

The effects of curcumin formulated in phytosomes on atherosclerosis induced by a high fat diet in New Zealand white rabbits were investigated by the group of Hatamipour M. et al. [152]. Curcumin phytosomes (Meriserin, Indena SpA, Milan, Italy) at two doses equivalent to 10 and 100 mg/kg of curcuminoids were administered for 4 weeks. The results showed a significant reduction in the atherosclerotic plaque histopathologically evaluated on sections of the aortic arch. In addition, the intima/media thickness ratio and the macrophage infiltration rate of the plaque were significantly decreased by the higher dose of curcumin phytosomes compared to the lower one, the measurement being performed on hematoxylin-eosine stained sections of the aortic arch [152].

The group of Poruba M. et al. [153] administered silymarin in different formulations (a standardized extract of silymarin, micronized silymarin and silymarin in the form of phytosome) to non-obese hereditary hyper-triglyceridemic rats as dietary supplements (1%) for 4 weeks. The results showed that all tested forms of silymarin significantly decreased the plasma levels of TG, TC and increased the HDL-C levels [153]. Silymarin formulated in phytosomes significantly increased the protein expression of cytochrome P450 4A (CYP4A), known as contributing to omega and omega-1 hydroxylation of fatty acids required for the synthesis of TG [153]. The silymarin in the form of phytosome had the best bioavailability [154]. All the three silymarin diets significantly increased the protein expression of cholesterol 7alpha-hydroxylase (CYP7A1), a hepatic enzyme responsible for metabolizing cholesterol into 7α-hydroxycholesterol, a rate-limiting step for the bile acids synthesis. Silymarin in the form of phytosome significantly increased the protein expression of ATP-binding cassette (ABC) transporters (ABCG5 and ABCG8), regulating the cholesterol efflux from the hepatocytes into the bile [153]. The positive effect of silymarin on plasma TC could be partly due to the higher excretion of cholesterol mediated by CYP7A1 and ABC transporters. The decreased plasma level of TG may be due to the increased liver TG metabolism through CYP4A. In this case, the formulation in phytosomes added therapeutic value to silymarin.

4.2.2. Clinical Studies

Bergamot (*Citrus bergamia*) offers a unique profile of flavonoids and flavonoid glycosides, such as neoeriocitrin, neohesperidin, naringin, rutin, neodesmin, rhoifolin and ponciarin [155]. Rondanelli M. et al. [156] aimed to evaluate the effect of bergamot phytoconstituents formulated in phytosomes on the lipid parameters in 64 overweight and obese class I subjects (BMI 25–35 kg/m^2) with diagnosed mild hypercholesterolemia (5.4–7.0 mmoL/L). Bergamot Phytosome (Vazguard, Indena SpA, Milan, Italy) is an innovative lecithin formulation of the bergamot enriched polyphenols fraction (BPF), the phospholipids (sunflower lecithin) being formulated with 40% in weight standardized BPF extract as described previously by Mollace V. et al. [93], in order to enhance the oral bioavailability of bergamot's main flavonoids. Tablets contain 500 mg of bergamot phytosomes (standardized to contain 11–19% of total flavanones). The bergamot phytosomes were administered for 12 weeks to overweight and obese subjects, and after the first 30 days of treatment the values of TC and LDL-C significantly decreased, while the level of HDL-C increased compared to the placebo group [156]. The complex composition of bergamot extract endowed the phytosomes with multiple mechanisms of action. Thus, the signaling pathways involved the direct stimulation of AMP-activated protein kinase (AMPK), and the inhibition of HMG-CoA reductase by some flavanones that have a hydroxyl mevalonate moiety [156].

4.3. Hepatic Disorders

The liver works like a central factory for the body metabolism, being the organ responsible for nutrients processing, synthesis and catabolism of numerous key proteins and lipids, as well as for drugs detoxification. Therefore, the health of the liver is very important for the health of the whole body. NAFLD or the metabolic-associated fatty liver disease (MAFLD) affects over 30% of the world population [157]. It arises from lipid accumulation in hepatocytes, a process that alters the liver's normal function. It is associated with obesity, dyslipidemia and insulin resistance, which are risk factors for type 2 DM (T2DM) and CVD [157,158]. Of interest, 75% of T2DM patients also display NAFLD [157]. To date, there is no specific treatment for NAFLD, but previous studies have shown that diets rich in antioxidants and anti-inflammatory phytochemicals, with little or no side effects, can be effective in treating NAFLD [159].

4.3.1. Preclinical Studies

The Ginkgoselect Phytosome® (Indena SpA, Milan, Italy), prepared from soy phospholipids and *Ginkgo biloba* extract, has been tested for hepatoprotective properties in Wistar rats with rifampicin-induced hepatotoxicity (500 mg/kg, for 30 days). Treatment with Ginkgoselect Phytosome® at 25 mg/kg and 50 mg/kg significantly lowered the plasma levels of alanin aminotransferase (ALT) and aspartate aminotransferase (AST) and increased the serum total proteins and albumin, the latter being indicators of the hepatoprotective effects. No differences between the groups treated with phytosome and those treated with 100 mg/kg silymarin were observed [96]. Similar, the group of Naik S.R. et al. [160] conducted a study on Wistar albino rats with carbon tetrachloride (CCl_4)-induced liver damage and intraperitoneally treated with *Ginkgo biloba* phytosomes (25 mg/kg and 50 mg/kg) before and during the CCl_4 treatment. The results show that the serum activity of ALT, AST and alkaline phosphatases (ALPs) were significantly decreased in a dose-dependent manner, while the serum total protein and albumin levels were increased in the phytosome-treated group compared to the untreated animals [160]. The hepatoprotective effect of *G. biloba* phytosomes has been confirmed by a histopathologic assay showing the regeneration of the liver cells after CCl_4-induced injury and centrilobular necrosis of the liver tissue. The beneficial effects of phytosomes have been comparable to those of silymarin, a known hepatoprotective drug. In addition, the *G. biloba* phytosomes treatment increased the hepatic level of GSH and the activity of the antioxidant enzymes SOD, CAT, GPx and GR, while the TBARS levels were decreased in a dose-dependent manner, compared to untreated animals [160].

Silybum marianum, known as milk thistle, is a recognized hepato-protectant used in the treatment of hepatitis C, hepatocarcinoma, NAFLD and gall bladder disorders [161–163]. Four isomers have been described within silymarin, such as silybin, isosilybin, silicristin and silidianin, the main active component being silybin. Like many other naturally occurring compounds, silymarin has limitations such as partial water-solubility, poor bioavailability and poor intestinal absorption. In order to increase the bioavailability and to enhance the beneficial effects of milk thistle extract, El-Gazayerly O.N. et al. [164] prepared phytosomes containing different molar ratios of soy lecithin/egg yolk and silybin, but the most suitable formula was that which contained 0.25:1 egg yolk and silybin. Milk thistle extract (equivalent to 200 mg silybin/kg, orally) and silybin phytosomes (equivalent to 200 mg/kg silybin, orally) were administered daily to male albino rats with CCl_4-induced liver injury for 10 days. Both the phytosomes and the milk thistle extract induced elevated SOD levels in the treated groups, but the phytosomes were more efficient than milk thistle extract in this respect. The phytosomes also proved to be more effective compared to the milk thistle extract in the case of ALT, whose level was more decreased in the phytosomes group [164]. In another study, Shriram R.G. et al. [47] investigated the efficacy of phospholipid-based sylimarin phytosomes in enhancing the absorption and the oral bioavailability of silymarin, as well as their hepatoprotective properties, in male Wistar rats. The animals were orally treated by an optimized silymarin phytosomal suspension (100 mg silymarin/kg/day) for 7 days, followed by a single i.p. dose of a mixture of CCl_4 and olive oil on the seventh day. The silymarin phytosomal formulation significantly improved silymarin oral bioavailability compared to pure silymarin, as indicated by a 6-fold increase in the systemic bioavailability. The results show that the treatment with silymarin phytosomes was most efficient in restoring liver SOD, CAT, GPx, glutathione S-transferase (GST), GR and GSH levels in rats, the increase in these enzymes' levels being more evident than in the group treated with plain silymarin. Pre-treatment with silymarin–phospholipid complexes significantly abrogated the CCl_4-induced increase in lipid peroxides measured as MDA levels, while pre-treatment with pure silymarin failed to protect the rats from CCl_4-triggered lipid peroxidation. Pre-treatment with pure silymarin resulted in a moderate hepatoprotective effect as evidenced by a decrease in fatty tissue degeneration and parenchymal cells damage. The silibinin accounts for 50–70% of the milk thistle extract, and it is the major bioactive flavonolignan in silymarin. Tang S. et al. [165] assessed the hepatoprotective mechanism of silibinin–phospholipids complex in the pathogenesis of acute liver injury and investigated how silibinin phytosomes modulate necroptosis-S100A9-necroinflammation signaling molecules. To achieve this, BALB/c mice treated with D-galactosamine (D-GalN)/LPS (in order to trigger liver injury) received by gavage silibinin (25 mg/kg) or silibinin–phospholipid complex (25 mg/kg) 24 h before and 2 h after acute liver insult. Serum activity of AST and ALT, as well as the hepatic pathology score, were significantly decreased in the unformulated and formulated silibinin-treated groups compared to the injured group, but there was no significant difference between free silibinin and phospholipid complex formulation treatment. Of interest, the silibinin–phospholipid complex treatment decreased the levels of necroptosis-signaling molecules, S100 calcium-binding protein A9 (S100A9) and necroinflammation signaling molecules, making it more effective compared to unformulated silibinin. In addition, the authors incubated macrophages isolated from the tibia and femur of mice with formulated silibinin, in order to evaluate whether silibinin–phospholipid complex treatments promote the polarization of macrophages toward an anti- or pro-inflammatory phenotype. Interestingly, they detected a reduction in M1 markers (such as inducible nitric oxide synthase-iNOS, CD86 and TNFα) and an increase in M2 markers (such as arginase 1-Arg1, CD206 and transforming growth factor-beta-TGF-β), the level of TGF-β being significantly higher in cells exposed to silibinin phytosomes compared to unformulated silibinin. This can be a mechanism responsible for the hepatoprotective effects of phytosomes formulation of silibinin, and all these results prove the advantages of this formulation for the therapeutic potential of silymarin.

Naringenin is a natural bioactive compound belonging to the flavanone class, possessing antioxidant, anti-inflammatory and lipid-regulatory effects [19]. Due to its rapid elimination, naringenin needs frequent administration to maintain an effective plasma level. The group of Mukherjee P.K. [166] prepared naringenin–phospholipid complexes and evaluated their antioxidant and hepatoprotective properties compared to free naringenin at a dose of 100 mg/kg in the model of CCl_4-injured rats. Their results indicated that formulation of naringenin in phytosomes increases its maximum concentration by over 60% and prolongs its life in circulation (more than double, from 10 h at maximum concentration to 25 h), compared to free naringenin. Thus, the phospholipid formulation of naringenin increases its half-life and decreases the clearance rate, making it more effective in protecting the liver against harmful CCl_4. In this manner, the pre-treatment of rats with naringenin phytosomes significantly reduced the plasma concentration of ALT, AST and bilirubin increased by CCl_4 administration, and increased the hepatic levels of the antioxidant enzymes GPx, SOD and CAT, compared to free naringenin which has no significant beneficial effects.

Catechin is a natural bioactive compound belonging to the flavonoids class that has been shown to be a ROS scavenger, a promoter of anti-oxidant enzymes, hepatoprotective and inhibitor of pro-oxidant enzymes [167,168]. The group of Athmouni, K. et al. [169] developed catechin–phospholipid complexes and evaluated their protective effect on cadmium-caused liver injuries in rats. They found that catechin (15 mg/kg body weight) absorption in rats increased by 40% following formulation in phytosomes, compared to the unformulated compound, and this could be related to its increased solubility. In addition, treatment of rats having cadmium-induced liver injuries with catechin phytosomes induced a significant decrease in plasma AST, ALT and bilirubin, and ameliorated the activities of the antioxidant enzymes SOD, CAT and GPx, compared to unformulated catechin.

Apigenin is a hydrophobic, polyphenolic flavonoid known for its antioxidant, anti-inflammatory, antidiabetic and anti-microbial potential [19]. The group of Telange D.R. et al. [43] developed apigenin–phospholipid phytosomes to improve the aqueous solubility, in vivo bioavailability and antioxidant activity of apigenin. The optimized formulation demonstrated a 36-fold higher aqueous solubility of apigenin, and a significant increase (over 40%) in the bioavailability up to 8–10 h, compared to that of free apigenin (at a dose of 100 mg apigenin/kg). The hepatoprotective role of apigenin phytosomes was assessed on the rat model of CCl_4-induced liver injury, and the results show that phytosomes containing 25 mg apigenin/kg significantly increased the levels of GSH, SOD CAT, and decreased the levels of lipid peroxides (TBARS), compared to free apigenin.

Ursolic acid is a pentacyclic triterpenoid, which is found either as a free acid or as an aglycone of saponins. It is reported to have several therapeutic activities including antihyperlipidemic effects by inhibiting the activity of pancreatic lipase [170] and it is also known for its hepatoprotective potential in both acute and chronic liver diseases [171] The major limitations of ursolic acid are its poor absorption, rapid elimination and hence low bioavailability. Therefore, the group of Biswas S. [72] prepared and characterized phospholipid complexes of ursolic acid in order to overcome these limitations. They investigated ursolic acid's hepatoprotective activity and bioavailability in CCl_4-injured Wistar rats. The animals were treated with free ursolic acid extract or formulated in phytosomes at doses of 10 and 20 mg/kg p.o. equivalent to pure ursolic acid, for 7 days. After this time, a single i.p. dose of a mixture of CCl_4 and olive oil was administered to rats, to induce liver injury. The results show that the phytosome formulation increased the serum bioavailability of ursolic acid by over 8-fold, and enhanced its elimination time by 12-fold as compared to the pure compound at the same dose. Both formulas had hepatoprotective actions in CCl_4-treated rats demonstrated by the decrease in serum AST, ALT and ALP activity, the effects being slightly increased in the phytosome group compared to those with free ursolic acid. Total bilirubin serum levels were significantly decreased only in the group that received ursolic acid formulated in phytosomes, compared to the CCl_4-treated group. The activity of the liver antioxidant enzymes SOD, CAT, GPx, GST and GR, the GSH levels and the total protein concentration in the liver were best stimulated by the administration of 20 mg/kg ursolic acid formulated in phytosomes. In addition, the architecture of the liver tissue was significantly improved by the administration of phytosomes with ursolic acid, compared to pure ursolic acid or to the CCl_4-treated group, as it was evidenced by the hematoxylin-eosin-stained sections.

All these preclinical studies bring solid arguments for the use of phytosomal formulation of bioactive compounds to treat hepatic disorders.

4.3.2. Clinical Studies

In the study conducted by Safari Z. et al. [172], patients with NAFLD received curcumin phytosomes (250 mg containing 20% curcuminoids and 20% phosphatidylserine, Indena SpA) or placebo pills daily for 12 weeks, followed by the evaluation of the lipid profile, fasting blood sugar, anthropometric indices, liver enzymes, fibrosis and steatosis. The results showed that the administration of phytosomal curcumin significantly improved the liver status by reducing fibrosis and steatosis in NAFLD patients compared to the placebo group, but there was no difference in the lipid profile (TC, TG, LDL-C, HDL-C) and fasting blood glucose between these groups [172]. Panahi Y. et al. [173] aimed to evaluate the efficacy and safety of supplementation with phytosomal curcumin (Meriva®, Indena SpA, Milan, Italy), which contained a complex of curcumin and soy phosphatidylcholine in a 1:2 weight ratio, in subjects with NAFLD. The administration of phytosomal curcumin (1000 mg/day in 2 divided doses) for 8 weeks to NAFLD patients induced a significant decrease in the body mass index (BMI) values, the lowering of hepatic AST and ALT activities as well as the reduction in the portal vein diameter and liver size as compared to the placebo group. An increase in the hepatic vein flow velocity was also observed between the two analyzed groups. Furthermore, ultrasonographic findings (decrease in the echogenicity of the liver parenchyma) were improved in 75% of subjects in the curcumin group, while the rate of improvement in the placebo group was 4.7%. Formulation into nanophytosomes containing piperine has been shown to improve the low bioavailability of curcumin by decreasing the conjugation of curcumin with glucuronic acid in the liver and consequently lowering its elimination in urine [138]. Using these types of nanophytosomes, Cicero A.F.G. et al. [174] conducted a study in which they administered curcumin-containing phytosomes (Curserin®, Indena SpA, Milan, Italy: 200 mg curcumin, 120 mg phosphatidylserine, 480 mg phosphatidylcholine and 8 mg piperine from *Piper nigrum* L. dry extract) for 8 weeks to overweight subjects with suboptimal fasting plasma glucose. The results showed that the treated group exhibited improved lipid profile (as demonstrated by the decrease of TG and increase of HDL-C levels) as compared to the placebo group. In addition, it was noticed the improvement of the hepatic function, reflected by the reduction in the activities of AST, ALT and gamma–glutamyl transferase, as well as in the fatty liver score [174].

Larger clinical studies are needed to consolidate the therapeutic potential of curcumin formulated in phytosomes for hepatic disorders.

4.4. Diabetes Mellitus

Diabetes is one of the 21st century's major health concerns, being one of the most encountered disorders nowadays, with a more than 50% increase since 2017 [175]. The alteration in the microvasculature or macrovasculature leading to cardiovascular problems, diabetic kidney disease, diabetic neuropathies or retinopathies determines increased morbidity and mortality in diabetic patients [175]. The hallmark of DM is the increased level of plasma glucose which appears as a consequence of an altered insulin metabolic pathway, either due to its decreased secretion (caused by the dysfunction or even loss of function of pancreatic beta cells, characteristic to type 1 DM), defective action (insulin resistance, characteristic to T2DM) or both [8]. Another characteristic of DM is the presence of dyslipidemia characterized by elevated fasting and postprandial TG, increased LDL-C levels and low levels of protective HDL-C, which also plays an important role in the development of diabetic vasculopathies [8]. Synthetic oral anti-hyperglycemic drugs such as insulin, sulfonylureas, thiazolidinediones and biguanides were successfully developed for diabetes treatment. Unfortunately, many of these drugs have significant side effects such as fatal hepatotoxicity, increased risk of myocardial infarction and increased cardiovascular mortality (reviewed in [14]). To overcome these problems, alternative or complementary therapeutic strategies with little side effects, such as phytotherapy, were developed [139]. Different complex mixtures or classes of bioactive compounds including alkaloids, flavonoids, polyphenols and triterpenes were used for the amelioration of diabetic symptoms.

4.4.1. Preclinical Studies

Rani A. et al. [51] tested phytosomes containing curry tree (*Murraya koenigii*) extract to assess their antidiabetic effects in vivo, using STZ-induced diabetic Wistar rats. The animals were treated for 21 days with glucose and with different doses of extract (200–400 mg/kg) or phytosomes (100–200 mg/kg). The animals treated with phytosomes exhibited a 40% reduction in serum glucose concentration at a lower dose, suggesting enhancement in its therapeutic efficacy compared to the group treated with the extract. The levels of urea and creatinine, important markers for renal disorder in DM, were restored to almost normal levels in the treated group, indicating an antidiabetic activity of curry tree phytosomes [51].

Crataegus aronia is used to treat DM [50]. Nanophytosomes encapsulating *C. aronia* leaf extract were developed very recently by the group of Altiti A. et al. [50] by mixing 1:1 phospholipid (lecithin) with *C. aronia* leaf ethanolic extract. The nanophytosomes (150 mg/kg or 250 mg/kg) had hypoglycemic effects at 14 and 21 days of treatment of STZ-induced diabetic Wistar albino rats. The effect was dose-dependent, slightly more efficient than that of the unformulated extract at the same doses, but not equipotent to metformin [50].

An interesting therapeutic approach designed to increase the beneficial effects of natural compounds was that in which a complex of more than one natural extract is encapsulated in the same phytosome. This approach was chosen by Rathee S. and Kamboj A. [176] who used extracts from fruits of *Citrullus colocynthis* (L.), *Momordica balsamina* and *Momordica dioica* to obtain antidiabetic phytosomes. The optimized formula for these phytosomes was obtained by using the three-level Box–Behnken design which considers parameters such as phospholipid: extract ratio, process temperature and reaction time. The resulting phytosomes were stable and had a very good entrapment efficiency, while the polyherbal extracts and phospholipids in the complex were joined by non-covalent-bonds and did not form a new compound. To test the anti-diabetic effects, the polyherbal phytosomal formulation was administered to STZ-induced diabetic Wistar rats in doses of 100 mg/kg and 250 mg/kg for 15 days. The results show that, although both concentrations are effective in decreasing the serum glucose level, the lower concentration is more efficient, its effect being comparable to that of 50 mg/kg metformin.

Chrysin is a flavonoid encountered in different plants, flowers and bee propolis. In the context of DM, in vivo studies demonstrated that chrysin has hypolipidemic, anti-inflammatory and anti-oxidant effects [177–179]. However, the decreased bioavailability of chrysin due to its poor solubility and short circulation half-life leads to the necessity to formulate it in an efficient delivery system. Recently, the group of Kim S.M. et al. [179] used chrysin-loaded phytosomes prepared with egg phospholipid at a 1:3 molar ratio (chrysin: phospholipid) to study the antidiabetic effects of this natural compound. After 9 weeks of nanophytosomes administration (100 mg chrysin equivalent/kg) to db/db mice, the study demonstrated a decrease in serum glucose, insulin levels and homeostatic model assessment for insulin resistance (HOMA-IR), similar to 200 mg/kg metformin treatment. The hypoglycemic effect of chrysin nanophytosomes was due to their capacity to inhibit the gluconeogenesis by down-regulating phosphoenolpyruvate carboxykinase (PEPCK) in the liver, while stimulating the glucose uptake in db/db mice by increasing glucose transporter type 4 (GLUT4) gene expression and translocation in the skeletal muscle. Compared to free chrysin, the chrysin nanophytosomes demonstrated an additional effect in modulating the glucose metabolism-related genes both in the liver (PEPCK, hexokinase 2) and skeletal muscle (GLUT4, hexokinase 2 and PPARγ) due to the increased bioavailability of the chrysin in the phytosome formulation [179].

Rutin is a citrus flavonoid glycoside found in different plants, including *Ruta graveolens* L. (Rutaceae), *Eucalyptus* spp. (Myrtaceae) or *Sophora japonica* L. (Fabaceae) [180]. Besides being a powerful antioxidant and anti-inflammatory agent, rutin is also known for its antidiabetic action. The mechanisms of rutin anti-diabetic effects include the reduction in carbohydrates absorption from the small intestine, the up-regulation of glucose uptake paralleled by the suppression of gluconeogenesis as well as the increase in insulin secretion from pancreatic beta cells [181]. To overcome the limitation of its low bioavailability, rutin was encapsulated by Amjadi S. et al. [182] into nanophytosomes in order to evaluate the therapeutic potency of this nanocarrier in STZ-induced diabetic Wistar rats. The administration of rutin-loaded nanophytosomes (25 mg rutin/kg per day) for 4 weeks to diabetic rats decreased the level of glucose and glycated hemoglobin in the blood and restored the diabetes-induced damages in the pancreas, liver and kidney (evidenced by the histopathological assay) in a more efficient manner than free rutin. This demonstrates that encapsulation into phytosomes is an efficient technique to enhance the rutin therapeutic potential in diabetic conditions. In addition, rutin nanophytosomes were more effective than free rutin to control the hyperlipidemia, measured as decreased TC, TG and increased HDL-C, to reduce the AST and ALT activities, and to attenuate the oxidative stress expressed as decreased MDA levels and increased total antioxidant potential due to the increased activity of SOD and GPx in the animal model.

Curcumin is a polyphenol with well-known anti-diabetic, lipid-lowering and hepatoprotective actions [183,184]. Studies have shown that curcumin possesses insulin-sensitizing actions through different pathways. It was demonstrated that the molecular mechanisms of action of curcumin in DM include the activation of insulin receptors, the increase in lipoprotein lipase activity, the stimulation of insulin-independent glucose uptake by pancreatic beta cells and anti-inflammatory effects in adipose tissue, in parallel with the enhancement of adipokines [139]. Recently, the group of Alhabashneh W. et al. [185] tested curcumin phytosomes effects on glycemic and lipid profile of STZ-induced Wistar diabetic rats. The phytosomes obtained by mixing 1:1 phosphatidylcholine (soybean lecithin) and curcumin were orally administered to diabetic rats at 150 and 250 mg/kg dose, for 3 weeks. The results show that curcumin phytosomes administration determines the decrease in blood glucose, TC, LDL-C and TG in parallel with the significant rise in HDL-C. The hypoglycemic and hypolipidemic effects were dose-dependent and the effects of curcumin phytosomes were higher than for those treated with free curcumin at the same dose [185].

Berberine is a multi-target natural product with beneficial effects in different pathologies. Studies in humans show that berberine has a beneficial effect on the expression of genes which ameliorate glucose levels (1 mg/day), regulate the cholesterol absorption (300 mg/day) or modulate the microbiota (500 mg/day) [186]. In the context of DM, berberine has positive effects due to is antioxidant properties and also, very importantly, because it targets AMPK, a protein involved in the regulation of glucose metabolism, fatty acid oxidation and insulin resistance [187]. To overcome the low bioavailability of free berberine, the group of Yu F. et al. [52] developed phytosomes loaded with berberine using soybean phosphatidylcholine and commercially available berberine in a mass ratio of 5:1. Pharmacokinetic studies demonstrated that the oral bioavailability of the berberine-loaded nanophytosomes in Wistar rats was improved 3-fold as compared to the orally administrated free berberine. The obtained phytosomes have also anti-diabetic effects, the study demonstrating that administration of berberine in nanophytosomes (100 mg/kg) for 4 weeks to diabetic db/db mice decreased the plasma fasting blood glucose and reverted the TG levels in the liver to a better extent than free berberine. The insulin levels were not modulated either by free berberine or by the phytosome formulation.

Gymnema inodorum was successfully used in alternative medicine for the amelioration of DM. Its antidiabetic properties are due to the presence of active phenolic acids, flavonoids, triterpenoid compounds and pregnane glycosides, this complex composition conferring the *G. inodorum* extract antiglycemic and antioxidant effects and insulin-mimetic properties [121,188–190]. The *G. inodorum* leaf extract formulated in phytosomes has been tested for its anti-insulin resistance activity by measuring the glucose uptake and lipolysis in LPS-treated 3T3-L1 adipocytes. The results evidence that LPS adipocytes exposed to phytosomes with *G. inodorum* extract take up more glucose compared to LPS adipocytes alone, but higher levels of phospholipid in phytosomes (mass ratio GI extract: PC = 1:2 versus 1:1) slightly interfered with the anti-insulin-resistant effects of the *G. inodorum* extract by decreasing the glucose uptake and increasing the lipid degradation, measured as glycerol release in the culture medium [26]. These data highlight that an increased percentage of phospholipids in phytosomes can invalidate their beneficial effects through the oxidation products they can generate.

Tripterine is a pentacyclic triterpenoid quinone with anti-diabetic and anti-inflammatory potential. The group of Zhu S. et al. [191] used selenized tripterine phytosomes (Se@Tri-PTs) to identify the mechanisms by which these nanostructures alleviate podocyte injury, a major contributor to diabetic nephropathy. The study showed that 5 µg/mL of selenized phytosomes improved the viability of podocytes in vitro. In addition, the phytosomes reduced NLRP3 expression, re-established the expression of proteins that regulate autophagic processes (Beclin-1, microtubule-associated protein 1A/1B-light chain 3-LC3 II/LC3I, ubiquitin-binding protein p62-p62 and SIRT-1) and decreased the apoptosis of podocytes exposed for 48 h to high glucose [191].

4.4.2. Clinical Studies

Quercetin is a flavonol found in various fruits, vegetables or leaves, with beneficial effects in human health. To overcome quercetin's highly variable bioavailability (0–50%) and rapid elimination (1–2 h half-life time), different innovative formulations to deliver this active compound were tested. Quercetin Phytosome® (Quercefit™, Indena SpA, Milan, Italy) is one of the quercetin formulations that demonstrated improved solubility in the solution that simulated gastrointestinal fluids and also increased absorption (20-fold) [192]. Using this formulation, Riva A. et al. [192] evaluated the interaction between Quercefit and anti-diabetic therapy, antiplatelet agents and anticoagulants, in healthy subjects. The topic is important, due to the fact that it is well known that the interaction between synthetic drugs with different natural active compounds exists, and it can have serious clinical outcomes [193,194]. The study involved 12 diabetic patients treated with antidiabetic metformin, 30 subjects with antiplatelet therapy (acetylsalicylic acid, ticlopidine or clopidogrel) and 20 subjects with anticoagulants (warfarin or dabigatran), all of them receiving supplementation with Quercetin Phytosome for at least 10 days. The Quercefit supplementation consisted in the oral administration of two tablets of phytosomes/day, corresponding to 200 mg/day of quercetin. The results showed that Quercefit administration did not induce significant differences in the fasting glycaemia or glycated hemoglobin (for the anti-diabetic medication), measured bleeding time (for subjects with antiplatelet therapy) or International Normalized Ratio (INR) level (for the subjects with anticoagulant therapy) [178]. This study proves that the administration of quercetin phytosome does not interfere with different classes of allopathic drugs, such as metformin, aspirin or warfarin.

Meriva curcumin phytosomes (Indena) were also used to evaluate the possible beneficial actions of curcumin to improve the kidney functions of subjects with temporary kidney dysfunction (TKD). This study included a total of 87 subjects with TKD divided into two groups: one following the standard management (hydration, a reduced intake of NaCl and other electrolytes, decreased intake of carbohydrates, abolition of drugs or compounds that potentially harm the kidneys and a moderate exercise program) and a group that followed the same standard management and received also a supplementation with Meriva® (1.5 g/day, delivering 300 mg highly bioavailable curcumin) divided into three administrations/day, for 4 weeks. The results of the study show that Meriva® reduced the albumin almost to normal levels in the urine of patients with microalbuminuria and macroalbuminuria, and decreased the oxidative stress measured as plasma free radicals. The tolerability to Meriva® and the compliance of the patients were good. These parameters were improved compared to those from the standard management group, suggesting that Meriva can safely ameliorate the TKD symptoms [195].

The group of Cicero A.F.G. et al. [174] recently studied the effect of curcumin phytosome containing piperine (Curserin®, Indena, SpA, Milan, Italy) on a placebo-controlled clinical trial including 40 overweight subjects who received Curserin® compared to 40 overweight subjects that received a placebo. The study showed that two capsules/day of Curserin® administration for 8 weeks have beneficial effects on the: (i)anthropometric parameters (decreased BMI and waist circumference) and (ii) metabolic characteristics (decreased HOMA-IR, fasting plasma glucose and fasting plasma insulin) as compared to the placebo group. Very interesting, the authors observed for the first time a statistically significant reduction in serum cortisol level in human subjects treated with Curserin®. In another study, Mirhafez S.R. et al. [196] investigated the therapeutic properties of lower doses of phospholipid formulation of curcumin on the lipid profile, hepatic enzymes and hepatic fat mass in patients with NAFLD in a randomized controlled clinical trial. Patients in the treated group received curcumin phytosome in a dose of 250 mg/day (Meriva, Indena SpA, Milan, Italy) for 2 months. The results show that AST levels in the serum of the phytosome-treated group were significantly lower, as well as the NAFLD grade, compared to the placebo group.

Berberine phytosome formulation (Indena SpA, Milan, Italy), containing berberine extract (28–34%), in combination with sunflower lecithin, pea protein and grape seed extract, was used in a recent pilot study to evaluate their possible beneficial effects in polycystic ovary syndrome (PCOS), a medical condition associated with insulin resistance. A group of 12 normal and overweight women received two daily oral doses of 550 mg berberine tablets for 60 days. The treatment determined the normalization of (i) the glycemic and insulin profiles, measured as decreased HOMA-IR index, insulin and glycemia; (ii) lipid profile, evidenced as a lowering of VLDL-C and TG levels and (iii) inflammatory status measured as a decrease in TNFα and CRP levels in the plasma. In addition, the authors observed the redistribution of adipose tissue with the reduction in the visceral fat and fat mass, without any changes in the diet [187]. Importantly, the tested product was well-tolerated, with no modifications in safety blood parameters as AST, ALT, gamma–glutamyl-transferase or bowel discomfort, the lack of side effects being very important, permitting the long-term use of berberine.

4.5. Metabolic Syndrome

The metabolic syndrome represents a condition including a cluster of risk factors that contribute to the inception and progression of cardiovascular diseases. The risk factors are dyslipidemia (high TC, LDL-C and TG levels, low HDL-C levels), abdominal obesity, impaired fasting glucose/insulin resistance and high blood pressure. Among the induced diseases, obesity is a complex disorder involving the excessive accumulation of fat in the body. It is the most common disorder worldwide, which leads to many complications such as DM, stroke and CVD. The above complications represent the leading causes of mortality worldwide [197]. The treatment of obesity is mostly based on equalizing calorie ingestion and energy consumption. Several natural compounds are used for the treatment of obesity.

4.5.1. Preclinical Studies

Callistemon citrinus has been described as antimicrobial, anti-inflammatory, anti-obesogenic, antioxidant and hepatoprotective [198,199]. The main bioactive components are terpenoids, phenolic acids and flavonoids (including eucalyptine, blumenol, gallic acid and protocatechuic acid) which have low oral bioavailability and absorption. The group of Ortega-Pérez L.G. et al. [200] prepared *Callistemon citrinus* leaf extract in phyto-phospholipid complexes aiming to use them (doses range 50–200 mg extract/kg) for weight gain prevention in Wistar rats fed with a hypercaloric diet. They obtained phytosomes with the *C. citrinus* extract of a small size, high entrapment efficiency, improved oral bioavailability and enhanced stability at 20 °C (over three months) [201,202]. The phytosomes and unformulated *C. citrinus* extract exhibited similar inhibitory activity against the free radicals assessed by 2,2-diphenyl-1-picrylhydrazyl (DPPH) and 2,2′-azino-bis(3-ethylbenzothiazoline-6-sulfonic acid) (ABTS) methods, and the ability to reduce ferric to ferrous ions. In addition, both products reduced excessive weight in the obese rats. The administration of *C. citrinus* phytosomes, even in low doses, further reduced the adiposity index and TG levels in obese rats, compared to the unformulated extract [200].

Soybean (*Glycine max*) is known to influence body weight due to its content of saponin, proteins and phosphatidylcholine [203,204]. The topical route to administer bioactive compounds has received considerable attention because it is a non-invasive path and is characterized by high bioavailability due to the direct drug delivery to the site of action, avoiding losses along the gastrointestinal tract [205]. Thus, the group of El-Menshawe S.F. et al. [69] investigated the anti-obesity effect of soybean extract formulated in phytosomes and included them into a thermogel to be applied on the abdomen of experimental male albino rats fed with high-fat diet in order to gain weight. Their results showed that, after a one-month treatment, the soybean phytosomal thermogel induced a decrease in body weight (10%), adipose tissue weight (27%) and food consumption (35%) compared to rats receiving thermogel with unformulated soybean extract. In addition, the animals with soybean phytosomal thermogel presented a significant decrease in plasma levels of TC, TG, LDL-C and VLDL-C, evidencing a slight systemic action of the formulated extract included in thermogel. Moreover, the animals treated with soybean phytosomal thermogel have shown a decreased size in the adipose cells in the epididymal adipose tissue, compared to the crude soy thermogel group [69]. Therefore, topical phytosomal application of plant extracts could be considered a promising formulation for future treatments.

4.5.2. Clinical Studies

The phyto-phospholipid formulation of curcumin was tested in human subjects diagnosed with metabolic syndrome to evaluate its ability to increase the vitamins levels, such as vitamin E. Thus, the group of Mohammadi A. et al. [206] conducted a study that involved 120 subjects with metabolic syndrome, part of them receiving unformulated curcumin, the others receiving lecithinized curcumin for 6 weeks in a dose of 200 mg active substance/day. The results evidenced that neither unformulated curcumin, nor the lecithinized form, have an effect on serum levels of vitamin E, suggesting that the antioxidant properties of curcumin are not driven on vitamins, but on the modulatory effects exerted on the antioxidant enzymes which further induce anti-inflammatory effects discussed in Section 4.1.2.

The group of Rondanelli M. et al. [156] evaluated the effect of bergamot phytoconstituents formulated in phytosomes (Bergamot Phytosome, Vazguard, Indena SpA) on visceral adipose tissue, as an indicator for the metabolic syndrome, DM and CVD [207,208] in overweight and obese class I subjects. After one month of treatment with bergamot phytosomes, the subjects showed a significant reduction in visceral adipose tissue compared to the placebo group [156]. These results are of interest because visceral adipose tissue is considered an endocrine organ able to influence the function of other organs such as liver, heart or blood vessels. Beside the lipid-lowering effects of bergamot formulated in phytosomes described in Section 4.2.2, its action as bodyweight regulator increases its therapeutic potential.

The capacity to induce weight loss of Greenselect Phytosome, a green tea extract devoid of caffeine and formulated in lecithin to improve the absorption of catechins, was evaluated in a single blind, controlled study on 50 asymptomatic subjects with borderline metabolic syndrome factors and with increased plasma oxidative stress. A group of 50 similar volunteers who took the blank formulation was considered as control group. Greenselect Phytosome in the form of coated tablets (150 mg/tablet) was administered for 24 weeks, and the results show that the phytosome formulation promoted weight loss (8%), reduced waist circumference (6%) and decreased the value of plasma free radicals by 33%, as compared to the control group [83]. This study confirms the efficacy of green tea extract formulated in phytosomes in inducing weight loss.

4.6. Cardiovascular Disorders

CVD represent the main cause of morbidity and mortality worldwide, and hypercholesterolemia, hypertension, obesity, left ventricular hypertrophy or DM represent common CVD risk factors [209]. CVD includes disorders such as heart failure, myocardial infarction (MI), pulmonary embolism and stroke [210]. The molecular mechanisms of CVD development have been extensively investigated in recent decades, the oxidative and inflammatory stress being identified as important players in the advancement of these disorders. Although important progresses were made, some of the current pharmacological therapies used for CVD treatment (including statins, antihypertensive, antithrombotic and anti-coagulation agents) present important side effects, the compliance of patients to the therapy being sometimes reduced. In the last decade, natural products based on concentrated mixtures of bioactive compounds with low side effects compared to pharmacological therapies were developed and experimentally evaluated in order to evaluate their potential to ameliorate CVD effects.

4.6.1. Preclinical Studies

Gymnema sylvestre has been reported as possessing antioxidant, hypolipidemic and antidiabetic properties, which have been attributed to its bioactive compounds, such as triterpene glycoside named gymnemic acid [211,212]. The cardioprotective potential of phospholipid–gymnemic acid complexes was evaluated in a rat model of cardiomyopathy induced by doxorubicin (30 mg/kg/i.p./single dose). Pre-treatment with gymnemic acid phytosomes (50 and 100 mg/Kg/p.o./day) for 30 days significantly reduced the cardiac toxicity induced by doxorubicin, including improvement in hemodynamic parameters and the ratio of heart weight to body weight. Moreover, the phytosome treatment decreased the concentration of Ca^{2+} and lactate dehydrogenase (LDH) in serum, as well as the levels of caspase-3 and TBARS in myocardium, compared to the untreated group. In addition, the gymnemic acid formulated in phytosomes increased the levels of Na^+/K^+ ATPase and antioxidant enzymes SOD, CAT and GPx, as compared to the pathogenic control group. The anti-apoptotic effect of phytosomes with gymnemic acid was confirmed by prevention of inter-nucleosomal DNA laddering on agarose gel electrophoresis [213].

The extracts from the leaves of *Ginkgo biloba* have been found to possess cardioprotective, antioxidant, hepatoprotective and antidiabetic properties [214,215]. The antioxidant and cardioprotective effects of *Ginkgo biloba* phytosomes (Ginkoselect Phytosome®, Indena) were investigated in rats with isoproterenol-induced cardiotoxicity (85 mg/kg). The oral treatment with phytosomes (100 mg and 200 mg/kg) for 21 days lowered the serum levels of AST, LDH and creatine phosphokinase (CPK) as markers of myocardial injury. Moreover, the levels of lipid peroxides decreased and those of GSH, SOD, CAT, GPx and GR increased in the myocardium of treated rats compared to untreated animals [216]. In addition to the hypoglycemic, hypolipidemic, immunomodulatory and hepatoprotective effects of *Ocimum sanctum* (Tulsi), good cardioprotective activity due to its antioxidant activity was reported [217–219]. The constituents of *O. sanctum*, such as flavonoids (orientin, vicenin), phenolic compounds (eugenol, cirsilineol, apigenin) and anthocyanins, have been shown to scavenge lipid peroxides [220]. The cardioprotective activity of Ginkoselect Phytosome® supplemented with *O. sanctum* leaf extract was tested in isoproterenol-induced myocardial necrosis in rats. The results show that the co-administration of phytosomes (100 mg/kg) and extract (50 and 75 mg/kg) for 30 days to rats with myocardial necrosis induces the decrease in serum enzymatic markers of stressed myocardium (AST, LDH and CPK) and reduced the level of myocardial MDA, as a lipid peroxidation marker. A significant restoration of isoproterenol-affected activities and levels of AST, LDH, CPK, GSH, SOD, CAT, GPx and GR in the hearts of treated rats was measured, the most effective combination being 100 mg/kg phytosomes plus 75 mg/kg extract. The combined treatment failed to enhance the cardioprotective activity of either herbs when used individually [221]. Thus, it was demonstrated that phytosome formulation and combination with *O. sanctum* extract augmented the cardioprotective and antioxidant properties of individual ingredients.

Withania somnifera, known as Ashwagandha, has medicinal potential as an anti-inflammatory, anti-platelet, antihypertensive, hypoglycemic and hypolipidemic agent. Phytosomal complexes of *W. somnifera* root extract have been developed as NMITLI-101, NMITLI-118 and NMITLI-128 products (CSIR, New Delhi, India). To test the neuroprotective potential against experimental stroke, a study was conducted on a middle cerebral artery occlusion (MCAO) model in rats. The phytosomal complex NMITLI118RT+ was orally administrated at the dose of 85 mg/kg, 1 h prior to ischemia and 6 h post reperfusion. The results evidence a reduction in the neurological deficit score (over 60%) and decrease in the infarct size (over 50%), along with a 35% reduction in MDA levels and over 50% increased of GSH level [222].

Carthamus tinctorius, known as safflower, has been widely used for the treatment of cardio-cerebrovascular diseases, particularly cerebral infarction or cerebral ischemia-reperfusion (CIR) injury [223,224]. The effect of safflower extract–phospholipid complexes delivered via nasal route was tested on a rat model of MCAO and compared to the effect of unformulated extract. The therapeutic effect of phytosomes was more effective on cerebral infarction and acts by improving the blood circulation in the central nervous system, reducing the inflammatory reaction and inhibiting apoptosis. The mechanism responsible for these beneficial effects involves the caspase 3-mediated TNF-α/MAPK signaling pathway [68]. This study provides additional proof that the formulation of plant extracts in phytosomes increases their therapeutic potential.

Silybin is obtained from silymarin and is used as hepatoprotective agent [225], but its water solubility is poor and requires frequent administration [226]. The mechanisms by which silybin–phosphatidylcholine phytosomes reduce liver damage include the diminution in oxidative stress, lipid peroxidation and collagen accumulation in animal models [227]. The neuroprotective action of the silybin phytosomes (20 mg/kg per oral) against CIR injury was investigated in Wistar rats by the group of Pasala P.K. et al. [228]. The CIR injury was induced after 14 days of silybin pre-treatment by occlusion of bilateral common carotid arteries for 30 min followed by 4 h of reperfusion. Phytosomes treatment significantly increases SOD and GSH levels, and decreases MDA, TNFα and IL-6 levels in the hippocampus and cortex of treated CIR-injured rats. Histopathological studies confirmed the beneficial effects of phytosomes treatment by the alleviation of cortex cell death. In silico studies for proteins (TNFα, IL-6) involved in cerebral ischemia revealed that phytosomes exhibit strong binding interaction with them compared to thalidomide (positive control). Silybin formulation in phytosome increases its bioavailability and improves its beneficial actions compared to treatment with silybin alone [228]. These data confirm the enhancement of the therapeutic properties of bioactive compounds through their formulation in phytosomes.

The phytosomes containing extracts of ginger rhizome and mulberry fruit have been shown to decrease oxidative stress and inflammation [229]. The neuroprotective effect against ischemic stroke of phytosomes with ginger and mulberry fruit extracts was studied in male Wistar rats with metabolic syndrome induced by high-carbohydrate high-fat diet. Various doses of phytosomes (50–200 mg/kg) have been administered for 21 days before and 14 days after occlusion of the right middle cerebral artery. The results evidence that phytosomes treatment significantly enhanced memory, decreased acetylcholinesterase (AChE), IL-6 and MDA levels, and increased SOD, CAT and GPx levels, neuron density and phosphorylation of extracellular signal-regulated kinase (ERK). These data suggest the cognitive enhancing effect of phytosomes. The possible underlying mechanisms may occur partly via the improvement in cholinergic function via the ERK pathway, together with the decrease in neurodegeneration induced by the reduction in oxidative stress and inflammation [230]. In another study, phytosomes with ginger and mulberry fruit extracts significantly improved brain infarction, brain edema and neurological deficit score. In addition, the reduction in DNA-methyltransferase 1 (DNMT-1), NF-κB, TNFα and CRP, together with the increased activity of the aforementioned antioxidant enzymes and PPARγ expression in the lesioned brain, were also measured. The possible underlying mechanism may occur partly via the suppression of DNMT-1, giving rise to the improvement in the signal transduction via PPARγ, resulting in the decrease in inflammation and oxidative stress [231].

L-Carnosine and Aloe vera are food supplements used to enhance the exercise performance of athletes and to manage DM based on their potential to scavenge free radical and to exert anti-inflammatory activities [232–235]. It was demonstrated that nanophytosomes with L-carnosine/Aloe vera (25:1 w/w ratio) protect human umbilical vein endothelial cells (HUVECs) against methylglyoxal-induced toxicity following 24–72 h exposure. Nanophytosome-treated HUVECs (500 µg/mL) exhibited a greater ability in free radical scavenging, NO synthesis, tube formation, wound healing and trans-well migration compared to cells treated with unformulated constituents. The proangiogenic effects of the nanophytosomes have been confirmed by the enhanced gene expression of the following proangiogenic proteins: hypoxia-inducible factor 1-alpha (HIF-1α), vascular endothelial growth factor A (VEGF-A), basic fibroblast growth factor (bFGF), vascular endothelial growth factor (VEGF) receptor 2 (KDR) and angiotensin II (Ang II) [236]. These data empower the dual L-carnosine/Aloe vera nanophytosomes as potential therapy to attenuate the T2DM-associated microvascular complications with a reduced angiogenesis.

The *Rauvolfia serpentina* root extract contains bioactive compounds, such as flavonoids, N-containing indole alkaloids and phenols, and is effective in the treatment of diseases connected with the central nervous system, such as hypertension, insomnia and epilepsy [237]. The constituents such as reserpine, ajamlicine, serpentine, ajmaline deserpidine and yohimbine alkaloids are responsible for its anti-hypertensive properties [238,239]. The nanoformulation of the *R. serpentina* crude extract shows a lower potential to block the angiotensin-converting enzyme compared to the unformulated extract (73.99% versus 83.11%) at 5 mg/mL concentration, but was non-hemolytic compared to the extract that shows 4.31% hemolysis, as was demonstrated on human erythrocytes [240]. Thus, the formulation in phytosomes made the *R. serpentine* extract safer, despite the 10% diminution in its efficacy.

4.6.2. Clinical Studies

Coenzyme Q10 (CoQ10) is able to prevent the injuries induced by free radicals and inflammatory processes, but it is known as having low bioavailability [241,242]. The formulation of coenzyme Q10 into phytosomes increased its bioavailability by three times versus standard pharmaceutical formulations and opened new opportunities for using it in clinical practice [242]. The effects of acute and chronic supplementation with CoQ10 phytosome on the endothelial reactivity and total antioxidant capacity were evaluated in a clinical study conducted in 20 healthy young non-smoking subjects. They received 150 mg CoQ10 phytosome (equivalent to 30 mg CoQ10; Ubiqsome®, Indena SpA) or placebo pills, once daily for the chronic group, and a double dose for the acute group. CoQ10 phytosome improved endothelial reactivity, mean arterial pressure and total antioxidant capacity compared to baseline or placebo [243]. Further clinical studies are needed to strengthen the therapeutic potential of CoQ10 formulated into phytosomes and to expand the pathologies that can be addressed with this treatment.

The confirmed beneficial effects of bioactive compounds formulated in phytosomes to improve the MD outcomes are schematically summarized in Figure 4.

The preclinical and clinical studies that evaluated the therapeutic potential of phytosomes and their mechanisms of action are summarized in Table 4.

Table 4. Preclinical and clinical studies evidencing the therapeutic potential of phytosomes with bioactive compounds for MD treatment.

Study Type	Disorder	Bioactive Compounds Formulated in Phytosomes; Beneficial Effects
Preclinical	Oxidative and Inflammatory stress	- *Ginkgo biloba* extract on Wistar rats with rifampicin-induced hepatotoxicity: ↓ plasma lipid peroxides; ↑ GSH, SOD, CAT, GPx, GR [96]; - Curcumin on mice with carrageenan-induced inflammation: ↑ SOD, CAT, GPx, GR [99]; - *Zingiber officinale* and *Rosa canina* extracts on C57Bl/6J mice with LPS-induced inflammation: ↓ gut and liver TNFα, IL-1β; ↑ plasma SOD2, PON1 [38] - Gallic acid on rats with valproic acid-induced oxidative stress: ↑ GPx, GR, GSH, SOD, CAT (Nrf2) [113] - Berberine on mice with inflammation: ↓ edema, local inflammation, capillary permeability [29] - *Allium ampeloprasum* extract on BALB/c mice with colon carcinoma: ↑ liver GPx and SOD mRNA; ↓ MDA [120] - *Gymnema inodorum* leaf extract on LPS-stimulated RAW 264.7 macrophages: ↓ NO [26] - Tripterine + selenium on J774A.1 macrophage: ↓ NRLP3 inflammasome, pyroptosis, gasdermin D, IL-1β [124]
	Dyslipidemia	- *Murraya koenigii* extract on STZ-induced diabetic Wistar rats: ↓ TC, TG, LDL-C, VLDL-C [51] - *Crataegus aronia* leaf extract on STZ-induced diabetic Wistar rats: ↓ TC, TG, LDL-C; ↑ HDL-C [50] - Caffeic acid on Sprague Dawley rats fed high-fat diet: ↓ TC, TG, LDL-C, VLDL-C; ↑ HDL-C [151] - Curcumin on New Zealand white rabbits fed high-fat diet: ↓ atheroma, intima/media thickness, macrophage infiltration [152] - Silymarin on hyper-triglyceridemic rats: ↓ TC, TG; ↑HDL-C, CYP4A, CYP7A1, ABCG5/8 [153]
	Hepatic disorders	- *Ginkgo biloba* extract on Wistar rats with rifampicin/CCl$_4$-induced hepatotoxicity: ↓ plasma ALT, AST, ALP, liver TBARS; ↑ serum total proteins, albumin, GSH, SOD, CAT, GPx, GR [96,160]; - *Silybum marianum* extract/Silybin/Silibinin on Wistar rats with CCl$_4$-induced hepatotoxicity or BALB/c mice with D-GalN/LPS: ↓ ALT, AST, MDA, S100A9, M1 macrophages; ↑liver SOD CAT, GPx, GST, GR, GSH, M2 macrophages [47,164,165] - Naringenin on Wistar rats with CCl$_4$-induced hepatotoxicity: ↓ plasma ALT, AST, bilirubin; ↑ hepatic GPx, SOD, CAT [166] - Catechin on Wistar rats with cadmium-induced hepatotoxicity: ↓ plasma AST, ALT, bilirubin; ↑ SOD, CAT, GPx [169] - Apigenin on Wistar rats with CCl$_4$-induced hepatotoxicity: ↓ TBARS; ↑ GSH, SOD, CAT [43] - Ursolic acid on Wistar rats with CCl$_4$-induced hepatotoxicity: ↓ serum AST, ALT, ALP, bilirubin; ↑ liver SOD, CAT, GPx, GST, GR, GSH, total protein [72]
	Diabetes mellitus	- *Murraya koenigii* extract on STZ-induced diabetic Wistar rats: ↓ serum glucose, urea, and creatinine [51] - *Crataegus aronia* leaf extract on STZ-induced diabetic Wistar rats: ↓ serum glucose [50] - *Citrullus colocynthis*, *Momordica balsamina*, *Momordica dioica* extract on STZ-induced diabetic Wistar rats: ↓ serum glucose [176] - Chrysin on db/db mice: ↓ serum glucose, insulin, HOMA-IR, hepatic PEPCK; ↑ GLUT4 [179] - Rutin on STZ-induced diabetic Wistar rats: ↓ serum glucose, HbA1C, TC, TG, AST, ALT, MDA; ↑ HDL-C, SOD, GPx [182] - Curcumin on STZ-induced diabetic Wistar rats: ↓ serum glucose, TC, TG, LDL-C; ↑ HDL-C [185] - Berberine on db/db mice: ↓ serum glucose, TG [52] - *Gymnema inodorum* leaf extract on LPS-treated 3T3-L1 adipocytes: ↑ glucose uptake [26] - Tripterine (selenized) on high glucose-exposed podocytes: ↑ viability; ↓ NLRP3, apoptosis [191]
	Metabolic syndrome	- *Callistemon citrinus* leaf extract on obese Wistar rats: ↓ body weight, adiposity index, TG [200] - Soybean (*Glycine max*) on Wistar rats with high-fat diet: ↓ body weight, adipose tissue weight, food consumption, plasma TC, TG, LDL-C, VLDL-C [69]

Table 4. Cont.

Study Type	Disorder	Bioactive Compounds Formulated in Phytosomes; Beneficial Effects
	Cardiovascular diseases	- **Gymnemic acid** on rat with cardiomyopathy doxorubicin-induced: ↓ serum LDH, myocardial caspase-3 and TBARS; ↑ Na+/K+ ATPase, SOD, CAT, GPx; improve hemodynamic parameters and heart weight/body weight ratio [213] - **Ginkgo biloba** (±**Ocimum sanctum**) on rats with isoproterenol-induced cardiotoxicity: ↓ AST, LDH, CPK; ↑ myocardial GSH, SOD, CAT, GPx, GR [216] - **Withania somnifera** root extract on MCAO rats: ↓ neurological deficit score, infarct size, MDA; ↑ GSH [222] - **Carthamus tinctorius** extract on MCAO rats: ↑ blood circulation in CNS; ↓ inflammation, apoptosis (caspase 3-TNF-α/MAPK) [68] - **Silybin** on CIR Wistar rats: ↑ SOD, GSH; ↓ MDA, TNFα, IL-6 in cortex and hippocampus [228] - **Zingiber officinale** rhizomes + **Morus** fruits extracts on Wistar with metabolic syndrome: ↑ memory, SOD, CAT G?x, neuron density, pERK; ↓ AChE, IL-6, MDA, [217]; ↑ neurological deficit score, PPARγ, ↓ DNMT-1, NF-κB, TNFα, CRP [231] - **L-Carnosine** + **Aloe vera** on methylglyoxal -HUVECs: ↑free radical scavenging, NO synthesis, tube formation, wound healing, trans-well migration, HIF-1α, VEGF-A, bFGF, VEGF receptor 2 (KDR), Ang II [236] - **Rauvolfia serpentina** root extract on human erythrocytes: ↓ hemolysis [237]
	Oxidative and Inflammatory stress	- **Grape seeds** extract on young healthy volunteers: ↑serum total antioxidant activity [132] - **Curcumin** on chronic kidney disease patients: ↓ plasma CCL-2, IFNγ, IL-4, TBARS, gut Escherichia-Shigella; ↑ gut Lachnoclostridium, Lactobacillaceae spp. [140]
	Dyslipidemia	- **Citrus bergamia** on overweight and obese class I subjects: ↓ TC, LDL-C; ↑ HDL-C [156]
	Hepatic disorders	- **Curcumin** (±**piperine**) on patients with NAFLD: ↓ fibrosis, liver parenchyma echogenicity, fatty liver score, AST, ALT, GGT, TG, BMI; ↑ HDL-C [172–174]
Clinical	Diabetes mellitus	- **Quercetin** on diabetic patients: does not interfere with antidiabetic or anticoagulant therapies [192] - **Curcumin** on kidney dysfunction, overweight or NAFLD subjects: ↓ plasma free radicals; ↑kidney function [195]; – serum glucose, insulin, HOMA-IR, cortisol [174]; ↓ AST, NAFLD grade [196] - **Berberine** on polycystic ovary syndrome patients: ↓ serum glucose, insulin, HOMA-IR, VLDL-C, TG, TNFα, CRP, visceral fat [187]
	Metabolic syndrome	- **Curcumin** on subjects with metabolic syndrome: ↑ antioxidant effects independent on vitamin E [206] - **Citrus bergamia** on overweight and obese class I subjects: ↓ visceral adipose tissue [156] - **Camellia sinensis** extract on subjects with metabolic syndrome: ↓ body weight, waist circumference, plasma free radicals [83]
	Cardiovascular diseases	- **Coenzyme Q10** on healthy young subjects: ↑ endothelial reactivity, arterial pressure, total antioxidant capacity [243]

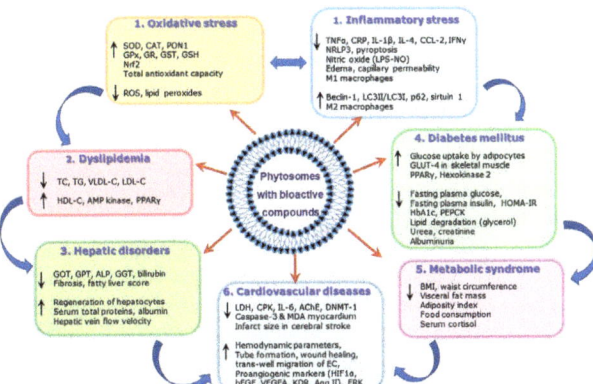

Figure 4. Validated beneficial effects and action mechanisms of bioactive compounds formulated in phytosomes to improve the metabolic disorder outcomes; upwards arrow (↑) represents increases; downwards arrow (↓) represents decreases.

5. Final Discussion

The phytosome formulation can save and amplify the therapeutic potential of phytochemicals, being a very promising delivery system that ensures the entrapment capacity and biocompatibility in safe conditions. In the present review, we documented and highlighted the studies which demonstrate the improved therapeutic qualities of the bioactive compounds formulated in phytosomes. They can be used to counteract risk factors that induce metabolic disorders, or to treat as complementary therapy the already installed diseases. Many products based on phytosome formulation of bioactive compounds have been prepared in the last two decades and proved the in vitro and in vivo enhanced bioavailability of the carried phytochemicals, which consequently manifested the enhanced therapeutic effects of the phytoconstituents.

The most investigated bioactive compounds formulated in phytosomes for their beneficial effects in the treatment of MD are curcumin, silymarin, ginkgo biloba extract, berberine and ginger extract. Their mechanisms of action involve the upregulation of antioxidant enzymes SOD, CAT and the GSH system, the increase in anti-inflammatory Nrf2 and NRLP3, the decrease in the pro-inflammatory cytokines, the induction of M2 macrophages, lipid-lowering effects, increase in glucose uptake, reduction in hepatic transaminases and regeneration of the liver tissue, all of which are associated with the decrease of visceral fat, improvement in the hemodynamic parameters, angiogenesis and significant recovery of infarcted tissues (Figure 4).

Remarkably, almost all reviewed studies demonstrate a good tolerability of the phytosome formulation. Many of them show significantly improved effects compared to the unformulated compounds or extracts, especially for those addressed to oxidative and inflammatory stress, hepatic disorders, dyslipidemia and CVD. Great care must be taken in future studies to establish the correct administered doses and the concentration of active principles when comparing the effects of compounds formulated in phytosomes with those unformulated. It is very important to verify the possible harmful effect of a high ratio of phospholipids, which may become a potential source of lipid peroxides.

The results obtained so far in human subjects are promising. It is mandatory to extend such studies on larger cohorts of subjects or patients or for longer periods of time. Thus, additional clinical trials are necessary, but with improved and standardized study design, with very well characterized formulations of the phytosomes in terms of concentration of the active compounds and deliverable doses. The encouraging results obtained following the use of phytosomes should stimulate scientists to further develop improved formulations of delivery for natural bioactive compounds to ensure their increased bioavailability and improve compliance of patients at risk for MD.

6. Conclusions

Many bioactive compounds or plant extracts are known to exert multiple health beneficial actions, having antioxidant, anti-inflammatory, lipid- or glucose-regulatory properties, but their low solubility and stability restrict the application of these compounds in therapy. In the present review, we emphasize the evidence supporting the use of the formulation of bioactive compounds in phytosomes with the aim of increasing their therapeutic potential. The encouraging results obtained in preclinical and clinical studies following the use of phytosomes with bioactive compounds should stimulate scientists to further discover and evaluate such products, and physicians to design larger trials in order to test them. This will strengthen the confidence of physicians and patients in the improved therapeutic effects of these phyto-phospholipid complexes. It is safe to say that treatment with bioactive compounds formulated in phytosomes should be encouraged as complementary therapy in MD patients, as well as in all subjects at risk.

Author Contributions: Conceptualization, M.D., A.V.S. and C.S.S.; writing—original draft preparation, L.T., G.M.S., T.B., L.Ș.N., M.D. and C.S.S.; writing—review and editing, L.T., C.S.S. and A.V.S. All authors have read and agreed to the published version of the manuscript.

Funding: This research was funded by the Romanian Academy and by the Romanian Ministry of Research, Innovation, and Digitization, CNCS/CCCDI-UEFISCDI, grant number PN-III-P2-2.1-PED-2021-1929, PN-III-P4-PCE-2021-0831, and CF 197-2022/PNRR-III-C9-2022-I8. The manuscript benefits from full waiver.

Institutional Review Board Statement: Not applicable.

Informed Consent Statement: Not applicable.

Data Availability Statement: Not applicable.

Conflicts of Interest: The authors declare no conflicts of interest.

References

1. Brønden, A.; Christensen, M.B.; Glintborg, D.; Snorgaard, O.; Kofoed-Enevoldsen, A.; Madsen, G.K.; Toft, K.; Kristensen, J.K.; Højlund, K.; Hansen, T.K.; et al. Effects of DPP-4 inhibitors, GLP-1 receptor agonists, SGLT-2 inhibitors and sulphonylureas on mortality, cardiovascular and renal outcomes in type 2 diabetes: A network meta-analyses-driven approach. *Diabet. Med.* **2023**, *40*, e15157. [CrossRef]
2. Tomlinson, B.; Wu, Q.Y.; Zhong, Y.M.; Li, Y.H. Advances in Dyslipidaemia Treatments: Focusing on ApoC3 and ANGPTL3 Inhibitors. *J. Lipid Atheroscler.* **2024**, *13*, 2–20. [CrossRef] [PubMed]
3. Bilson, J.; Mantovani, A.; Byrne, C.D.; Targher, G. Steatotic liver disease, MASLD and risk of chronic kidney disease. *Diabetes Metab.* **2024**, *50*, 101506. [CrossRef] [PubMed]
4. Habibullah, M.; Jemmieh, K.; Ouda, A.; Haider, M.Z.; Malki, M.I.; Elzouki, A.N. Metabolic-associated fatty liver disease: A selective review of pathogenesis, diagnostic approaches, and therapeutic strategies. *Front. Med.* **2024**, *11*, 1291501. [CrossRef] [PubMed]
5. Wang, Y.; Fleishman, J.S.; Li, T.; Li, Y.; Ren, Z.; Chen, J.; Ding, M. Pharmacological therapy of metabolic dysfunction-associated steatotic liver disease-driven hepatocellular carcinoma. *Front. Pharmacol.* **2023**, *14*, 1336216. [CrossRef] [PubMed]
6. Filipovic, B.; Marjanovic-Haljilji, M.; Mijac, D.; Lukic, S.; Kapor, S.; Kapor, S.; Starcevic, A.; Popovic, D.; Djokovic, A. Molecular Aspects of MAFLD-New Insights on Pathogenesis and Treatment. *Curr. Issues Mol. Biol.* **2023**, *45*, 9132–9148. [CrossRef]
7. Kasper, P.; Martin, A.; Lang, S.; Kütting, F.; Goeser, T.; Demir, M.; Steffen, H.M. NAFLD and cardiovascular diseases: A clinical review. *Clin. Res. Cardiol.* **2021**, *110*, 921–937. [CrossRef] [PubMed]
8. Jia, G.; Bai, H.; Mather, B.; Hill, M.A.; Jia, G.; Sowers, J.R. Diabetic Vasculopathy: Molecular Mechanisms and Clinical Insights. *Int. J. Mol. Sci.* **2024**, *25*, 804. [CrossRef]
9. Powell-Wiley, T.M.; Poirier, P.; Burke, L.E.; Després, J.P.; Gordon-Larsen, P.; Lavie, C.J.; Lear, S.A.; Ndumele, C.E.; Neeland, I.J.; Sanders, P.; et al. Obesity and Cardiovascular Disease: A Scientific Statement From the American Heart Association. *Circulation* **2021**, *143*, e984–e1010. [CrossRef]
10. Toma, L.; Stancu, C.S.; Sima, A.V. Endothelial Dysfunction in Diabetes Is Aggravated by Glycated Lipoproteins; Novel Molecular Therapies. *Biomedicines* **2020**, *9*, 18. [CrossRef]

11. Vellasamy, S.; Murugan, D.; Abas, R.; Alias, A.; Seng, W.Y.; Woon, C.K. Biological Activities of Paeonol in Cardiovascular Diseases: A Review. *Molecules* **2021**, *26*, 4976. [CrossRef] [PubMed]
12. Sando, K.R.; Knight, M. Nonstatin therapies for management of dyslipidemia: A review. *Clin. Ther.* **2015**, *37*, 2153–2179. [CrossRef] [PubMed]
13. Uehara, Y.; Chiesa, G.; Saku, K. High-Density Lipoprotein-Targeted Therapy and Apolipoprotein A-I Mimetic Peptides. *Circ. J.* **2015**, *79*, 2523–2528. [CrossRef] [PubMed]
14. Ghadge, A.A.; Kuvalekar, A.A. Controversy of oral hypoglycemic agents in type 2 diabetes mellitus: Novel move towards combination therapies. *Diabetes Metab. Syndr.* **2017**, *11* (Suppl. S1), S5–S13. [CrossRef] [PubMed]
15. Yeung, A.W.K.; Tzvetkov, N.T.; Durazzo, A.; Lucarini, M.; Souto, E.B.; Santini, A.; Gan, R.Y.; Jozwik, A.; Grzybek, W.; Horbańczuk, J.O.; et al. Natural products in diabetes research: Quantitative literature analysis. *Nat. Prod. Res.* **2021**, *35*, 5813–5827. [CrossRef] [PubMed]
16. Hu, Y.; Chen, X.; Hu, M.; Zhang, D.; Yuan, S.; Li, P.; Feng, L. Medicinal and edible plants in the treatment of dyslipidemia: Advances and prospects. *Chin. Med.* **2022**, *17*, 113. [CrossRef] [PubMed]
17. Mancak, M.; Altintas, D.; Balaban, Y.; Caliskan, U.K. Evidence-based herbal treatments in liver diseases. *Hepatol. Forum* **2024**, *5*, 50–60. [CrossRef] [PubMed]
18. Barani, M.; Sangiovanni, E.; Angarano, M.; Rajizadeh, M.A.; Mehrabani, M.; Piazza, S.; Gangadharappa, H.V.; Pardakhty, A.; Mehrbani, M.; Dell'Agli, M.; et al. Phytosomes as Innovative Delivery Systems for Phytochemicals: A Comprehensive Review of Literature. *Int. J. Nanomed.* **2021**, *16*, 6983–7022. [CrossRef] [PubMed]
19. Toma, L.; Sanda, G.M.; Niculescu, L.S.; Deleanu, M.; Sima, A.V.; Stancu, C.S. Phenolic Compounds Exerting Lipid-Regulatory, Anti-Inflammatory and Epigenetic Effects as Complementary Treatments in Cardiovascular Diseases. *Biomolecules* **2020**, *10*, 641. [CrossRef]
20. Rui, R.; Yang, H.; Liu, Y.; Zhou, Y.; Xu, X.; Li, C.; Liu, S. Effects of Berberine on Atherosclerosis. *Front. Pharmacol.* **2021**, *12*, 764175. [CrossRef]
21. Huang, P. Proanthocyanidins may be potential therapeutic agents for the treatment of carotid atherosclerosis: A review. *J. Int. Med. Res.* **2023**, *51*, 3000605231167314. [CrossRef] [PubMed]
22. Rasouli, H.; Yarani, R.; Pociot, F.; Popović-Djordjević, J. Anti-diabetic potential of plant alkaloids: Revisiting current findings and future perspectives. *Pharmacol. Res.* **2020**, *155*, 104723. [CrossRef] [PubMed]
23. Deka, H.; Choudhury, A.; Dey, B.K. An Overview on Plant Derived Phenolic Compounds and Their Role in Treatment and Management of Diabetes. *J. Pharmacopunct.* **2022**, *25*, 199–208. [CrossRef] [PubMed]
24. Nguyen, H.N.; Ullevig, S.L.; Short, J.D.; Wang, L.; Ahn, Y.J.; Asmis, R. Ursolic Acid and Related Analogues: Triterpenoids with Broad Health Benefits. *Antioxidants* **2021**, *10*, 1161. [CrossRef] [PubMed]
25. Ekor, M. The growing use of herbal medicines: Issues relating to adverse reactions and challenges in monitoring safety. *Front. Pharmacol.* **2014**, *4*, 177. [CrossRef] [PubMed]
26. Nuchuchua, O.; Inpan, R.; Srinuanchai, W.; Karinchai, J.; Pitchakarn, P.; Wongnoppavich, A.; Imsumran, A. Phytosome Supplements for Delivering Gymnema inodorum Phytonutrients to Prevent Inflammation in Macrophages and Insulin Resistance in Adipocytes. *Foods* **2023**, *12*, 2257. [CrossRef] [PubMed]
27. Azzi, A. Antioxidants: Wonder drugs or quackery? *Biofactors* **2017**, *43*, 785–788. [CrossRef] [PubMed]
28. Pan-On, S.; Dilokthornsakul, P.; Tiyaboonchai, W. Trends in advanced oral drug delivery system for curcumin: A systematic review. *J. Control. Release* **2022**, *348*, 335–345. [CrossRef] [PubMed]
29. Güngör Ak, A.; Akkol, E.K.; Aksu, B.; Karataş, A. Preparation and optimization of berberine phospholipid complexes using QbD approach and in vivo evaluation for anti-inflammatory, analgesic and antipyretic activity. *J. Res. Pharm.* **2022**, *26*, 370–382. [CrossRef]
30. Lu, M.; Qiu, Q.; Luo, X.; Liu, X.; Sun, J.; Wang, C.; Lin, X.; Deng, Y.; Song, Y. Phyto-phospholipid complexes (phytosomes): A novel strategy to improve the bioavailability of active constituents. *Asian J. Pharm. Sci.* **2019**, *14*, 265–274. [CrossRef]
31. Rai, S.; Pandey, V.; Rai, G. Transfersomes as versatile and flexible nano-vesicular carriers in skin cancer therapy: The state of the art. *Nano Rev. Exp.* **2017**, *8*, 1325708. [CrossRef] [PubMed]
32. Khan, S.; Sharma, A.; Jain, V. An Overview of Nanostructured Lipid Carriers and its Application in Drug Delivery through Different Routes. *Adv. Pharm. Bull.* **2023**, *13*, 446–460. [CrossRef]
33. Umar, H.; Wahab, H.A.; Gazzali, A.M.; Tahir, H.; Ahmad, W. Cubosomes: Design, Development, and Tumor-Targeted Drug Delivery Applications. *Polymers* **2022**, *14*, 3118. [CrossRef] [PubMed]
34. Kumari, S.; Goyal, A.; Sönmez Gürer, E.; Algın Yapar, E.; Garg, M.; Sood, M.; Sindhu, R.K. Bioactive Loaded Novel Nano-Formulations for Targeted Drug Delivery and Their Therapeutic Potential. *Pharmaceutics* **2022**, *14*, 1091. [CrossRef]
35. Teja, P.K.; Mithiya, J.; Kate, A.S.; Bairwa, K.; Chauthe, S.K. Herbal nanomedicines: Recent advancements, challenges, opportunities and regulatory overview. *Phytomedicine* **2022**, *96*, 153890. [CrossRef]
36. Li, J.; Wang, X.; Zhang, T.; Wang, C.; Huang, Z.; Luo, X.; Deng, Y. A review on phospholipids and their main applications in drug delivery systems. *Asian J. Pharm. Sci.* **2015**, *10*, 81–98. [CrossRef]
37. Khan, J.; Alexander, A.; Ajazuddin; Saraf, S.; Saraf, S. Recent advances and future prospects of phyto-phospholipid complexation technique for improving pharmacokinetic profile of plant actives. *J. Control. Release* **2013**, *168*, 50–60. [CrossRef]

38. Deleanu, M.; Toma, L.; Sanda, G.M.; Barbălată, T.; Niculescu, L.; Sima, A.V.; Deleanu, C.; Săcărescu, L.; Suciu, A.; Alexandru, G.; et al. Formulation of Phytosomes with Extracts of Ginger Rhizomes and Rosehips with Improved Bioavailability, Antioxidant and Anti-Inflammatory Effects In Vivo. *Pharmaceutics* **2023**, *15*, 1066. [CrossRef]
39. Tripathy, S.; Patel, D.; Baro, L.; Nair, S.K. A review on phytosomes, their characterization, advancement and potential for transdermal application. *J. Drug Deliv. Ther.* **2013**, *3*, 147–152. [CrossRef]
40. Gaikwad, S.S.; Morade, Y.Y.; Kothule, A.M.; Kshirsagar, S.J.; Laddha, U.D.; Salunkhe, K.S. Overview of phytosomes in treating cancer: Advancement, challenges, and future outlook. *Heliyon* **2023**, *9*, e16561. [CrossRef]
41. Karpuz, M.; Silindir Gunay, M.; Ozer, Y. Liposomes and phytosomes for phytoconstituents. In *Advances and Avenues in the Development of Novel Carriers for Bioactives and Biological Agents*; Academic Press: Cambridge, MA, USA, 2020; pp. 525–553.
42. Freag, M.S.; Elnaggar, Y.S.; Abdallah, O.Y. Lyophilized phytosomal nanocarriers as platforms for enhanced diosmin delivery: Optimization and ex vivo permeation. *Int. J. Nanomed.* **2013**, *8*, 2385–2397. [CrossRef]
43. Telange, D.R.; Patil, A.T.; Pethe, A.M.; Fegade, H.; Anand, S.; Dave, V.S. Formulation and characterization of an apigenin-phospholipid phytosome (APLC) for improved solubility, in vivo bioavailability, and antioxidant potential. *Eur. J. Pharm. Sci.* **2017**, *108*, 36–49. [CrossRef] [PubMed]
44. Singh, R.P.; Narke, R. Preparation and Evaluation of Phytosome of Lawsone. *Int. J. Pharm. Sci. Res.* **2015**, *6*, 5217–5226. [CrossRef]
45. Magdy, N. Phytosomes: A Novel Approach for Delivery of Herbal Constituents. *J. Nutr. Diet. Probiotics* **2018**, *1*, 180007.
46. Fuior, E.V.; Mocanu, C.A.; Deleanu, M.; Voicu, G.; Anghelache, M.; Rebleanu, D.; Simionescu, M.; Calin, M. Evaluation of VCAM-1 Targeted Naringenin/Indocyanine Green-Loaded Lipid Nanoemulsions as Theranostic Nanoplatforms in Inflammation. *Pharmaceutics* **2020**, *12*, 1066. [CrossRef] [PubMed]
47. Shriram, R.G.; Moin, A.; Alotaibi, H.F.; Khafagy, E.S.; Al Saqr, A.; Abu Lila, A.S.; Charyulu, R.N. Phytosomes as a Plausible Nano-Delivery System for Enhanced Oral Bioavailability and Improved Hepatoprotective Activity of Silymarin. *Pharmaceuticals* **2022**, *15*, 790. [CrossRef] [PubMed]
48. Perrie, Y.; Ali, H.; Kirby, D.J.; Mohammed, A.U.; McNeil, S.E.; Vangala, A. Environmental Scanning Electron Microscope Imaging of Vesicle Systems. *Methods Mol. Biol.* **2017**, *1522*, 131–143. [CrossRef] [PubMed]
49. Rathor, S.; Bhatt, D.C. Novel Glibenclamide–Phospholipid Complex for Diabetic Treatment: Formulation, Physicochemical Characterization, and in-vivo Evaluation. *Indian J. Pharm. Educ. Res.* **2022**, *56*, 697–705. [CrossRef]
50. Altiti, A.J.; Khleifat, K.M.; Alqaraleh, M.; Shraim, A.S.; Qinna, N.; Al-Tawarah, N.M.; Al-Qaisi, T.S.; Aldmour, R.H.; Al-Tarawneh, A.; Qaralleh, H. Protective Role of Combined Crataegus Aronia Ethanol Extract and Phytosomes against Hyperglycemia and Hyperlipidemia in Streptozotocin-Induced Diabetic Rat. *Biointerface Res. Appl. Chem.* **2023**, *13*, 1–14. [CrossRef]
51. Rani, A.; Kumar, S.; Khar, R. Murraya koenigii Extract Loaded Phytosomes Prepared using Antisolvent Precipitation Technique for Improved Antidiabetic and Hypolidemic Activity. *Indian J. Pharm. Educ. Res.* **2022**, *56*, s326–s338. [CrossRef]
52. Yu, F.; Li, Y.; Chen, Q.; He, Y.; Wang, H.; Yang, L.; Guo, S.; Meng, Z.; Cui, J.; Xue, M.; et al. Monodisperse microparticles loaded with the self-assembled berberine-phospholipid complex-based phytosomes for improving oral bioavailability and enhancing hypoglycemic efficiency. *Eur. J. Pharm. Biopharm.* **2016**, *103*, 136–148. [CrossRef] [PubMed]
53. Benne, N.; Leboux, R.J.T.; Glandrup, M.; van Duijn, J.; Lozano Vigario, F.; Neustrup, M.A.; Romeijn, S.; Galli, F.; Kuiper, J.; Jiskoot, W.; et al. Atomic force microscopy measurements of anionic liposomes reveal the effect of liposomal rigidity on antigen-specific regulatory T cell responses. *J. Control. Release* **2020**, *318*, 246–255. [CrossRef]
54. Lee, S.H.; Sato, Y.; Hyodo, M.; Harashima, H. Size-Dependency of the Surface Ligand Density of Liposomes Prepared by Post-insertion. *Biol. Pharm. Bull.* **2017**, *40*, 1002–1009. [CrossRef] [PubMed]
55. Smith, M.C.; Crist, R.M.; Clogston, J.D.; McNeil, S.E. Zeta potential: A case study of cationic, anionic, and neutral liposomes. *Anal. Bioanal. Chem.* **2017**, *409*, 5779–5787. [CrossRef] [PubMed]
56. Chibowski, E.; Szcześ, A. Zeta potential and surface charge of DPPC and DOPC liposomes in the presence of PLC enzyme. *Adsorption* **2016**, *22*, 755–765. [CrossRef]
57. Solomon, D.; Gupta, N.; Mulla, N.S.; Shukla, S.; Guerrero, Y.A.; Gupta, V. Role of In Vitro Release Methods in Liposomal Formulation Development: Challenges and Regulatory Perspective. *AAPS J.* **2017**, *19*, 1669–1681. [CrossRef] [PubMed]
58. Simion, V.; Stan, D.; Constantinescu, C.A.; Deleanu, M.; Dragan, E.; Tucureanu, M.M.; Gan, A.M.; Butoi, E.; Constantin, A.; Manduteanu, I.; et al. Conjugation of curcumin-loaded lipid nanoemulsions with cell-penetrating peptides increases their cellular uptake and enhances the anti-inflammatory effects in endothelial cells. *J. Pharm. Pharmacol.* **2016**, *68*, 195–207. [CrossRef] [PubMed]
59. Varga, Z.; Fehér, B.; Kitka, D.; Wacha, A.; Bóta, A.; Berényi, S.; Pipich, V.; Fraikin, J.L. Size Measurement of Extracellular Vesicles and Synthetic Liposomes: The Impact of the Hydration Shell and the Protein Corona. *Colloids Surf. B Biointerfaces* **2020**, *192*, 111053. [CrossRef] [PubMed]
60. Tutkus, M.; Akhtar, P.; Chmeliov, J.; Görföl, F.; Trinkunas, G.; Lambrev, P.H.; Valkunas, L. Fluorescence Microscopy of Single Liposomes with Incorporated Pigment-Proteins. *Langmuir* **2018**, *34*, 14410–14418. [CrossRef]
61. Jain, P.; Soni, A.; Jain, P.; Bhawsar, J. Phytochemical analysis of Mentha spicata plant extract using UV-VIS, FTIR and GC/MS technique. *J. Chem. Pharm. Res.* **2016**, *2016*, 1–6.
62. Mazumder, A.; Dwivedi, A.; du Preez, J.L.; du Plessis, J. In vitro wound healing and cytotoxic effects of sinigrin-phytosome complex. *Int. J. Pharm.* **2016**, *498*, 283–293. [CrossRef] [PubMed]

63. Peleg-Shulman, T.; Gibson, D.; Cohen, R.; Abra, R.; Barenholz, Y. Characterization of sterically stabilized cisplatin liposomes by nuclear magnetic resonance. *Biochim. Biophys. Acta* **2001**, *1510*, 278–291. [CrossRef] [PubMed]
64. de Azambuja Borges, C.R.L.; Silva, N.O.; Rodrigues, M.R.; Germani Marinho, M.A.; de Oliveira, F.S.; Cassiana, M.; Horn, A.P.; Parize, A.L.; Flores, D.C.; Clementin, R.M.; et al. Dimiristoylphosphatidylcholine/genistein molecular interactions: A physico-chemical approach to anti-glioma drug delivery systems. *Chem. Phys. Lipids* **2019**, *225*, 104828. [CrossRef] [PubMed]
65. Ghanbarzadeh, B.; Babazadeh, A.; Hamishehkar, H. Nano-phytosome as a potential food-grade delivery system. *Food Biosci.* **2016**, *15*, 126–135. [CrossRef]
66. Wang, H.; Cui, Y.; Fu, Q.; Deng, B.; Li, G.; Yang, J.; Wu, T.; Xie, Y. A phospholipid complex to improve the oral bioavailability of flavonoids. *Drug Dev. Ind. Pharm.* **2015**, *41*, 1693–1703. [CrossRef]
67. Purpura, M.; Lowery, R.P.; Wilson, J.M.; Mannan, H.; Münch, G.; Razmovski-Naumovski, V. Analysis of different innovative formulations of curcumin for improved relative oral bioavailability in human subjects. *Eur. J. Nutr.* **2018**, *57*, 929–938. [CrossRef] [PubMed]
68. Wang, Y.; Shi, Y.; Zou, J.; Zhang, X.; Wang, M.; Guo, D.; Lv, G.; Su, J.; Wang, T. The intranasal administration of *Carthamus tinctorius* L. extract/phospholipid complex in the treatment of cerebral infarction via the TNF-α/MAPK pathway. *Biomed. Pharmacother.* **2020**, *130*, 110563. [CrossRef] [PubMed]
69. El-Menshawe, S.F.; Ali, A.A.; Rabeh, M.A.; Khalil, N.M. Nanosized soy phytosome-based thermogel as topical anti-obesity formulation: An approach for acceptable level of evidence of an effective novel herbal weight loss product. *Int. J. Nanomed.* **2018**, *13*, 307–318. [CrossRef] [PubMed]
70. Marczylo, T.H.; Verschoyle, R.D.; Cooke, D.N.; Morazzoni, P.; Steward, W.P.; Gescher, A.J. Comparison of systemic availability of curcumin with that of curcumin formulated with phosphatidylcholine. *Cancer Chemother. Pharmacol.* **2007**, *60*, 171–177. [CrossRef]
71. Zhou, Y.; Dong, W.; Ye, J.; Hao, H.; Zhou, J.; Wang, R.; Liu, Y. A novel matrix dispersion based on phospholipid complex for improving oral bioavailability of baicalein: Preparation, in vitro and in vivo evaluations. *Drug Deliv.* **2017**, *24*, 720–728. [CrossRef]
72. Biswas, S.; Mukherjee, P.K.; Harwansh, R.K.; Bannerjee, S.; Bhattacharjee, P. Enhanced bioavailability and hepatoprotectivity of optimized ursolic acid-phospholipid complex. *Drug Dev. Ind. Pharm.* **2019**, *45*, 946–958. [CrossRef] [PubMed]
73. Gausuzzaman, S.A.L.; Saha, M.; Dip, S.J.; Alam, S.; Kumar, A.; Das, H.; Sharker, S.M.; Rashid, M.A.; Kazi, M.; Reza, H.M. A QbD Approach to Design and to Optimize the Self-Emulsifying Resveratrol-Phospholipid Complex to Enhance Drug Bioavailability through Lymphatic Transport. *Polymers* **2022**, *14*, 3220. [CrossRef] [PubMed]
74. Jager, R.; Lowery, R.P.; Calvanese, A.V.; Joy, J.M.; Purpura, M.; Wilson, J.M. Comparative absorption of curcumin formulations. *Nutr. J.* **2014**, *13*, 11. [CrossRef]
75. Petrangolini, G.; Ronchi, M.; Frattini, E.; De Combarieu, E.; Allegrini, P.; Riva, A. A New Food-grade Coenzyme Q10 Formulation Improves Bioavailability: Single and Repeated Pharmacokinetic Studies in Healthy Volunteers. *Curr. Drug Deliv.* **2019**, *16*, 759–767. [CrossRef] [PubMed]
76. Riva, A.; Ronchi, M.; Petrangolini, G.; Bosisio, S.; Allegrini, P. Improved Oral Absorption of Quercetin from Quercetin Phytosome®, a New Delivery System Based on Food Grade Lecithin. *Eur. J. Drug Metab. Pharmacokinet.* **2019**, *44*, 169–177. [CrossRef] [PubMed]
77. Flory, S.; Sus, N.; Haas, K.; Jehle, S.; Kienhofer, E.; Waehler, R.; Adler, G.; Venturelli, S.; Frank, J. Increasing Post-Digestive Solubility of Curcumin Is the Most Successful Strategy to Improve its Oral Bioavailability: A Randomized Cross-Over Trial in Healthy Adults and In Vitro Bioaccessibility Experiments. *Mol. Nutr. Food Res.* **2021**, *65*, e2100613. [CrossRef]
78. Petrangolini, G.; Corti, F.; Ronchi, M.; Arnoldi, L.; Allegrini, P.; Riva, A. Development of an Innovative Berberine Food-Grade Formulation with an Ameliorated Absorption: In Vitro Evidence Confirmed by Healthy Human Volunteers Pharmacokinetic Study. *Evid. Based Complement. Altern. Med.* **2021**, *2021*, 7563889. [CrossRef]
79. Riva, A.; Allegrini, P.; Franceschi, F.; Togni, S.; Giacomelli, L.; Eggenhoffner, R. A novel boswellic acids delivery form (Casperome®) in the management of musculoskeletal disorders: A review. *Eur. Rev. Med. Pharmacol. Sci.* **2017**, *21*, 5258–5263. [CrossRef]
80. Drobnic, F.; Riera, J.; Appendino, G.; Togni, S.; Franceschi, F.; Valle, X.; Pons, A.; Tur, J. Reduction of delayed onset muscle soreness by a novel curcumin delivery system (Meriva®): A randomised, placebo-controlled trial. *J. Int. Soc. Sports Nutr.* **2014**, *11*, 31. [CrossRef]
81. Di Pierro, F.; Menghi, A.B.; Barreca, A.; Lucarelli, M.; Calandrelli, A. Greenselect Phytosome as an adjunct to a low-calorie diet for treatment of obesity: A clinical trial. *Altern. Med. Rev.* **2009**, *14*, 154–160.
82. Gilardini, L.; Pasqualinotto, L.; Di Pierro, F.; Risso, P.; Invitti, C. Effects of Greenselect Phytosome® on weight maintenance after weight loss in obese women: A randomized placebo-controlled study. *BMC Complement. Altern. Med.* **2016**, *16*, 233. [CrossRef]
83. Belcaro, G.; Ledda, A.; Hu, S.; Cesarone, M.R.; Feragalli, B.; Dugall, M. Greenselect phytosome for borderline metabolic syndrome. *Evid. Based Complement. Altern. Med.* **2013**, *2013*, 869061. [CrossRef]
84. Suryawanshi, J. Phytosome: An emerging trend in herbal drug treatment. *J. Med. Genet. Genom.* **2011**, *3*, 109–114.
85. Alexander, A.; Ajazuddin; Patel, R.J.; Saraf, S.; Saraf, S. Recent expansion of pharmaceutical nanotechnologies and targeting strategies in the field of phytopharmaceuticals for the delivery of herbal extracts and bioactives. *J. Control. Release* **2016**, *241*, 110–124. [CrossRef]
86. Vigna, G.B.; Costantini, F.; Aldini, G.; Carini, M.; Catapano, A.; Schena, F.; Tangerini, A.; Zanca, R.; Bombardelli, E.; Morazzoni, P.; et al. Effect of a standardized grape seed extract on low-density lipoprotein susceptibility to oxidation in heavy smokers. *Metabolism* **2003**, *52*, 1250–1257. [CrossRef]
87. Kiefer, D.; Pantuso, T. Panax ginseng. *Am. Fam. Physician* **2003**, *68*, 1539–1542.

88. Yu, Z.; Liu, X.; Chen, H.; Zhu, L. Naringenin-Loaded Dipalmitoylphosphatidylcholine Phytosome Dry Powders for Inhaled Treatment of Acute Lung Injury. *J. Aerosol Med. Pulm. Drug Deliv.* **2020**, *33*, 194–204. [CrossRef]
89. Cesarone, M.R.; Belcaro, G.; Hu, S.; Dugall, M.; Hosoi, M.; Ledda, A.; Feragalli, B.; Maione, C.; Cotellese, R. Supplementary prevention and management of asthma with quercetin phytosome: A pilot registry. *Minerva Med.* **2019**, *110*, 524–529. [CrossRef]
90. Kidd, P.; Head, K. A review of the bioavailability and clinical efficacy of milk thistle phytosome: A silybin-phosphatidylcholine complex (Siliphos). *Altern. Med. Rev.* **2005**, *10*, 193–203.
91. Sindhumol, P.G.; Thomas, M.; Mohanachandran, P.S. Phytosomes: A novel dosage form for enhancement of bioavailability of botanicals and neutraceuticals. *Int. J. Pharm. Pharm. Sci.* **2010**, *2*, 10–14.
92. Riva, A.; Longo, V.; Berlanda, D.; Allegrini, P.; Masetti, G.; Botti, S.; Petrangolini, G. Healthy Protection Of Bergamot Is Linked to the Modulation of Microbiota. *Appl. Microb. Res.* **2020**, *3*, 45–51. [CrossRef]
93. Mollace, V.; Scicchitano, M.; Paone, S.; Casale, F.; Calandruccio, C.; Gliozzi, M.; Musolino, V.; Carresi, C.; Maiuolo, J.; Nucera, S.; et al. Hypoglycemic and Hypolipemic Effects of a New Lecithin Formulation of Bergamot Polyphenolic Fraction: A Double Blind, Randomized, Placebo-Controlled Study. *Endocr. Metab. Immune Disord. Drug Targets* **2019**, *19*, 136–143. [CrossRef]
94. Bombardelli, E.; Currì, S.B.; Loggia, R.D.; Del Negro, P.; Gariboldi, P.; Tubaro, A. Anti-inflammatory activity of 18-ß-glycyrrhetinic acid in phytosome form. *Fitoterapia* **1989**, *60*, 29–37.
95. Di Renzo, G. Ginkgo biloba and the central nervous system. *Fitoterapia* **2000**, *71* (Suppl. S1), S43–S47. [CrossRef]
96. Naik, S.R.; Panda, V.S. Hepatoprotective effect of Ginkgoselect Phytosome in rifampicin induced liver injury in rats: Evidence of antioxidant activity. *Fitoterapia* **2008**, *79*, 439–445. [CrossRef]
97. Menon, V.P.; Sudheer, A.R. Antioxidant and anti-inflammatory properties of curcumin. *Adv. Exp. Med. Biol.* **2007**, *595*, 105–125. [CrossRef]
98. Soltani, A.; Salmaninejad, A.; Jalili-Nik, M.; Soleimani, A.; Javid, H.; Hashemy, S.I.; Sahebkar, A. 5′-Adenosine monophosphate-activated protein kinase: A potential target for disease prevention by curcumin. *J. Cell. Physiol.* **2019**, *234*, 2241–2251. [CrossRef]
99. Baradaran, S.; Hajizadeh Moghaddam, A.; Khanjani Jelodar, S.; Moradi-Kor, N. Protective Effects of Curcumin and its Nano-Phytosome on Carrageenan-Induced Inflammation in Mice Model: Behavioral and Biochemical Responses. *J. Inflamm. Res.* **2020**, *13*, 45–51. [CrossRef]
100. Hosseinzadeh, A.; Bahrampour Juybari, K.; Fatemi, M.J.; Kamarul, T.; Bagheri, A.; Tekiyehmaroof, N.; Sharifi, A.M. Protective Effect of Ginger (*Zingiber officinale* Roscoe) Extract against Oxidative Stress and Mitochondrial Apoptosis Induced by Interleukin-1β in Cultured Chondrocytes. *Cells Tissues Organs* **2017**, *204*, 241–250. [CrossRef]
101. Ballester, P.; Cerdá, B.; Arcusa, R.; Marhuenda, J.; Yamedjeu, K.; Zafrilla, P. Effect of Ginger on Inflammatory Diseases. *Molecules* **2022**, *27*, 7223. [CrossRef]
102. Barbalata, T.; Deleanu, M.; Carnuta, M.G.; Niculescu, L.S.; Raileanu, M.; Sima, A.V.; Stancu, C.S. Hyperlipidemia Determines Dysfunctional HDL Production and Impedes Cholesterol Efflux in the Small Intestine: Alleviation by Ginger Extract. *Mol. Nutr. Food Res.* **2019**, *63*, e1900029. [CrossRef]
103. Ebrahimzadeh, A.; Ebrahimzadeh, A.; Mirghazanfari, S.M.; Hazrati, E.; Hadi, S.; Milajerdi, A. The effect of ginger supplementation on metabolic profiles in patients with type 2 diabetes mellitus: A systematic review and meta-analysis of randomized controlled trials. *Complement. Ther. Med.* **2022**, *65*, 102802. [CrossRef]
104. Carnuta, M.G.; Deleanu, M.; Barbalata, T.; Toma, L.; Raileanu, M.; Sima, A.V.; Stancu, C.S. Zingiber officinale extract administration diminishes steroyl-CoA desaturase gene expression and activity in hyperlipidemic hamster liver by reducing the oxidative and endoplasmic reticulum stress. *Phytomedicine* **2018**, *48*, 62–69. [CrossRef]
105. Kiyama, R. Nutritional implications of ginger: Chemistry, biological activities and signaling pathways. *J. Nutr. Biochem.* **2020**, *86*, 108486. [CrossRef]
106. Zhu, J.; Chen, H.; Song, Z.; Wang, X.; Sun, Z. Effects of Ginger (*Zingiber officinale* Roscoe) on Type 2 Diabetes Mellitus and Components of the Metabolic Syndrome: A Systematic Review and Meta-Analysis of Randomized Controlled Trials. *Evid. Based Complement. Altern. Med.* **2018**, *2018*, 5692962. [CrossRef]
107. Ayati, Z.; Amiri, M.S.; Ramezani, M.; Delshad, E.; Sahebkar, A.; Emami, S.A. Phytochemistry, Traditional Uses and Pharmacological Profile of Rose Hip: A Review. *Curr. Pharm. Des.* **2018**, *24*, 4101–4124. [CrossRef]
108. Boscaro, V.; Rivoira, M.; Sgorbini, B.; Bordano, V.; Dadone, F.; Gallicchio, M.; Pons, A.; Benetti, E.; Rosa, A.C. Evidence-Based Anti-Diabetic Properties of Plant from the Occitan Valleys of the Piedmont Alps. *Pharmaceutics* **2022**, *14*, 2371. [CrossRef]
109. Adachi, Y.; Shimoyama, R. Triplet repeat primed pcr for japanese patients with myotonic dystrophy type 1. *J. Neurol. Sci.* **2015**, *357*, e235. [CrossRef]
110. de Cristo Soares Alves, A.; Mainardes, R.M.; Khalil, N.M. Nanoencapsulation of gallic acid and evaluation of its cytotoxicity and antioxidant activity. *Mater. Sci. Eng. C Mater. Biol. Appl.* **2016**, *60*, 126–134. [CrossRef]
111. Peng, Y.; Zhang, H.; Liu, R.; Mine, Y.; McCallum, J.; Kirby, C.; Tsao, R. Antioxidant and anti-inflammatory activities of pyranoanthocyanins and other polyphenols from staghorn sumac (*Rhus hirta* L.) in Caco-2 cell models. *J. Funct. Foods* **2016**, *20*, 139–147. [CrossRef]
112. Dehghani, M.A.; Shakiba Maram, N.; Moghimipour, E.; Khorsandi, L.; Atefi Khah, M.; Mahdavinia, M. Protective effect of gallic acid and gallic acid-loaded Eudragit-RS 100 nanoparticles on cisplatin-induced mitochondrial dysfunction and inflammation in rat kidney. *Biochim. Biophys. Acta Mol. Basis Dis.* **2020**, *1866*, 165911. [CrossRef] [PubMed]

113. Abbasalipour, H.; Hajizadeh Moghaddam, A.; Ranjbar, M. Sumac and gallic acid-loaded nanophytosomes ameliorate hippocampal oxidative stress via regulation of Nrf2/Keap1 pathway in autistic rats. *J. Biochem. Mol. Toxicol.* **2022**, *36*, e23035. [CrossRef] [PubMed]
114. Bellezza, I.; Giambanco, I.; Minelli, A.; Donato, R. Nrf2-Keap1 signaling in oxidative and reductive stress. *Biochim. Biophys. Acta Mol. Cell Res.* **2018**, *1865*, 721–733. [CrossRef] [PubMed]
115. Sut, S.; Faggian, M.; Baldan, V.; Poloniato, G.; Castagliuolo, I.; Grabnar, I.; Perissutti, B.; Brun, P.; Maggi, F.; Voinovich, D.; et al. Natural Deep Eutectic Solvents (NADES) to Enhance Berberine Absorption: An In Vivo Pharmacokinetic Study. *Molecules* **2017**, *22*, 1921. [CrossRef] [PubMed]
116. Liang, Y.; Xu, X.; Yin, M.; Zhang, Y.; Huang, L.; Chen, R.; Ni, J. Effects of berberine on blood glucose in patients with type 2 diabetes mellitus: A systematic literature review and a meta-analysis. *Endocr. J.* **2019**, *66*, 51–63. [CrossRef] [PubMed]
117. Zhao, Z.; Wei, Q.; Hua, W.; Liu, Y.; Liu, X.; Zhu, Y. Hepatoprotective effects of berberine on acetaminophen-induced hepatotoxicity in mice. *Biomed. Pharmacother.* **2018**, *103*, 1319–1326. [CrossRef] [PubMed]
118. Godugu, C.; Patel, A.R.; Doddapaneni, R.; Somagoni, J.; Singh, M. Approaches to improve the oral bioavailability and effects of novel anticancer drugs berberine and betulinic acid. *PLoS ONE* **2014**, *9*, e89919. [CrossRef]
119. Alam, A.; Al Arif Jahan, A.; Bari, M.S.; Khandokar, L.; Mahmud, M.H.; Junaid, M.; Chowdhury, M.S.; Khan, M.F.; Seidel, V.; Haque, M.A. Allium vegetables: Traditional uses, phytoconstituents, and beneficial effects in inflammation and cancer. *Crit. Rev. Food Sci. Nutr.* **2023**, *63*, 6580–6614. [CrossRef] [PubMed]
120. Shoeibi, A.; Karimi, E.; Zareian, M.; Oskoueian, E. Enhancing Healthcare Outcomes and Modulating Apoptosis- and Antioxidant-Related Genes through the Nano-Phytosomal Delivery of Phenolics Extracted from Allium ampeloprasum. *Genes* **2023**, *14*, 1547. [CrossRef]
121. An, J.P.; Park, E.J.; Ryu, B.; Lee, B.W.; Cho, H.M.; Doan, T.P.; Pham, H.T.T.; Oh, W.K. Oleanane Triterpenoids from the Leaves of Gymnema inodorum and Their Insulin Mimetic Activities. *J. Nat. Prod.* **2020**, *83*, 1265–1274. [CrossRef]
122. Dunkhunthod, B.; Talabnin, C.; Murphy, M.; Thumanu, K.; Sittisart, P.; Eumkeb, G. Gymnema inodorum (Lour.) Decne. Extract Alleviates Oxidative Stress and Inflammatory Mediators Produced by RAW264.7 Macrophages. *Oxidative Med. Cell. Longev.* **2021**, *2021*, 8658314. [CrossRef] [PubMed]
123. Zhu, S.; Luo, C.; Feng, W.; Li, Y.; Zhu, M.; Sun, S.; Zhang, X. Selenium-deposited tripterine phytosomes ameliorate the antiarthritic efficacy of the phytomedicine via a synergistic sensitization. *Int. J. Pharm.* **2020**, *578*, 119104. [CrossRef] [PubMed]
124. Liu, S.; Chen, Q.; Yan, L.; Ren, Y.; Fan, J.; Zhang, X.; Zhu, S. Phytosomal tripterine with selenium modification attenuates the cytotoxicity and restrains the inflammatory evolution via inhibiting NLRP3 inflammasome activation and pyroptosis. *Int. Immunopharmacol.* **2022**, *108*, 108871. [CrossRef] [PubMed]
125. Zhang, X.; Zhang, T.; Zhou, X.; Liu, H.; Sun, H.; Ma, Z.; Wu, B. Enhancement of oral bioavailability of tripterine through lipid nanospheres: Preparation, characterization, and absorption evaluation. *J. Pharm. Sci.* **2014**, *103*, 1711–1719. [CrossRef]
126. Zhao, J.; Chen, X.; Ho, K.-H.; Cai, C.; Li, C.-W.; Yang, M.; Yi, C. Nanotechnology for diagnosis and therapy of rheumatoid arthritis: Evolution towards theranostic approaches. *Chin. Chem. Lett.* **2021**, *32*, 66–86. [CrossRef]
127. Cui, Y.; Zhu, T.; Zhang, X.; Chen, J.; Sun, F.; Li, Y.; Teng, L. Oral delivery of superoxide dismutase by lipid polymer hybrid nanoparticles for the treatment of ulcerative colitis. *Chin. Chem. Lett.* **2022**, *33*, 4617–4622. [CrossRef]
128. Wree, A.; Eguchi, A.; McGeough, M.D.; Pena, C.A.; Johnson, C.D.; Canbay, A.; Hoffman, H.M.; Feldstein, A.E. NLRP3 inflammasome activation results in hepatocyte pyroptosis, liver inflammation, and fibrosis in mice. *Hepatology* **2014**, *59*, 898–910. [CrossRef] [PubMed]
129. Iskender, H.; Dokumacioglu, E.; Sen, T.M.; Ince, I.; Kanbay, Y.; Saral, S. The effect of hesperidin and quercetin on oxidative stress, NF-κB and SIRT1 levels in a STZ-induced experimental diabetes model. *Biomed. Pharmacother.* **2017**, *90*, 500–508. [CrossRef] [PubMed]
130. Kamisli, S.; Ciftci, O.; Kaya, K.; Cetin, A.; Kamisli, O.; Ozcan, C. Hesperidin protects brain and sciatic nerve tissues against cisplatin-induced oxidative, histological and electromyographical side effects in rats. *Toxicol. Ind. Health* **2015**, *31*, 841–851. [CrossRef]
131. Kalita, B.; Patwary, B.N. Formulation and in vitro Evaluation of Hesperidin-Phospholipid Complex and its Antioxidant Potential. *Curr. Drug Ther.* **2020**, *15*, 28–36. [CrossRef]
132. Nuttall, S.L.; Kendall, M.J.; Bombardelli, E.; Morazzoni, P. An evaluation of the antioxidant activity of a standardized grape seed extract, Leucoselect. *J. Clin. Pharm. Ther.* **1998**, *23*, 385–389. [CrossRef] [PubMed]
133. Fine, A.M. Oligomeric proanthocyanidin complexes: History, structure, and phytopharmaceutical applications. *Altern. Med. Rev.* **2000**, *5*, 144–151. [PubMed]
134. Zhang, X.Y.; Li, W.G.; Wu, Y.J.; Bai, D.C.; Liu, N.F. Proanthocyanidin from grape seeds enhances doxorubicin-induced antitumor effect and reverses drug resistance in doxorubicin-resistant K562/DOX cells. *Can. J. Physiol. Pharmacol.* **2005**, *83*, 309–318. [CrossRef] [PubMed]
135. Wahlström, B.; Blennow, G. A study on the fate of curcumin in the rat. *Acta Pharmacol. Toxicol.* **1978**, *43*, 86–92. [CrossRef] [PubMed]
136. Pan, M.H.; Huang, T.M.; Lin, J.K. Biotransformation of curcumin through reduction and glucuronidation in mice. *Drug Metab. Dispos.* **1999**, *27*, 486–494. [PubMed]

137. Ireson, C.; Orr, S.; Jones, D.J.; Verschoyle, R.; Lim, C.K.; Luo, J.L.; Howells, L.; Plummer, S.; Jukes, R.; Williams, M.; et al. Characterization of metabolites of the chemopreventive agent curcumin in human and rat hepatocytes and in the rat in vivo, and evaluation of their ability to inhibit phorbol ester-induced prostaglandin E2 production. *Cancer Res.* **2001**, *61*, 1058–1064. [PubMed]
138. Pivari, F.; Mingione, A.; Brasacchio, C.; Soldati, L. Curcumin and Type 2 Diabetes Mellitus: Prevention and Treatment. *Nutrients* **2019**, *11*, 1837. [CrossRef] [PubMed]
139. Bahloul, B.; Castillo-Henríquez, L.; Jenhani, L.; Aroua, N.; Ftouh, M.; Kalboussi, N.; Vega-Baudrit, J.; Mignet, N. Nanomedicine-based potential phyto-drug delivery systems for diabetes. *J. Drug Deliv. Sci. Technol.* **2023**, *82*, 104377. [CrossRef]
140. Pivari, F.; Mingione, A.; Piazzini, G.; Ceccarani, C.; Ottaviano, E.; Brasacchio, C.; Dei Cas, M.; Vischi, M.; Cozzolino, M.G.; Fogagnolo, P.; et al. Curcumin Supplementation (Meriva®) Modulates Inflammation, Lipid Peroxidation and Gut Microbiota Composition in Chronic Kidney Disease. *Nutrients* **2022**, *14*, 231. [CrossRef]
141. Pirillo, A.; Casula, M.; Olmastroni, E.; Norata, G.D.; Catapano, A.L. Global epidemiology of dyslipidaemias. *Nat. Rev. Cardiol.* **2021**, *18*, 689–700. [CrossRef]
142. Miao, J.; Zang, X.; Cui, X.; Zhang, J. Autophagy, Hyperlipidemia, and Atherosclerosis. *Adv. Exp. Med. Biol.* **2020**, *1207*, 237–264. [CrossRef] [PubMed]
143. Michaeli, D.T.; Michaeli, J.C.; Albers, S.; Boch, T.; Michaeli, T. Established and Emerging Lipid-Lowering Drugs for Primary and Secondary Cardiovascular Prevention. *Am. J. Cardiovasc. Drugs* **2023**, *23*, 477–495. [CrossRef]
144. Lagace, T.A. PCSK9 and LDLR degradation: Regulatory mechanisms in circulation and in cells. *Curr. Opin. Lipidol.* **2014**, *25*, 387–393. [CrossRef] [PubMed]
145. Ward, N.C.; Watts, G.F.; Eckel, R.H. Statin Toxicity. *Circ. Res.* **2019**, *124*, 328–350. [CrossRef] [PubMed]
146. Ramsewak, R.S.; Nair, M.G.; Strasburg, G.M.; DeWitt, D.L.; Nitiss, J.L. Biologically active carbazole alkaloids from Murraya koenigii. *J. Agric. Food Chem.* **1999**, *47*, 444–447. [CrossRef]
147. Xie, W.; Zhao, Y.; Du, L. Emerging approaches of traditional Chinese medicine formulas for the treatment of hyperlipidemia. *J. Ethnopharmacol.* **2012**, *140*, 345–367. [CrossRef]
148. Pirmoghani, A.; Salehi, I.; Moradkhani, S.; Karimi, S.A.; Salehi, S. Effect of Crataegus extract supplementation on diabetes induced memory deficits and serum biochemical parameters in male rats. *IBRO Rep.* **2019**, *7*, 90–96. [CrossRef] [PubMed]
149. Shahidi, F.; Ambigaipalan, P. Phenolics and polyphenolics in foods, beverages and spices: Antioxidant activity and health effects—A review. *J. Funct. Foods* **2015**, *18*, 820–897. [CrossRef]
150. Fathi, M.; Mirlohi, M.; Varshosaz, J.; Madani, G. Novel Caffeic Acid Nanocarrier: Production, Characterization, and Release Modeling. *J. Nanomater.* **2013**, *2013*, 434632. [CrossRef]
151. Mangrulkar, S.; Shah, P.; Navnage, S.; Mazumdar, P.; Chaple, D. Phytophospholipid Complex of Caffeic Acid: Development, In vitro Characterization, and In Vivo Investigation of Antihyperlipidemic and Hepatoprotective Action in Rats. *AAPS PharmSciTech* **2021**, *22*, 28. [CrossRef]
152. Hatamipour, M.; Jamialahmadi, T.; Ramezani, M.; Tabassi, S.A.S.; Simental-Mendía, L.E.; Sarborji, M.R.; Banach, M.; Sahebkar, A. Protective Effects of Curcumin Phytosomes against High-Fat Diet-Induced Atherosclerosis. *Adv. Exp. Med. Biol.* **2021**, *1308*, 37–44. [CrossRef] [PubMed]
153. Poruba, M.; Kazdová, L.; Oliyarnyk, O.; Malinská, H.; Matusková, Z.; Tozzi di Angelo, I.; Skop, V.; Vecera, R. Improvement bioavailability of silymarin ameliorates severe dyslipidemia associated with metabolic syndrome. *Xenobiotica* **2015**, *45*, 751–756. [CrossRef] [PubMed]
154. Patel, J.; Patel, R.; Khambholja, K.; Patel, N. An overview of phytosomes as an advanced herbal drug delivery system. *Asian J. Pharm. Sci.* **2009**, *4*, 363–371.
155. Watson, R.R.; Preedy, V.R.; Zibadi, S. *Polyphenols in Human Health and Disease*; Academic Press: Cambridge, MA, USA, 2013; Volume 1, pp. 1–1419.
156. Rondanelli, M.; Peroni, G.; Riva, A.; Petrangolini, G.; Allegrini, P.; Fazia, T.; Bernardinelli, L.; Naso, M.; Faliva, M.A.; Tartara, A.; et al. Bergamot phytosome improved visceral fat and plasma lipid profiles in overweight and obese class I subject with mild hypercholesterolemia: A randomized placebo controlled trial. *Phytother. Res.* **2021**, *35*, 2045–2056. [CrossRef] [PubMed]
157. Ezhilarasan, D.; Lakshmi, T. A Molecular Insight into the Role of Antioxidants in Nonalcoholic Fatty Liver Diseases. *Oxidative Med. Cell. Longev.* **2022**, *2022*, 9233650. [CrossRef] [PubMed]
158. Friedman, S.L.; Neuschwander-Tetri, B.A.; Rinella, M.; Sanyal, A.J. Mechanisms of NAFLD development and therapeutic strategies. *Nat. Med.* **2018**, *24*, 908–922. [CrossRef] [PubMed]
159. Saeed, N.; Nadeau, B.; Shannon, C.; Tincopa, M. Evaluation of Dietary Approaches for the Treatment of Non-Alcoholic Fatty Liver Disease: A Systematic Review. *Nutrients* **2019**, *11*, 3064. [CrossRef] [PubMed]
160. Naik, S.R.; Panda, V.S. Antioxidant and hepatoprotective effects of Ginkgo biloba phytosomes in carbon tetrachloride-induced liver injury in rodents. *Liver Int.* **2007**, *27*, 393–399. [CrossRef]
161. Bares, J.M.; Berger, J.; Nelson, J.E.; Messner, D.J.; Schildt, S.; Standish, L.J.; Kowdley, K.V. Silybin treatment is associated with reduction in serum ferritin in patients with chronic hepatitis C. *J. Clin. Gastroenterol.* **2008**, *42*, 937–944. [CrossRef]
162. Freedman, N.D.; Curto, T.M.; Morishima, C.; Seeff, L.B.; Goodman, Z.D.; Wright, E.C.; Sinha, R.; Everhart, J.E. Silymarin use and liver disease progression in the Hepatitis C Antiviral Long-Term Treatment against Cirrhosis trial. *Aliment. Pharmacol. Ther.* **2011**, *33*, 127–137. [CrossRef]

163. Federico, A.; Dallio, M.; Loguercio, C. Silymarin/Silybin and Chronic Liver Disease: A Marriage of Many Years. *Molecules* **2017**, *22*, 191. [CrossRef] [PubMed]
164. El-Gazayerly, O.N.; Makhlouf, A.I.; Soelm, A.M.; Mohmoud, M.A. Antioxidant and hepatoprotective effects of silymarin phytosomes compared to milk thistle extract in CCl4 induced hepatotoxicity in rats. *J. Microencapsul.* **2014**, *31*, 23–30. [CrossRef] [PubMed]
165. Tang, S.; Zhang, X.; Duan, Z.; Xu, M.; Kong, M.; Zheng, S.; Bai, L.; Chen, Y. The novel hepatoprotective mechanisms of silibinin-phospholipid complex against d-GalN/LPS-induced acute liver injury. *Int. Immunopharmacol.* **2023**, *116*, 109808. [CrossRef] [PubMed]
166. Maiti, K.; Mukherjee, K.; Gantait, A.; Saha, B.P.; Mukherjee, P.K. Enhanced therapeutic potential of naringenin-phospholipid complex in rats. *J. Pharm. Pharmacol.* **2006**, *58*, 1227–1233. [CrossRef] [PubMed]
167. Liu, J.; Lu, J.F.; Wen, X.Y.; Kan, J.; Jin, C.H. Antioxidant and protective effect of inulin and catechin grafted inulin against CCl4-induced liver injury. *Int. J. Biol. Macromol.* **2015**, *72*, 1479–1484. [CrossRef] [PubMed]
168. Raffa, D.; Maggio, B.; Raimondi, M.V.; Plescia, F.; Daidone, G. Recent discoveries of anticancer flavonoids. *Eur. J. Med. Chem.* **2017**, *142*, 213–228. [CrossRef] [PubMed]
169. Athmouni, K.; Mkadmini Hammi, K.; El Feki, A.; Ayadi, H. Development of catechin-phospholipid complex to enhance the bioavailability and modulatory potential against cadmium-induced oxidative stress in rats liver. *Arch. Physiol. Biochem.* **2020**, *126*, 82–88. [CrossRef] [PubMed]
170. Kazmi, I.; Afzal, M.; Rahman, S.; Iqbal, M.; Imam, F.; Anwar, F. Antiobesity potential of ursolic acid stearoyl glucoside by inhibiting pancreatic lipase. *Eur. J. Pharmacol.* **2013**, *709*, 28–36. [CrossRef]
171. Liu, J. Oleanolic acid and ursolic acid: Research perspectives. *J. Ethnopharmacol.* **2005**, *100*, 92–94. [CrossRef]
172. Safari, Z.; Bagheriya, M.; Khoram, Z.; Ebrahimi Varzaneh, A.; Heidari, Z.; Sahebkar, A.; Askari, G. The effect of curcumin on anthropometric indices, blood pressure, lipid profiles, fasting blood glucose, liver enzymes, fibrosis, and steatosis in non-alcoholic fatty livers. *Front. Nutr.* **2023**, *10*, 1163950. [CrossRef]
173. Panahi, Y.; Kianpour, P.; Mohtashami, R.; Jafari, R.; Simental-Mendía, L.E.; Sahebkar, A. Efficacy and Safety of Phytosomal Curcumin in Non-Alcoholic Fatty Liver Disease: A Randomized Controlled Trial. *Drug Res.* **2017**, *67*, 244–251. [CrossRef] [PubMed]
174. Cicero, A.F.G.; Sahebkar, A.; Fogacci, F.; Bove, M.; Giovannini, M.; Borghi, C. Effects of phytosomal curcumin on anthropometric parameters, insulin resistance, cortisolemia and non-alcoholic fatty liver disease indices: A double-blind, placebo-controlled clinical trial. *Eur. J. Nutr.* **2020**, *59*, 477–483. [CrossRef] [PubMed]
175. Cole, J.B.; Florez, J.C. Genetics of diabetes mellitus and diabetes complications. *Nat. Rev. Nephrol.* **2020**, *16*, 377–390. [CrossRef]
176. Rathee, S.; Kamboj, A. Optimization and development of antidiabetic phytosomes by the Box–Behnken design. *J. Liposome Res.* **2018**, *28*, 161–172. [CrossRef] [PubMed]
177. El-Dassoasy, H.M.; Abo-Warda, S.M.; Fahmy, A. Chrysin and luteolin alleviate vascular complications associated with insulin resistance mainly through PPAR-γ activation. *Am. J. Chin. Med.* **2014**, *42*, 1153–1167. [CrossRef] [PubMed]
178. Andrade, N.; Andrade, S.; Silva, C.; Rodrigues, I.; Guardão, L.; Guimarães, J.T.; Keating, E.; Martel, F. Chronic consumption of the dietary polyphenol chrysin attenuates metabolic disease in fructose-fed rats. *Eur. J. Nutr.* **2020**, *59*, 151–165. [CrossRef] [PubMed]
179. Kim, S.M.; Imm, J.Y. The Effect of Chrysin-Loaded Phytosomes on Insulin Resistance and Blood Sugar Control in Type 2 Diabetic db/db Mice. *Molecules* **2020**, *25*, 5503. [CrossRef]
180. Gullón, B.; Lú-Chau, T.A.; Moreira, M.T.; Lema, J.M.; Eibes, G. Rutin: A review on extraction, identification and purification methods, biological activities and approaches to enhance its bioavailability. *Trends Food Sci. Technol.* **2017**, *67*, 220–235. [CrossRef]
181. Al-Ishaq, R.K.; Abotaleb, M.; Kubatka, P.; Kajo, K.; Büsselberg, D. Flavonoids and Their Anti-Diabetic Effects: Cellular Mechanisms and Effects to Improve Blood Sugar Levels. *Biomolecules* **2019**, *9*, 430. [CrossRef]
182. Amjadi, S.; Shahnaz, F.; Shokouhi, B.; Azarmi, Y.; Siahi-Shadbad, M.; Ghanbarzadeh, S.; Kouhsoltani, M.; Ebrahimi, A.; Hamishehkar, H. Nanophytosomes for enhancement of rutin efficacy in oral administration for diabetes treatment in streptozotocin-induced diabetic rats. *Int. J. Pharm.* **2021**, *610*, 121208. [CrossRef]
183. Panahi, Y.; Khalili, N.; Sahebi, E.; Namazi, S.; Simental-Mendía, L.E.; Majeed, M.; Sahebkar, A. Effects of Curcuminoids Plus Piperine on Glycemic, Hepatic and Inflammatory Biomarkers in Patients with Type 2 Diabetes Mellitus: A Randomized Double-Blind Placebo-Controlled Trial. *Drug Res.* **2018**, *68*, 403–409. [CrossRef]
184. Yeung, S.; Soliternik, J.; Mazzola, N. Nutritional supplements for the prevention of diabetes mellitus and its complications. *J. Nutr. Intermed. Metab.* **2018**, *14*, 16–21. [CrossRef]
185. Alhabashneh, W.; Khleifat, K.; Alqaraleh, M.; Alomari, L.; Qinna, N.; Allimoun, M.; Qaralleh, H.; Farah, H.; Alqais, T. Evaluation of the Therapeutic Effect of Curcumin Phytosomes on Streptozotocin-Induced Diabetic Rats. *Trop. J. Nat. Prod. Res.* **2022**, *6*, 529–536. [CrossRef]
186. Ilyas, Z.; Perna, S.; Al-Thawadi, S.; Alalwan, T.A.; Riva, A.; Petrangolini, G.; Gasparri, C.; Infantino, V.; Peroni, G.; Rondanelli, M. The effect of Berberine on weight loss in order to prevent obesity: A systematic review. *Biomed. Pharmacother.* **2020**, *127*, 110137. [CrossRef]

187. Rondanelli, M.; Riva, A.; Petrangolini, G.; Allegrini, P.; Giacosa, A.; Fazia, T.; Bernardinelli, L.; Gasparri, C.; Peroni, G.; Perna, S. Berberine Phospholipid Is an Effective Insulin Sensitizer and Improves Metabolic and Hormonal Disorders in Women with Polycystic Ovary Syndrome: A One-Group Pretest-Post-Test Explanatory Study. *Nutrients* **2021**, *13*, 3665. [CrossRef] [PubMed]
188. Panyadee, P.; Balslev, H.; Wangpakapattanawong, P.; Inta, A. Medicinal plants in homegardens of four ethnic groups in Thailand. *J. Ethnopharmacol.* **2019**, *239*, 111927. [CrossRef] [PubMed]
189. Srinuanchai, W.; Nooin, R.; Pitchakarn, P.; Karinchai, J.; Suttisansanee, U.; Chansriniyom, C.; Jarussophon, S.; Temviriyanukul, P.; Nuchuchua, O. Inhibitory effects of *Gymnema inodorum* (Lour.) Decne leaf extracts and its triterpene saponin on carbohydrate digestion and intestinal glucose absorption. *J. Ethnopharmacol.* **2021**, *266*, 113398. [CrossRef] [PubMed]
190. Jeytawan, N.; Yadoung, S.; Jeeno, P.; Yana, P.; Sutan, K.; Naksen, W.; Wongkaew, M.; Sommano, S.R.; Hongsibsong, S. Antioxidant and Phytochemical Potential of and Phytochemicals in *Gymnema inodorum* (Lour.) Decne in Northern Thailand. *Plants* **2022**, *11*, 3498. [CrossRef]
191. Zhu, S.; Liu, Q.; Chang, Y.; Luo, C.; Zhang, X.; Sun, S. Integrated Network Pharmacology and Cellular Assay to Explore the Mechanisms of Selenized Tripterine Phytosomes (Se@Tri-PTs) Alleviating Podocyte Injury in Diabetic Nephropathy. *Curr. Pharm. Des.* **2023**, *29*, 3073–3086. [CrossRef]
192. Riva, A.; Corti, A.; Belcaro, G.; Cesarone, M.R.; Dugall, M.; Vinciguerra, G.; Feragalli, B.; Zuccarini, M.; Eggenhoffner, R.; Giacomelli, L. Interaction study between antiplatelet agents, anticoagulants, diabetic therapy and a novel delivery form of quercetin. *Minerva Cardioangiol.* **2019**, *67*, 79–83. [CrossRef]
193. Di Minno, A.; Frigerio, B.; Spadarella, G.; Ravani, A.; Sansaro, D.; Amato, M.; Kitzmiller, J.P.; Pepi, M.; Tremoli, E.; Baldassarre, D. Old and new oral anticoagulants: Food, herbal medicines and drug interactions. *Blood Rev.* **2017**, *31*, 193–203. [CrossRef] [PubMed]
194. Gupta, R.C.; Chang, D.; Nammi, S.; Bensoussan, A.; Bilinski, K.; Roufogalis, B.D. Interactions between antidiabetic drugs and herbs: An overview of mechanisms of action and clinical implications. *Diabetol. Metab. Syndr.* **2017**, *9*, 59. [CrossRef] [PubMed]
195. Ledda, A.; Belcaro, G.; Feragalli, B.; Hosoi, M.; Cacchio, M.; Luzzi, R.; Dugall, M.; Cotellese, R. Temporary kidney dysfunction: Supplementation with Meriva® in initial, transient kidney micro-macro albuminuria. *Panminerva Med.* **2019**, *61*, 444–448. [CrossRef] [PubMed]
196. Mirhafez, S.R.; Azimi-Nezhad, M.; Dehabeh, M.; Hariri, M.; Naderan, R.D.; Movahedi, A.; Abdalla, M.; Sathyapalan, T.; Sahebkar, A. The Effect of Curcumin Phytosome on the Treatment of Patients with Non-alcoholic Fatty Liver Disease: A Double-Blind, Randomized, Placebo-Controlled Trial. *Adv. Exp. Med. Biol.* **2021**, *1308*, 25–35. [CrossRef] [PubMed]
197. Vaduganathan, M.; Mensah, G.A.; Turco, J.V.; Fuster, V.; Roth, G.A. The Global Burden of Cardiovascular Diseases and Risk: A Compass for Future Health. *J. Am. Coll. Cardiol.* **2022**, *80*, 2361–2371. [CrossRef]
198. Sowndhararajan, K.; Deepa, P.; Kim, S. A review of the chemical composition and biological activities of *Callistemon lanceolatus* (Sm.) Sweet. *J. Appl. Pharm. Sci.* **2021**, *11*, 065–073. [CrossRef]
199. Ortega-Pérez, L.G.; Piñón-Simental, J.S.; Magaña-Rodríguez, O.R.; López-Mejía, A.; Ayala-Ruiz, L.A.; García-Calderón, A.J.; Godínez-Hernández, D.; Rios-Chavez, P. Evaluation of the toxicology, anti-lipase, and antioxidant effects of *Callistemon citrinus* in rats fed with a high fat-fructose diet. *Pharm. Biol.* **2022**, *60*, 1384–1393. [CrossRef] [PubMed]
200. Ortega-Pérez, L.G.; Ayala-Ruiz, L.A.; Magaña-Rodríguez, O.R.; Piñón-Simental, J.S.; Aguilera-Méndez, A.; Godínez-Hernández, D.; Rios-Chavez, P. Development and Evaluation of Phytosomes Containing *Callistemon citrinus* Leaf Extract: A Preclinical Approach for the Treatment of Obesity in a Rodent Model. *Pharmaceutics* **2023**, *15*, 2178. [CrossRef] [PubMed]
201. Chakhtoura, M.; Haber, R.; Ghezzawi, M.; Rhayem, C.; Tcheroyan, R.; Mantzoros, C.S. Pharmacotherapy of obesity: An update on the available medications and drugs under investigation. *EClinicalMedicine* **2023**, *58*, 101882. [CrossRef]
202. Tham, K.W.; Lim, A.Y.L.; Baur, L.A. The global agenda on obesity: What does this mean for Singapore? *Singap. Med. J.* **2023**, *64*, 182–187. [CrossRef]
203. Velasquez, M.T.; Bhathena, S.J. Role of dietary soy protein in obesity. *Int. J. Med. Sci.* **2007**, *4*, 72–82. [CrossRef] [PubMed]
204. Lee, H.S.; Nam, Y.; Chung, Y.H.; Kim, H.R.; Park, E.S.; Chung, S.J.; Kim, J.H.; Sohn, U.D.; Kim, H.C.; Oh, K.W.; et al. Beneficial effects of phosphatidylcholine on high-fat diet-induced obesity, hyperlipidemia and fatty liver in mice. *Life Sci.* **2014**, *118*, 7–14. [CrossRef] [PubMed]
205. Elnaggar, Y.S.; El-Refaie, W.M.; El-Massik, M.A.; Abdallah, O.Y. Lecithin-based nanostructured gels for skin delivery: An update on state of art and recent applications. *J. Control. Release* **2014**, *180*, 10–24. [CrossRef] [PubMed]
206. Mohammadi, A.; Sadeghnia, H.R.; Saberi-Karimian, M.; Safarian, H.; Ferns, G.A.; Ghayour-Mobarhan, M.; Sahebkar, A. Effects of Curcumin on Serum Vitamin E Concentrations in Individuals with Metabolic Syndrome. *Phytother. Res.* **2017**, *31*, 657–662. [CrossRef] [PubMed]
207. Cesaro, A.; De Michele, G.; Fimiani, F.; Acerbo, V.; Scherillo, G.; Signore, G.; Rotolo, F.P.; Scialla, F.; Raucci, G.; Panico, D.; et al. Visceral adipose tissue and residual cardiovascular risk: A pathological link and new therapeutic options. *Front. Cardiovasc. Med.* **2023**, *10*, 1187735. [CrossRef] [PubMed]
208. Kim, J.; Kim, K. CT-based measurement of visceral adipose tissue volume as a reliable tool for assessing metabolic risk factors in prediabetes across subtypes. *Sci. Rep.* **2023**, *13*, 17902. [CrossRef] [PubMed]
209. Wong, N.D. Epidemiological studies of CHD and the evolution of preventive cardiology. *Nat. Rev. Cardiol.* **2014**, *11*, 276–289. [CrossRef] [PubMed]

210. Abbas, A.; Raza, A.; Ullah, M.; Hendi, A.A.; Akbar, F.; Khan, S.U.; Zaman, U.; Saeed, S.; Ur Rehman, K.; Sultan, S.; et al. A Comprehensive Review: Epidemiological Strategies, Catheterization and Biomarkers used as a Bioweapon in Diagnosis and Management of Cardio Vascular Diseases. *Curr. Probl. Cardiol.* **2023**, *48*, 101661. [CrossRef]
211. Galletto, R.; Siqueira, V.L.D.; Ferreira, E.B.; de Oliveira, A.J.B.; Bazotte, R.B. Absence of antidiabetic and hypolipidemic effect of Gymnema sylvestre in non-diabetic and alloxan-diabetic rats. *Braz. Arch. Biol. Technol.* **2004**, *47*, 545. [CrossRef]
212. Ohmori, R.; Iwamoto, T.; Tago, M.; Takeo, T.; Unno, T.; Itakura, H.; Kondo, K. Antioxidant activity of various teas against free radicals and LDL oxidation. *Lipids* **2005**, *40*, 849–853. [CrossRef]
213. Pathan, R.A.; Bhandari, U.; Javed, S.; Nag, T.C. Anti-apoptotic potential of gymnemic acid phospholipid complex pretreatment in Wistar rats with experimental cardiomyopathy. *Indian J. Exp. Biol.* **2012**, *50*, 117–127. [PubMed]
214. Naik, S.R.; Pilgaonkar, V.W.; Panda, V.S. Neuropharmacological evaluation of Ginkgo biloba phytosomes in rodents. *Phytother. Res.* **2006**, *20*, 901–905. [CrossRef] [PubMed]
215. DeFeudis, F.V.; Papadopoulos, V.; Drieu, K. Ginkgo biloba extracts and cancer: A research area in its infancy. *Fundam. Clin. Pharmacol.* **2003**, *17*, 405–417. [CrossRef]
216. Panda, V.S.; Naik, S.R. Cardioprotective activity of Ginkgo biloba Phytosomes in isoproterenol-induced myocardial necrosis in rats: A biochemical and histoarchitectural evaluation. *Exp. Toxicol. Pathol.* **2008**, *60*, 397–404. [CrossRef] [PubMed]
217. Sharma, M.; Kishore, K.; Gupta, S.K.; Joshi, S.; Arya, D.S. Cardioprotective potential of ocimum sanctum in isoproterenol induced myocardial infarction in rats. *Mol. Cell. Biochem.* **2001**, *225*, 75–83. [CrossRef] [PubMed]
218. Arya, D.S.; Nandave, M.; Ojha, S.K.; Kumari, S.; Joshi, S.; Mohanty, I. Myocardial salvaging effects of Ocimum sanctum in experimental model of myocardial necrosis: A haemodynamic, biochemical and histoarchitectural assessment. *Curr. Sci.* **2006**, *91*, 667–672.
219. Gupta, S.K.; Prakash, J.; Srivastava, S. Validation of traditional claim of Tulsi, Ocimum sanctum Linn. as a medicinal plant. *Indian. J. Exp. Biol.* **2002**, *40*, 765–773. [PubMed]
220. Uma Devi, P.; Ganasoundari, A.; Vrinda, B.; Srinivasan, K.K.; Unnikrishnan, M.K. Radiation protection by the ocimum flavonoids orientin and vicenin: Mechanisms of action. *Radiat. Res.* **2000**, *154*, 455–460. [CrossRef] [PubMed]
221. Panda, V.S.; Naik, S.R. Evaluation of cardioprotective activity of Ginkgo biloba and Ocimum sanctum in rodents. *Altern. Med. Rev.* **2009**, *14*, 161–171.
222. Ahmad, H.; Arya, A.; Agrawal, S.; Samuel, S.S.; Singh, S.K.; Valicherla, G.R.; Sangwan, N.; Mitra, K.; Gayen, J.R.; Paliwal, S.; et al. Phospholipid complexation of NMITLI118RT+: Way to a prudent therapeutic approach for beneficial outcomes in ischemic stroke in rats. *Drug Deliv.* **2016**, *23*, 3606–3618. [CrossRef]
223. Zhang, L.L.; Tian, K.; Tang, Z.H.; Chen, X.J.; Bian, Z.X.; Wang, Y.T.; Lu, J.J. Phytochemistry and Pharmacology of *Carthamus tinctorius* L. *Am. J. Chin. Med.* **2016**, *44*, 197–226. [CrossRef] [PubMed]
224. Sun, B.; Cai, X.; Wu, T.; Chen, L. Protective effect of Honghua (safflower) extract on cerebral ischemia-reperfusion injury in mice. *Chin. J. Tradit. Med. Sci. Technol.* **2018**, *25*, 205–207.
225. Yuan, Z.W.; Li, Y.Z.; Liu, Z.Q.; Feng, S.L.; Zhou, H.; Liu, C.X.; Lin, L.; Xie, Y. Role of tangeretin as a potential bioavailability enhancer for silybin: Pharmacokinetic and pharmacological studies. *Pharmacol. Res.* **2018**, *128*, 153–166. [CrossRef] [PubMed]
226. Xu, P.; Zhou, H.; Li, Y.Z.; Yuan, Z.W.; Liu, C.X.; Liu, L.; Xie, Y. Baicalein Enhances the Oral Bioavailability and Hepatoprotective Effects of Silybin Through the Inhibition of Efflux Transporters BCRP and MRP2. *Front. Pharmacol.* **2018**, *9*, 1115. [CrossRef] [PubMed]
227. Yanyu, X.; Yunmei, S.; Zhipeng, C.; Qineng, P. The preparation of silybin-phospholipid complex and the study on its pharmacokinetics in rats. *Int. J. Pharm.* **2006**, *307*, 77–82. [CrossRef] [PubMed]
228. Pasala, P.K.; Uppara, R.K.; Rudrapal, M.; Zothantluanga, J.H.; Umar, A.K. Silybin phytosome attenuates cerebral ischemia-reperfusion injury in rats by suppressing oxidative stress and reducing inflammatory response: In vivo and in silico approaches. *J. Biochem. Mol. Toxicol.* **2022**, *36*, e23073. [CrossRef] [PubMed]
229. Palachai, N.; Wattanathorn, J.; Muchimapura, S.; Thukham-Mee, W. Antimetabolic Syndrome Effect of Phytosome Containing the Combined Extracts of Mulberry and Ginger in an Animal Model of Metabolic Syndrome. *Oxidative Med. Cell. Longev.* **2019**, *2019*, 5972575. [CrossRef]
230. Wattanathorn, J.; Palachai, N.; Thukham-Mee, W.; Muchimapura, S. Memory-Enhancing Effect of a Phytosome Containing the Combined Extract of Mulberry Fruit and Ginger in an Animal Model of Ischemic Stroke with Metabolic Syndrome. *Oxidative Med. Cell. Longev.* **2020**, *2020*, 3096826. [CrossRef]
231. Palachai, N.; Wattanathorn, J.; Muchimapura, S.; Thukham-Mee, W. Phytosome Loading the Combined Extract of Mulberry Fruit and Ginger Protects against Cerebral Ischemia in Metabolic Syndrome Rats. *Oxidative Med. Cell. Longev.* **2020**, *2020*, 5305437. [CrossRef]
232. Hobson, R.M.; Saunders, B.; Ball, G.; Harris, R.C.; Sale, C. Effects of β-alanine supplementation on exercise performance: A meta-analysis. *Amino Acids* **2012**, *43*, 25–37. [CrossRef]
233. Teplicki, E.; Ma, Q.; Castillo, D.E.; Zarei, M.; Hustad, A.P.; Chen, J.; Li, J. The Effects of Aloe vera on Wound Healing in Cell Proliferation, Migration, and Viability. *Wounds* **2018**, *30*, 263–268. [PubMed]
234. de Courten, B.; Jakubova, M.; de Courten, M.P.; Kukurova, I.J.; Vallova, S.; Krumpolec, P.; Valkovic, L.; Kurdiova, T.; Garzon, D.; Barbaresi, S.; et al. Effects of carnosine supplementation on glucose metabolism: Pilot clinical trial. *Obesity* **2016**, *24*, 1027–1034. [CrossRef] [PubMed]

235. Okyar, A.; Can, A.; Akev, N.; Baktır, G.; Sütlüpinar, N. Effect of Aloe vera leaves on blood glucose level in type I and type II diabetic rat models. *Phytother. Res.* **2001**, *15*, 157–161. [CrossRef] [PubMed]
236. Darvishi, B.; Dinarvand, R.; Mohammadpour, H.; Kamarul, T.; Sharifi, A.M. Dual l-Carnosine/Aloe vera Nanophytosomes with Synergistically Enhanced Protective Effects against Methylglyoxal-Induced Angiogenesis Impairment. *Mol. Pharm.* **2021**, *18*, 3302–3325. [CrossRef] [PubMed]
237. Prakash, P.; Rajakani, R.; Gupta, V. Transcriptome-wide identification of Rauvolfia serpentina microRNAs and prediction of their potential targets. *Comput. Biol. Chem.* **2016**, *61*, 62–74. [CrossRef] [PubMed]
238. Panja, S.; Chaudhuri, I.; Khanra, K.; Bhattacharyya, N. Biological application of green silver nanoparticle synthesized from leaf extract of Rauvolfia serpentina Benth. *Asian Pac. J. Trop. Dis.* **2016**, *6*, 549–556. [CrossRef]
239. Gantait, S.; Kundu, S.; Yeasmin, L.; Ali, M.N. Impact of differential levels of sodium alginate, calcium chloride and basal media on germination frequency of genetically true artificial seeds of *Rauvolfia serpentina* (L.) Benth. ex Kurz. *J. Appl. Res. Med. Aromat. Plants* **2017**, *4*, 75–81. [CrossRef]
240. Touqeer, S.I.; Jahan, N.; Abbas, N.; Ali, A. Formulation and Process Optimization of Rauvolfia serpentina Nanosuspension by HPMC and In Vitro Evaluation of ACE Inhibitory Potential. *J. Funct. Biomater.* **2022**, *13*, 268. [CrossRef] [PubMed]
241. Raizner, A.E.; Quiñones, M.A. Coenzyme Q(10) for Patients with Cardiovascular Disease: JACC Focus Seminar. *J. Am. Coll. Cardiol.* **2021**, *77*, 609–619. [CrossRef]
242. Martelli, A.; Testai, L.; Colletti, A.; Cicero, A.F.G. Coenzyme Q(10): Clinical Applications in Cardiovascular Diseases. *Antioxidants* **2020**, *9*, 341. [CrossRef]
243. Cicero, A.F.G.; Fogacci, F.; Di Micoli, A.; Veronesi, M.; Borghi, C. Noninvasive instrumental evaluation of coenzyme Q(10) phytosome on endothelial reactivity in healthy nonsmoking young volunteers: A double-blind, randomized, placebo-controlled crossover clinical trial. *Biofactors* **2022**, *48*, 1160–1165. [CrossRef] [PubMed]

Disclaimer/Publisher's Note: The statements, opinions and data contained in all publications are solely those of the individual author(s) and contributor(s) and not of MDPI and/or the editor(s). MDPI and/or the editor(s) disclaim responsibility for any injury to people or property resulting from any ideas, methods, instructions or products referred to in the content.

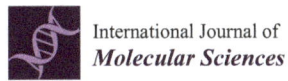

Article

Autumn Olive (*Elaeagnus umbellata* Thunb.) Berries Improve Lipid Metabolism and Delay Aging in Middle-Aged *Caenorhabditis elegans*

Yebin Kim [1], Seonghyeon Nam [2], Jongbin Lim [2] and Miran Jang [1,3,*]

[1] Department of Institute of Digital Anti-Aging Healthcare, Inje University, Gimhae 50834, Republic of Korea; dpqls1812@oasis.inje.ac.kr

[2] Department of Food Bioengineering, Jeju National University, Jeju 63243, Republic of Korea; seonghyeon_n@stu.jejunu.ac.kr (S.N.); jongbinlim@jejunu.ac.kr (J.L.)

[3] Department of Food Technology and Nutrition, Inje University, Gimhae 50834, Republic of Korea

* Correspondence: mrjang@inje.ac.kr; Tel.: +82-55-320-3234

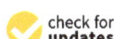

Citation: Kim, Y.; Nam, S.; Lim, J.; Jang, M. Autumn Olive (*Elaeagnus umbellata* Thunb.) Berries Improve Lipid Metabolism and Delay Aging in Middle-Aged *Caenorhabditis elegans*. *Int. J. Mol. Sci.* **2024**, *25*, 3418. https://doi.org/10.3390/ijms25063418

Academic Editors: Marilena Gilca and Adelina Vlad

Received: 28 December 2023
Revised: 7 March 2024
Accepted: 14 March 2024
Published: 18 March 2024

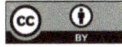

Copyright: © 2024 by the authors. Licensee MDPI, Basel, Switzerland. This article is an open access article distributed under the terms and conditions of the Creative Commons Attribution (CC BY) license (https://creativecommons.org/licenses/by/4.0/).

Abstract: This study evaluated the positive effects of autumn olive berries (AOBs) extract on delaying aging by improving lipid metabolism in middle-aged *Caenorhabditis elegans* that had become obese due to a high-glucose (GLU) diet. The total phenolic content and DPPH radical scavenging abilities of freeze-dried AOBs (FAOBs) or spray-dried AOBs (SAOBs) were examined, and FAOBs exhibited better antioxidant activity. HPLC analysis confirmed that catechin is the main phenolic compound of AOBs; its content was 5.95 times higher in FAOBs than in SAOBs. Therefore, FAOBs were used in subsequent in vivo experiments. FAOBs inhibited lipid accumulation in both the young adult and middle-aged groups in a concentration-dependent manner under both normal and 2% GLU conditions. Additionally, FAOBs inhibited ROS accumulation in a concentration-dependent manner under normal and 2% GLU conditions in the middle-aged worms. In particular, FAOB also increased body bending and egg production in middle-aged worms. To confirm the intervention of genetic factors related to lipid metabolism from the effects of FAOB, body lipid accumulation was confirmed using worms deficient in the daf-16, atgl-1, aak-1, and akt-1 genes. Regarding the effect of FAOB on reducing lipid accumulation, the impact was nullified in daf-16-deficient worms under the 2% GLU condition, and nullified in both the daf-16 and atgl-1-deficient worms under fasting conditions. In conclusion, FAOB mediated daf-16 and atgl-1 to regulate lipogenesis and lipolysis in middle-aged worms. Our findings suggest that FAOB improves lipid metabolism in metabolically impaired middle-aged worms, contributing to its age-delaying effect.

Keywords: autumn olive (*Elaeagnus umbellata* Thunb.); middle-aged *C. elegans*; lipid metabolism; delaying aging

1. Introduction

The prevalence of obesity is increasing at an alarming rate worldwide, especially in recent decades [1]. The rise in obesity is also associated with an increased incidence of significant health risk factors and diseases, including insulin resistance, type 2 diabetes, non-alcoholic fatty liver disease, atherosclerosis, and certain cancers [2]. Obesity is influenced by the processes of lipogenesis and lipolysis [3,4]. *Caenorhabditis elegans* is considered an excellent multicellular organism model for studying the mechanisms of aging because it has a short lifespan, rapid progeny reproduction, and well-defined genetic pathways [5]. Furthermore, molecular pathways involved in energy metabolism in mammals, including humans, are strongly conserved in *C. elegans* [6]. Dietary glucose influences physiological and molecular processes in *C. elegans*, making it a valuable model for understanding human hyperglycemia and obesity. It has been reported that high-glucose diets (HGD) result in lipid accumulation, alter membrane fluidity, affect lifespan and progeny, and increase cellular levels of reactive oxygen species (ROS) and protein glycosylation [7,8].

Indeed, middle-aged people who have maintained unhealthy eating habits are susceptible to a variety of negative health outcomes [9]. Obesity in middle age is more sensitive to arteriosclerosis than obesity in youth [10]. In particular, in the case of middle-aged women who have reached menopause, abdominal and hepatic fat accumulation as well as waist circumference increase due to changes in hormonal and metabolic profiles. Middle-aged women with metabolic disturbances have an increased risk of cardiovascular disease and acute coronary artery disease due to excessive production of very low-density lipoprotein (VLDL), and even have a poorer prognosis than men [11]. However, although there are many reports of short-term diet effects with test periods set to days or weeks in in vivo studies, few studies have experimentally investigated accumulating dietary effects over middle age.

Autumn olive (*Elaeagnus umbellata* Thunb.) is one of the wild spiny branched shrubs, and is a plant in the Elaeagnaceae family that is native to Asia [10,11]. Autumn olive berries (AOBs) mature between September and November to an edible dark red color, and are sweet, sour, and juicy [12–14]. AOBs are known to contain a lot of catechins, lutein, gallic acid, caffeic acid, phytoene, phytofluene, β-cryptoxanthin, β-carotene, and α-cryptoxanthin [15,16]. Phytochemicals in AOBs, and particularly catechins, have been reported to exhibit antidiabetic effects by regulating glucose levels [17–19]. On the other hand, there are few studies on their anti-obesity effects related to lipid metabolism. Multiple reports explained that catechins are the main compounds of AOBs; meanwhile, such catechins are well-known compounds that have anti-obesity effects [20]. Thus, we hypothesized that catechins of AOBs might show an inhibitory effect on lipid accumulation.

In this experiment, AOBs were prepared for use as the main ingredients for powdered tea, and the following were investigated. First, we assessed the effect of AOBs on lipid accumulation in nematodes fed a high-glucose diet by middle age. Second, we evaluated the effect of autumn olive berries on menopausal symptoms (reduced behavior, decreased fertility, ROS accumulation) in middle age. Finally, we studied whether the autumn olive berries effect was affected by the intervention of lipid metabolism (lipogenesis and lipolysis)-related genetic factors.

2. Results

2.1. Confirmation of the Antioxidant Activity and Polyphenol Contents of FAOBs and SAOBs

The total phenolic contents (TPC) of freeze-dried AOBs (FAOBs) and spray-dried AOBs (SAOBs) were 258.23 ± 1.00 mg GAE/100 g and 63.02 ± 2.00 mg GAE/100 g, respectively (Table 1). The DPPH scavenging capacity of FAOB and SAOB were 3842.23 ± 294.91 mg AA/100 g and 3151.78 ± 395.08 mg AA/100 g, respectively (Table 1).

Table 1. TPC and DPPH values of freeze-dried AOBs (FAOBs) and spray-dried AOBs (SAOBs).

Samples	TPC (mg GAE/100 g)	DPPH (mg AA/100 g)
FAOB	258.23 ± 1.00	3842.23 ± 294.91
SAOB	63.02 ± 2.00	3151.78 ± 395.08
p-value *	0.05	0.03

TPC: total phenolic contents, GAE: gallic acid equivalent, and AA: ascorbic acid. All values represent the means ± SDs of three separate experiments. *: Statistical analyses were performed using Student's *t*-test (unpaired and two-tailed).

2.2. Catechin Identification

The HPLC chromatograms of FAOB and SAOB are shown in Figure 1. The results show that catechin was the key compound of FAOB. Interestingly, the catechin peak appeared high in FAOB and low in SAOB. The SAOB results almost coincided with the chromatogram of methanol used as the mobile phase. Quantification of catechin in FAOB and SAOB showed that they contained 154.02 ± 5.29 and 27.53 ± 3.05 mg/100 g, respectively (Table 2).

There were statistically significant differences in the catechin content of FAOB and SAOB (p-value = 0.002), suggesting that differences in the physiological activities of FAOB and SAOB might be attributed to the catechin content. Based on the previously indicated polyphenol and catechin contents and antioxidant capacity results, we considered that FAOB has more potential, and thus decided to use FAOB for further experiments.

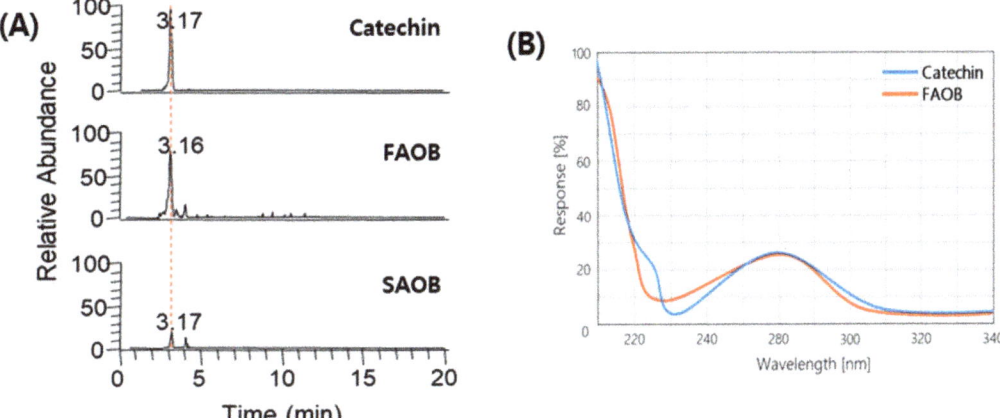

Figure 1. HPLC chromatograms of freeze-dried AOB (FAOB) and spray-dried AOB (SAOB). (**A**) HPLC chromatograms of catechin and two AOB extract samples. (**B**) Respective DAD spectra of the peaks with the same retention time. The red dotted line on the HPLC chromatogram represents the same retention time.

Table 2. Catechin contents of freeze-dried AOB (FAOB) and spray-dried AOB (SAOB).

Samples	Catechin (mg/100 g)
FAOB	154.02 ± 5.29
SAOB	27.53 ± 3.05
p-value *	0.002

All values represent the means ± SDs of three separate experiments. *: Statistical analyses were performed using Student's t-test (unpaired and two-tailed).

2.3. Safety of FAOB in C. elegans

To determine the safe concentrations of AOB, an acute toxicity test was conducted with different concentrations (31.25–1000 μg/mL) of AOB. As a result, various tested concentrations of FAOB did not statistically show any difference in survival rates. However, survival rates decreased by 2% and 4% at 500 and 1000 μg/mL FAOB, respectively. Thus, safe concentrations (62.5, 125, and 250 μg/mL) of FAOB were used in subsequent experiments (Figure 2A). Also, FAOB at 250 μg/mL did not affect the survival of nematodes compared to the control, even under oxidative and heat stress conditions (Figure 2B,C).

2.4. FAOB Inhibits Lipid Accumulation in C. elegans

We examined the effect of AOB on fat accumulation in young and middle-aged adult worms. AOB showed a concentration-dependent decrease in total fat accumulation compared to the control under normal and 2% GLU diet conditions in young adult worms (Figure 3B).

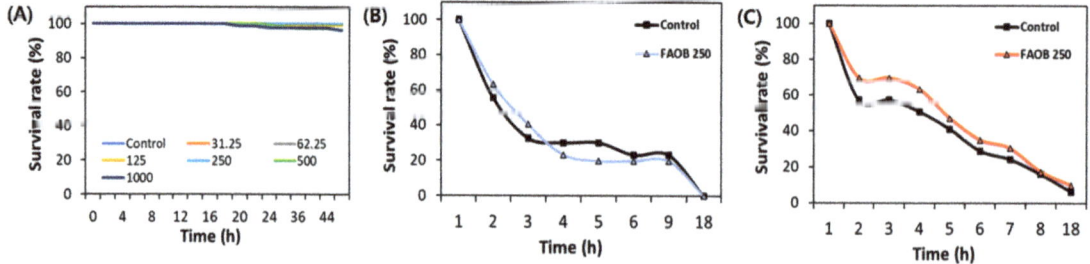

Figure 2. Safety of FAOB under various conditions. (**A**) The effect of AOB at different concentrations (31.25–1000 μg/mL) under normal conditions (50 worms were used in each group). The effect of FAOB at 250 μg/mL under (**B**) oxidative stress and (**C**) heat stress (n = 3 plates and 10 randomly selected worms were used).

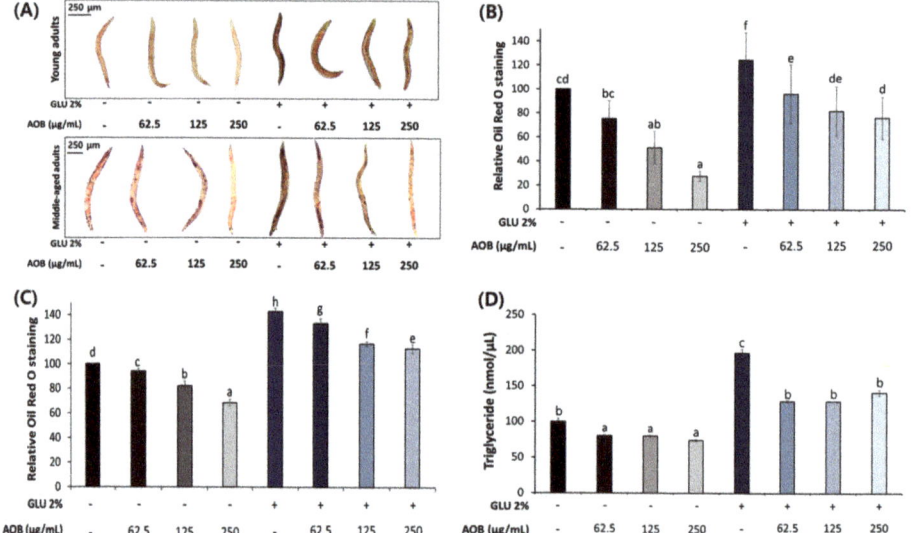

Figure 3. Inhibitory effect of AOB on lipid accumulation. (**A**) Images of stored body fat in young-aged and middle-aged worms under normal and 2% GLU conditions. Quantification results of total lipids in (**B**) young adult and (**C**) middle-aged worms under normal and 2% GLU dietary conditions. (**D**) Triglyceride (TG) contents of middle-aged worms under normal and 2% GLU conditions. Bars represent the means ± SDs of three separate experiments (for ORO assay, n = 3 plates and 10 randomly selected worms were used. More than 2000 worms were used in each group for TG assay). Different letters above the bars mean statistically significant differences ($p < 0.05$). "-" means untreated, and "+" means treated.

The inhibitory effect of FAOB on total fat accumulation was also confirmed in middle-aged worms (Figure 3C). Also, the triglyceride (TG) content in the AOB-treated group was reduced compared to the control under normal and 2% GLU diet conditions in the middle-aged group (Figure 3D).

2.5. AOB Reduces Reactive Oxygen Species (ROS) Accumulation in Middle-Aged C. elegans

ROS are metabolites that cause aging, and it has been reported in previous studies that a high-GLU diet causes ROS accumulation [21]. FAOB exhibited a reduction effect on ROS production in both young and middle-aged worms (Figure 4).

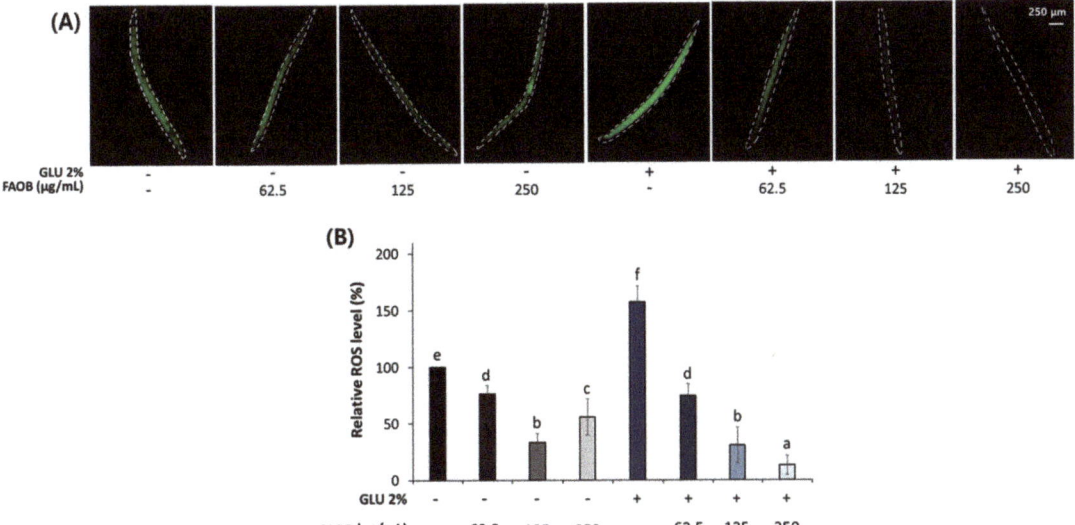

Figure 4. Inhibitory effect of FAOB on reactive oxygen species (ROS) accumulation. (**A**) Images of produced body ROS in middle-aged worms under normal and 2% GLU conditions. (**B**) Quantification results of ROS contents in middle-aged worms under normal and 2% GLU dietary conditions. Bars represent the means ± SDs of three separate experiments (n = 3 plates and 10 randomly selected worms were used). Different letters above the bars mean statistically significant differences ($p < 0.05$). "-" means untreated, and "+" means treated.

2.6. FAOB Exhibits an Age-Delaying Effect in C. elegans

In aging studies using nematodes, behavioral changes and offspring production ability are identified as biomarkers [22]. In our results, FAOB increased locomotion ability and fertility that were reduced by aging (Figure 5).

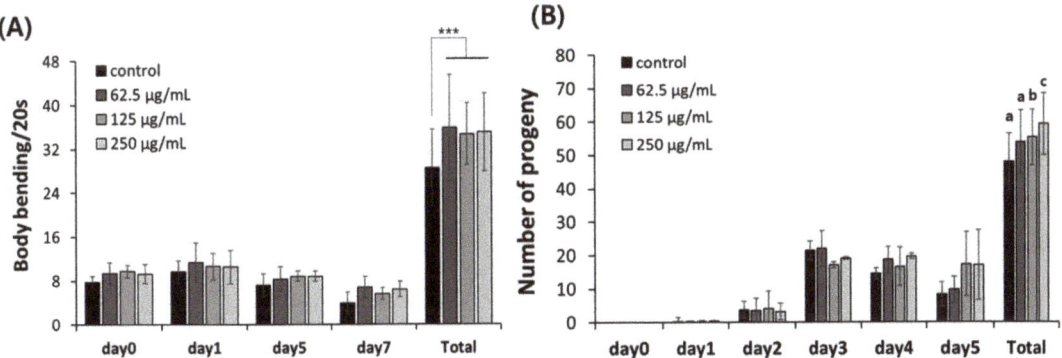

Figure 5. Age-delaying effects of AOB. (**A**) Bending and (**B**) reproduction abilities. Bars represent the means ± SDs of three separate experiments (n = 3 plates and 10 randomly selected worms were used). (**A**) Statistical analyses were performed using Student's t-test (unpaired and two tailed). *** $p < 0.001$, (**B**) Statistical analysis was performed using one-way ANOVA followed by Tukey's post hoc test. Different letters above the bars mean statistically significant differences ($p < 0.05$).

2.7. FAOB Regulates Lipid Accumulation by Daf-16 under 2% GLU Dietary Conditions

To investigate whether AOB regulates lipid metabolism in middle-aged worms under GLU feeding conditions, the total fat contents were analyzed using N2, daf-16, aak-1, akt-1, and atgl-1 knockdown worms. Although body fat reduction was found in the FAOB-treated group in wild-type N2 worms, such an effect of FAOB was not seen in daf-16 worms (Figure 6). Other worm strains had statistically reduced body fat by FAOB treatment, similar to N2. This means that the inhibitory effect of FAOB on body fat accumulation from a GLU diet depends on daf-16.

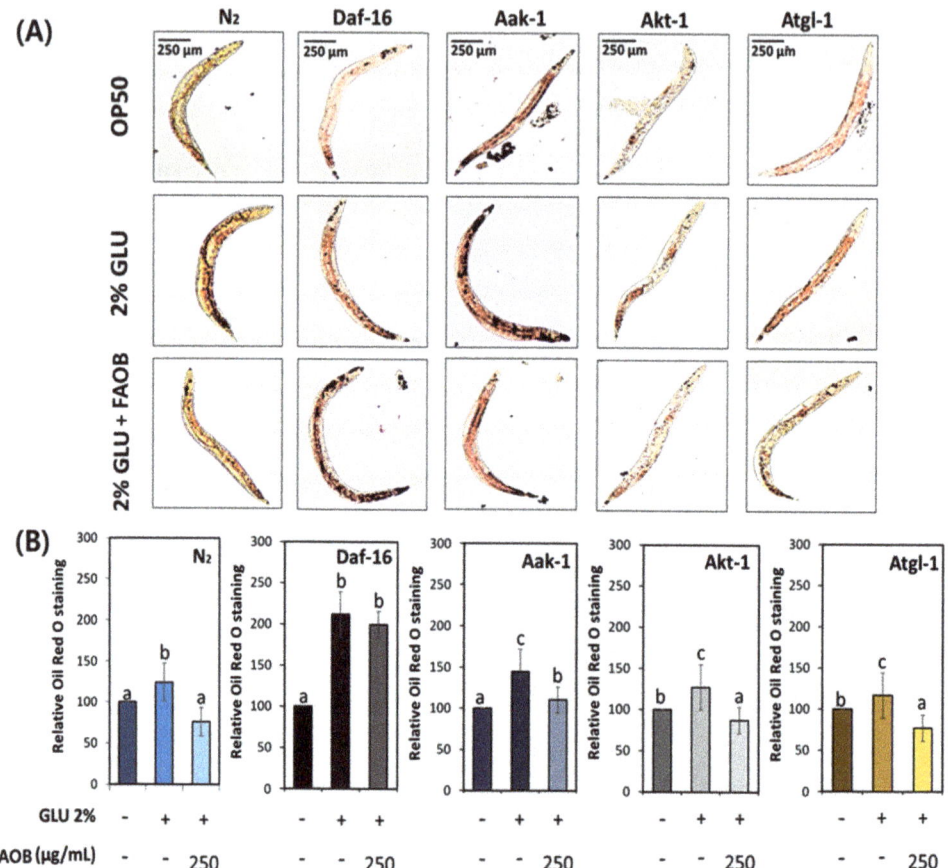

Figure 6. The effect of FAOB on lipid levels alters depending on lipid metabolism-related factors under 2% GLU dietary conditions. (**A**) Images of stored body fat in various worm strains under 2% GLU conditions. (**B**) Quantification results of total lipids in various worm strains under 2% GLU conditions. Bars represent the means ± SDs of three separate experiments (n = 3 plates and 10 randomly selected worms were used). Different letters above the bars mean statistically significant differences ($p < 0.05$). "-" means untreated, and "+" means treated.

2.8. FAOB Is Involved in Lipolysis Signaling Pathway under Fasting Conditions

To investigate whether FAOB is involved in lipolysis in middle-aged worms during fasting, the total fat contents were analyzed using N2, daf-16, aak-1, akt-1, and atgl-1 knockdown worms. Body fat reduction was found in the FAOB treatment group compared to the control in wild-type N2 worms under fasting conditions (Figure 7). This effect of FAOB has not been seen in daf-16 and atgl-1 worms (Figure 7). In other worm strains, the body fat was statistically reduced by FAOB treatment, similarly to N2. Daf-16 and atgl-1 are factors involved in lipolysis signaling, and our results indicate that FAOB depends on daf-16 and atgl-1 to intervene in lipolysis.

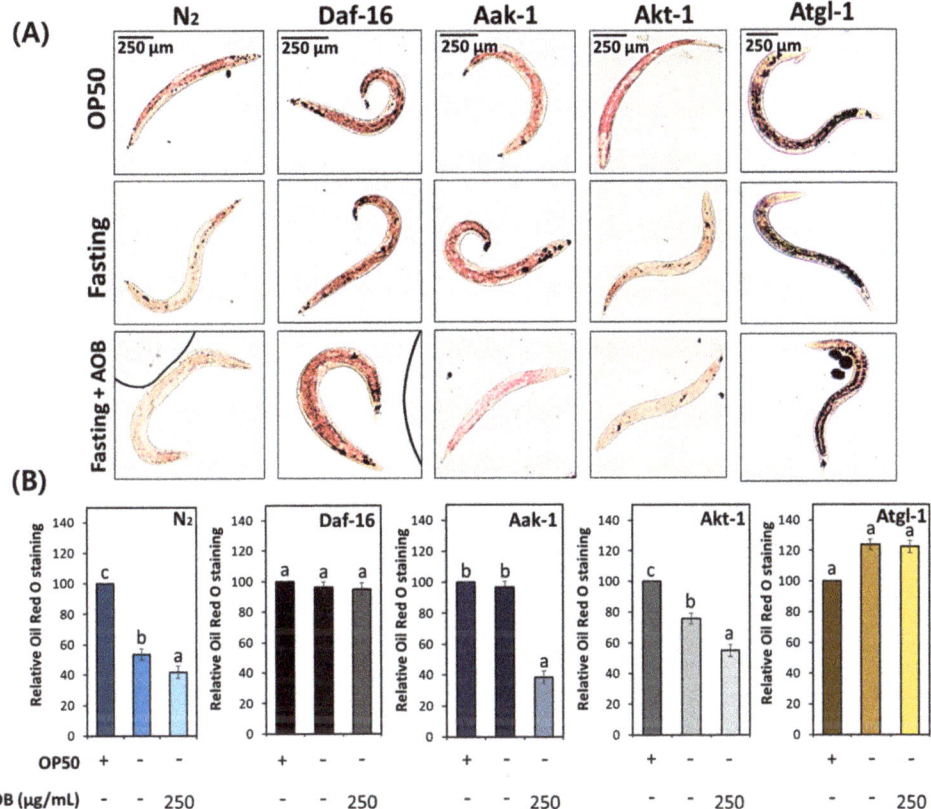

Figure 7. The effect of AOB on lipolysis alters depending on lipid metabolism-related factors under fasting conditions. (**A**) Images of stored body fat in various worm strains under fasting conditions. (**B**) Quantification results of total lipids in various worm strains under fasting conditions. Bars represent the means ± SDs of three separate experiments (n = 3 plates and 10 randomly selected worms were used). Different letters above the bars mean statistically significant differences ($p < 0.05$). "-" means untreated, and "+" means treated.

3. Discussion

AOB is a red fruit that is reported to contain high levels of bioactive compounds such as carotenoids, organic acids, cinnamic acids, benzoic acids, flavonols, anthocyanins, tannins, and catechins [15–17]. We noted phenolic compounds among the bioactive substances in AOBs. Phenolic substances reported to be present in AOBs, including catechins, caffeic acid, chlorogenic acid, gallic acid, quercetin, and lutein, were used as reference compounds for the HPLC analysis. As a result, catechin was detected as the single main substance of AOBs we used, and the catechin content of FAOB was 5.95-fold higher than that of SAOB (Figure 1, Table 2). It has been reported that the phenolic contents and antioxidant activity of AOBs depend on the drying temperature during oven drying [15]. AOB was reported to have different contents of sugars, organic acids, and proteins depending on maturity [23]. Also, the content of minerals and organic acids differed depending on the presence or absence of the berry peels of *Ellaegnus angustifolia* L. [24]. In addition to AOB-related research, many studies have demonstrated that plant materials differ in their internal and external quality factors and potency as a result of their cultivation characteristics and post-harvest management [22,25]. On the other hand, plant extracts used in many studies are extracted using alcoholic solvents to obtain phenolic substances [26]; however, we performed water extraction because we intended to utilize AOB as a tea product. Taken together, it is sufficiently predictable that different pretreatment variables (post-harvest quality control, extraction, drying, and processing methods) of AOBs induce changes in their functionality. Therefore, further research is needed on the relationship between the composition profile and bioactivity of AOBs under different pretreatment conditions.

Catechins, widely recognized as the main functional components of tea and wine, include catechin, epicatechin, epigallocatechin (EGC), epicatechin-3-gallate (ECG), epigallocatechin-3-gallate (EGCG), and gallocatechin gallate (GCG) [27]. Catechins exhibit anti-cancer, anti-obesity, anti-diabetic, anti-cardiovascular, anti-infection, liver-protective, and nerve-protective properties [28,29]. In particular, catechin has antioxidant activity that scavenges ROS and at the same time can positively regulate lipid metabolism [28–30]. Therefore, it is believed that AOBs containing catechin as the abundant ingredient have the potential to effectively prevent obesity and related chronic degenerative diseases.

Lipid metabolism disorders and aging show close associations [21]. In particular, increased lipotoxicity under specific conditions, such as aging, may contribute to a variety of age-related diseases, including cardiovascular disease, cancer, arthritis, type 2 diabetes, and Alzheimer's disease [21,31–35]. Recent studies have described the mechanisms of changes in lipolysis during aging [36,37]. However, although they can explain system-level changes in lipid metabolism, how these changes influence aging and aging-related diseases has not been verified [31]. Our results showed that during obesity induction with a high-GLU diet, middle-aged and young worms accumulated 20% and 40% lipid, respectively (Figure 3). It has been verified that more lipids accumulate with age when given the same high-GLU diet over the same period.

There is an opinion that obesity, especially in middle age, can be caused not only by changes in the metabolic system, but also by a decrease in physical activity [38]. In the present study, day 7 worms were observed to experience a decline of more than 50% in physical activity compared to day 1 worms (Figure 5A). This result is consistent with the view that there is a decline in behavior in middle age that may lead to obesity. However, further research is required, as we have not confirmed whether the metabolic system at the molecular level has changed.

Lipid metabolism is regulated by lipid synthesis (lipogenesis) and lipid degradation (lipolysis and beta-oxidation) [4,5]. These processes are intertwined at the molecular level and require a logical understanding to gain insight. Crucial in lipid metabolism is the working of daf-16/FOXO and atgl-1/ATGL [39–41]. In particular, FOXO is a key transcription factor in lipid metabolism that controls the balance of lipogenesis and lipolysis by downregulating ATGL, and is involved in lipid accumulation in mammals [41]. However, there are only a few reports on the interaction between daf-16/FOXO and atgl-1/ATGL in C. elegans.

We prepared worms under a high-GLU diet or fasting conditions to clearly define the role of daf-16 and atgl-1 concerning the FAOB effect. As a result of FAOB administration, it was confirmed that the effect seen in wild-type worms disappeared in daf-16 knockdown worms under both GLU feeding and fasting conditions (Figures 6 and 7). This indicates that FAOB is dependent on daf-16 related to lipogenesis and lipolysis. In addition, the effect of FAOB seen in N2 was lost in atgl-1 knockdown worms under fasting conditions, indicating that FAOB cooperates with atgl-1 under certain lipolytic conditions such as fasting. Previous studies have shown that daf-16 and atgl-1 can be regulated by akt-1/AKT and aak-1/AMPK [42–45]. However, our results confirmed that the FAOB effect is dependent on daf-16 and atgl-1, but is not related to akt-1 and aak-1 (Figures 6 and 7). In other words, this suggests that FAOB acts directly on daf-16 or atgl-1, rather than daf-16 and atgl-1 being involved by regulating the upstream factors akt-1 or aak-1. Although daf-16 is upstream of atgl-1, further gene expression analysis is needed to clarify their upper and lower relationships for the effects of FAOB.

4. Materials and Methods

4.1. Preparation of AOB Extracts

The AOB samples used in this study were provided by NutriAdvisor (Seong-Nam, Gyeonggi-do, Republic of Korea). AOBs were grown in Hapcheon, Gyeongsangsam-do, Korea, and mature fruits were purchased in fresh condition and immediately freeze-dried or spray-dried. FAOBs were dried in a vacuum at $-20\ °C$ for 72 h with a freeze dryer (Ilshin Lab. Co., Gyeonggi-do, Republic of Korea). SAOBs were produced using a spray dryer (Fisher Scientific, Vernon Hills, IL, USA). The spray drying conditions were set to an injection temperature of 150 °C, an emission temperature of 100 °C, and a rotation speed of 14,000 rpm. Since the AOB samples were prepared for use as the main material for the tea powder, they were extracted under reflux at 80 °C with 100% distilled water (1:10 w/v) without using an organic solvent. After that, the extracts were evaporated to remove the solvent, and then made into powder. AOB samples were dissolved in DMSO to prepare a 15 mg/mL stock solution, and were stored at $-80\ °C$ and then diluted fresh in distilled water to an appropriate concentration right before the experiment.

4.2. Reagents

All of the reagents used in our studies were HPLC or molecular biology grade. Reagents, unless otherwise specified, were obtained from Sigma Chemical Co. (St. Louis, MO, USA).

4.3. HPLC Analysis

To profile the phenolic compounds in AOB, information on the equipment, column, and analysis methods required for HPLC operation are presented in Table 3. The catechin used was D-catechin (CAS no. 154-23-4), which was dissolved in distilled water immediately before analysis. The catechin contents of the AOB samples were calculated using a catechin (5–50 µg/mL) calibration curve.

Table 3. HPLC analysis conditions.

\multicolumn{2}{c}{HPLC (UltiMate 3000, Thermo Scientific, Sunnyvale, CA, USA)}	
Column	Waters symmetry C18 column (4.6 × 150 mm, 5 µm)
Mobile phase	(A) 0.1% (v/v) aqueous phosphoric acid (B) Acetonitrile (Duksan, Ansan-si, Gyeonggi-do, Republic of Korea) Gradient method: 50–90% solvent B for 1 min, 90–85% solvent B for 2 min, 85–80% solvent B for 2 min, 80–70% solvent B for 3 min, 70–30% solvent B for 3 min, and a linear step from 30 to 10% solvent B for 9 min.
Flow rate	0.8 mL/min
Inject volume	20 µL
Detector	Diode array detector (DAD)
Wavelength	280 nm

4.4. Total Phenolic Contents (TPC) of AOB

The total phenolic contents (TPC) in the AOBs were determined using the Folin–Ciocalteu (FC) method. Simply, 700 µL of the sample (mixed with FC in a 1:1 ratio) was combined with 700 µL of sodium carbonate and left in the dark for 1 h. The absorbance reading was performed at 720 nm. The total phenolic contents of the sample were calculated using the equation derived from the gallic acid standard curve. The results were expressed as gallic acid equivalents (GAE) per one hundred grams.

4.5. DPPH Radical Scavenging Capacity

In a simple procedure, a sample of the same volume was mixed with a DPPH solution (0.2 mM) and left at room temperature for 30 min. Then, the reaction mixture was measured at 517 nm using a microplate reader (SYNERGY HTX, Biotek, Santa Clara, CA, USA).

The DPPH radical-scavenging activity was calculated using the following formula:

$$\text{radical scavenging activity (\%)} = [1 - (\text{sample O.D.}/\text{blank O.D.})] \times 100$$

Furthermore, we determined the value of the antioxidant capacity, which was calculated using an ascorbic acid (AA) calibration curve and expressed in micrograms of AA one hundred per gram of sample dry weight (DW).

4.6. Worm Study

4.6.1. Worm Culture

To conduct the in vivo experiments, we use *C. elegans* strain N2 (wild-type) and its derivative mutant strains; daf-16 (tm5030), atgl-1 (tm12352), aak-1 (tm1944), and akt-1 (tm399) were obtained from the National BioResource Project (NBRP) of Japan.

Maintenance of the worms was applied by modifying what was recorded in the WormBook [46] to properly conduct our experiments. All of these strains were maintained on nematode growth medium (NGM) plates that were spread with *E. coli* OP50 and maintained at a temperature of 20 °C throughout the entire duration of the experiment. Age synchronization of the nematodes was achieved by separating the eggs from gravid adults using a solution comprising 6% sodium hypochlorite (Yuhanclorox, Seoul, Republic of Korea) and 5 M NaOH.

4.6.2. Acute Toxicity

Toxicity assessments were performed with modifications to those recorded by the Organization for Economic Co-operation and Development (OECD) (2016) [47]. Synchronized L4 was washed twice with M9 buffer and suspended in M9 buffer containing cholesterol. Subsequently, 1 mL of this suspension was transferred to each well of a 24-well plate (20–30 worms per well) and combined with 10 µL of various concentrations of FAOB and SAOB. Then, the plates were incubated at 20 °C for 24 h. The acute toxicity results were quantified as percent survival after counting living worms.

4.6.3. Determination of Stress Resistance

In the context of thermal and oxidative stress analysis, 50 synchronized N2 L1 larvae were prepared as follows: OP50 and FAOB were combined, and the mixture was seeded on NGM plates. The worm plate was first maintained at 20 °C for 60 h to assess the impact of thermal stress. Subsequently, it was incubated at 35 °C for 18 h. To investigate the effect on oxidative stress, the pretreated worms were transferred to a 24-well plate containing a 100 µM juglone (5-hydroxy-1,4-naphthoquinone) solution and incubated at 20 °C.

4.6.4. Oil Red O Staining

The oil red O assay was modified by Kim et al. [21]. L1 worms were exposed to different concentrations of extracts for 7 days, and cultivated worms were fixed in 4% formaldehyde for 24 h, then dehydrated with 60% isopropanol at −70 °C for 15 min. The dehydrated worms were washed three times with M9 buffer and dyed with an oil red O solution for 3 h. The stained worms were washed with M9 buffer, then observed under a microscope (Nikon, Seoul, Republic of Korea). The relative strength of the stained lipid droplets in the worms was quantified using Image J software (1.8.0, Joonas Regalis Rikkonen, Barcelona, Spain).

4.6.5. Triglyceride (TG) Quantification Assay

The adult worms that were in culture were suspended in 500 μL of M9 buffer containing a 0.05% Tween-20 solution. Then, they were homogenized on ice for 5 min using a glass homogenizer (ALLSHENG, Hangzhou, China) to collect the pellet, which was subsequently centrifuged at $1000\times g$ for 5 min. The obtained supernatant was analyzed for TG content. The TG content was measured via absorbance at 570 nm using a TG kit (Biomax, Gyeonggi-do, Republic of Korea).

4.6.6. Reproduction and Pumping Rates

To count the number of progenies, the worms were transferred to fresh NGM plates daily throughout their reproductive period, and eggs were left on plates to hatch. The offspring of each worm were counted when they reached the L2 or L3 stage. The test was performed three times.

To evaluate behavior activity, we counted the number of pharyngeal pumps on 0, 1, 5, and 7 days. Specifically, 10 nematodes were randomly selected for each concentration and age point, and the pumping frequency was determined three times for 20 s. This test was conducted three times.

4.6.7. Determination of ROS Level

L1 worms were maintained in different concentrations of extracts for 7 days, and then incubated with 100 μM H_2DCF-DA in the dark for 3 h. Subsequently, the nematodes were fixed on microscope slides using NAN3 (2%). These slides were observed using a Nikon ECLIPS Ci fluorescence microscope. The fluorescence intensities were examined using Image J software. An average of 10 worms per group was chosen for quantification.

4.7. Statistical Analysis

The results are presented as the means ± standard deviations (SD) of three independent replicates. The significance of intergroup differences was determined via one-way analysis of variance (ANOVA) followed by Tukey's multiple range test. SPSS 27.0 was used for all statistical analyses except lifespan. p-values < 0.05 were considered to be significant. The survival results were analyzed with the Kaplan–Meier method, using the OASIS application (https://sbi.postech.ac.kr/oasis/, accessed on 29 November 2023). p-values of survival differences were determined with the log-rank test. Statistical analyses were performed using Student's t test (unpaired, two tailed) with at least three replicates, unless otherwise indicated. Statistical analyses were performed in SPSS 27.0.

5. Conclusions

This study investigated the relationship between obesity and aging in midlife, and examined the positive effects of AOB. The bio-activity of plants can vary depending on the drying method [24,48], and FAOB showed more effective radical scavenging ability compared to SAOB, which is believed to be because FAOB contained more polyphenols, including catechin. In the *C. elegans* study, treatment with FAOB significantly reduced lipid accumulation in both the young and the middle-aged groups. In addition, FAOB inhibited ROS accumulation in middle-aged worms under 2% GLU conditions. Interestingly, FAOB attenuated aging symptoms, including increasing the movement and reproductive capacity of aged worms. To understand the inhibitory effect of FAOB on lipid accumulation at the molecular level, we performed further investigations on the daf-16, aak-1, akt-1, and atgl-1 genes, which are related to lipid metabolism. The lipid accumulation reduction effect of FAOB was nullified under a high-GLU condition in the daf-16 knockdown mutant. The FAOB effect under fasting conditions was also nullified in the daf-16 and atgl-1 knockdown mutants. This suggests that these two factors are involved in the in vivo anti-obesity activity of FAOB in middle-aged worms, and further suggests its potential for anti-aging benefits. In summary, AOB acts on lipogenesis and lipolysis by regulating daf-16 and atgl-1 in middle-aged worms and alleviates aging symptoms. These results suggest that AODs are a valuable material with the potential to delay aging by modulating lipid metabolism.

Author Contributions: Conceptualization, M.J.; methodology, Y.K. and S.N.; software, Y.K. and S.N.; validation, Y.K.; formal analysis, J.L.; writing—original draft preparation, Y.K.; writing—review and editing, M.J.; visualization, Y.K.; supervision, M.J.; project administration, M.J.; funding acquisition, M.J. All authors have read and agreed to the published version of the manuscript.

Funding: This research was supported by a project for Collabo R&D between Industry, Academy, and Research Institute-funded Korea Ministry of SMEs and Startups in 2023 (project No. G21002258981) and the 'Leading University for Industry-Academia Cooperation 3.0' project supported by the Ministry of Education and the National Research Foundation of Korea.

Institutional Review Board Statement: Not applicable.

Informed Consent Statement: Not applicable.

Data Availability Statement: The data presented in this study are available on request from the corresponding author.

Conflicts of Interest: The authors declare no conflicts of interest.

References

1. Ng, M.; Fleming, T.; Robinson, M.; Thomson, B.; Graetz, N.; Margono, C.; Mullany, E.C.; Biryukov, S.; Abbafati, C.; Abera, S.F. Global, regional, and national prevalence of overweight and obesity in children and adults during 1980–2013: A systematic analysis for the Global Burden of Disease Study 2013. *Lancet* **2014**, *384*, 766–781. [CrossRef] [PubMed]
2. Geng, J.; Ni, Q.; Sun, W.; Li, L.; Feng, X. The links between gut microbiota and obesity and obesity related diseases. *Biomed. Pharmacother.* **2022**, *147*, 112678. [CrossRef] [PubMed]
3. Lodhi, I.J.; Yin, L.; Jensen-Urstad, A.P.; Funai, K.; Coleman, T.; Baird, J.H.; El Ramahi, M.K.; Razani, B.; Song, H.; Fu-Hsu, F. Inhibiting adipose tissue lipogenesis reprograms thermogenesis and PPARγ activation to decrease diet-induced obesity. *Cell Metab.* **2012**, *16*, 189–201. [CrossRef] [PubMed]
4. Arner, P. Catecholamine-induced lipolysis in obesity. *Int. J. Obes.* **1999**, *23*, S10–S13. [CrossRef] [PubMed]
5. Guarente, L.; Kenyon, C. Genetic pathways that regulate ageing in model organisms. *Nature* **2000**, *408*, 255–262. [CrossRef]
6. Silverman, G.A.; Luke, C.J.; Bhatia, S.R.; Long, O.S.; Vetica, A.C.; Perlmutter, D.H.; Pak, S.C. Modeling molecular and cellular aspects of human disease using the nematode Caenorhabditis elegans. *Pediatr. Res.* **2009**, *65*, 10–18. [CrossRef] [PubMed]
7. Svensk, E.; Devkota, R.; Ståhlman, M.; Ranji, P.; Rauthan, M.; Magnusson, F.; Hammarsten, S.; Johansson, M.; Borén, J.; Pilon, M. Caenorhabditis elegans PAQR-2 and IGLR-2 protect against glucose toxicity by modulating membrane lipid composition. *PLoS Genet.* **2016**, *12*, e1005982.
8. Alcántar-Fernández, J.; González-Maciel, A.; Reynoso-Robles, R.; Pérez Andrade, M.E.; Hernández-Vázquez, A.D.J.; Velázquez-Arellano, A.; Miranda-Ríos, J. High-glucose diets induce mitochondrial dysfunction in Caenorhabditis elegans. *PLoS ONE* **2019**, *14*, e0226652. [CrossRef]
9. Ory, M.G.; Anderson, L.A.; Friedman, D.B.; Pulczinski, J.C.; Eugene, N.; Satariano, W.A. Cancer prevention among adults aged 45–64 years: Setting the stage. *Am. J. Prev. Med.* **2014**, *46*, S1–S6. [CrossRef]
10. Strasser, B.; Arvandi, M.; Pasha, E.; Haley, A.; Stanforth, P.; Tanaka, H. Abdominal obesity is associated with arterial stiffness in middle-aged adults. *Nutr. Metab. Cardiovasc. Dis.* **2015**, *25*, 495–502. [CrossRef]
11. Hodson, L.; Banerjee, R.; Rial, B.; Arlt, W.; Adiels, M.; Boren, J.; Marinou, K.; Fisher, C.; Mostad, I.L.; Stratton, I.M. Menopausal status and abdominal obesity are significant determinants of hepatic lipid metabolism in women. *J. Am. Heart Assoc.* **2015**, *4*, e002158. [CrossRef] [PubMed]
12. Pei, R.; Yu, M.; Bruno, R.; Bolling, B.W. Phenolic and tocopherol content of autumn olive (*Elaeagnus umbellate*) berries. *J. Funct. Foods* **2015**, *16*, 305–314. [CrossRef]
13. Ahmad, S.D.; Sabir, M.S.; Juma, M.; Asad, H.S. Morphological and biochemical variations in *Elaeagnus umbellata* Thunb. from mountains of Pakistan. *Acta Bot. Croat.* **2005**, *64*, 121–128.
14. Ishaq, S.; Rathore, H.A.; Sabir, S.M.; Maroof, M.S. Antioxidant properties of *Elaeagnus umbellata* berry solvent extracts against lipid peroxidation in mice brain and liver tissues. *Food Sci. Biotechnol.* **2015**, *24*, 673–679. [CrossRef]
15. Zannou, O.; Pashazadeh, H.; Ghellam, M.; Hassan, A.M.; Koca, I. Optimization of drying temperature for the assessment of functional and physical characteristics of autumn olive berries. *J. Food Process. Preserv.* **2021**, *45*, e15658. [CrossRef]
16. Fordham, I.M.; Clevidence, B.A.; Wiley, E.R.; Zimmerman, R.H. Fruit of autumn olive: A rich source of lycopene. *HortScience* **2001**, *36*, 1136–1137. [CrossRef]
17. Gamba, G.; Donno, D.; Mellano, M.G.; Riondato, I.; De Biaggi, M.; Randriamampionona, D.; Beccaro, G.L. Phytochemical characterization and bioactivity evaluation of autumn olive (*Elaeagnus umbellata* Thunb.) pseudodrupes as potential sources of health-promoting compounds. *Appl. Sci.* **2020**, *10*, 4354. [CrossRef]

18. Nazir, N.; Zahoor, M.; Nisar, M.; Khan, I.; Karim, N.; Abdel-Halim, H.; Ali, A. Phytochemical analysis and antidiabetic potential of *Elaeagnus umbellata* (Thunb.) in streptozotocin-induced diabetic rats: Pharmacological and computational approach. *BMC Complement. Altern. Med.* **2018**, *18*, 332. [CrossRef]
19. Kim, J.-I.; Baek, H.-J.; Han, D.-W.; Yun, J.-A. Autumn olive (*Elaeagnus umbellata* Thunb.) berry reduces fasting and postprandial glucose levels in mice. *Nutr. Res. Pract.* **2019**, *13*, 11–16. [CrossRef]
20. Nazir, N.; Zahoor, M.; Ullah, L.; Ezzeldin, E.; Mostafa, G.A.E. Curative effect of catechin isolated from *Elaeagnus umbellata* thunb. berries for diabetes and related complications in streptozotocin-induced diabetic rats model. *Molecules* **2020**, *26*, 137. [CrossRef]
21. Kim, Y.; Lee, S.-b.; Cho, M.; Choe, S.; Jang, M. Indian almond (*Terminalia catappa* linn.) leaf extract extends lifespan by improving lipid metabolism and antioxidant activity dependent on AMPK signaling pathway in *Caenorhabditis elegans* under high-glucose-diet conditions. *Antioxidants* **2023**, *13*, 14. [CrossRef]
22. Cho, M.; Kim, Y.; You, S.; Hwang, D.Y.; Jang, M. Chlorogenic acid of *Cirsium japonicum* resists oxidative stress caused by aging and prolongs healthspan via SKN-1/Nrf2 and DAF-16/FOXO in *Caenorhabditis elegans*. *Metabolites* **2023**, *13*, 224. [CrossRef]
23. Wu, M.-C.; Hu, H.-T.; Yang, L.; Yang, L. Proteomic analysis of up-accumulated proteins associated with fruit quality during autumn olive (*Elaeagnus umbellata*) fruit ripening. *J. Agric. Food Chem.* **2011**, *59*, 577–583. [CrossRef]
24. Sahan, Y.; Gocmen, D.; Cansev, A.; Celik, G.; Aydin, D.; Dundar, A.N.; Dulger, D. Chemical and techno-functional properties of flours from peeled and unpeeled oleaster (*Elaeagnus angustifolia* L.). *J. Appl. Bot. Food Qual.* **2015**, *88*, 34–41.
25. Jang, M.; Kim, K.-H.; Kim, G.-H. Antioxidant capacity of thistle (*Cirsium japonicum*) in various drying methods and their protection effect on neuronal PC12 cells and *Caenorhabditis elegans*. *Antioxidants* **2020**, *9*, 200. [CrossRef]
26. Jang, M.; Choi, H.-Y.; Kim, G.-H. Inhibitory effects of *Orostachys malacophyllus* var. iwarenge extracts on reactive oxygen species production and lipid accumulation during 3T3-L1 adipocyte differentiation. *Food Sci. Biotechnol.* **2019**, *28*, 227–236. [CrossRef]
27. Cyboran, S.; Strugała, P.; Włoch, A.; Oszmiański, J.; Kleszczyńska, Y. Concentrated green tea supplement: Biological activity and molecular mechanisms. *Life Sci.* **2015**, *126*, 1–9. [CrossRef]
28. Murase, T.; Nagasawa, A.; Suzuki, J.; Hase, T.; Tokimitsu, I. Beneficial effects of tea catechins on diet-induced obesity: Stimulation of lipid catabolism in the liver. *Int. J. Obes.* **2002**, *26*, 1459–1464. [CrossRef] [PubMed]
29. Isemura, M. Catechin in human health and disease. *Molecules* **2019**, *24*, 528. [CrossRef] [PubMed]
30. Jiang, Y.; Ding, S.; Li, F.; Zhang, C.; Sun-Waterhouse, D.; Chen, Y.; Li, D. Effects of (+)-catechin on the differentiation and lipid metabolism of 3T3-L1 adipocytes. *J. Funct. Foods* **2019**, *62*, 103558. [CrossRef]
31. Chung, K.W. Advances in understanding of the role of lipid metabolism in aging. *Cells* **2021**, *10*, 880. [CrossRef] [PubMed]
32. Kao, Y.-C.; Ho, P.-C.; Tu, Y.-K.; Jou, I.-M.; Tsai, K.-J. Lipids and Alzheimer's disease. *Int. J. Mol. Sci.* **2020**, *21*, 1505. [CrossRef] [PubMed]
33. Sato, N.; Morishita, R. The roles of lipid and glucose metabolism in modulation of β-amyloid, tau, and neurodegeneration in the pathogenesis of Alzheimer disease. *Front. Aging Neurosci.* **2015**, *7*, 199. [CrossRef] [PubMed]
34. Luo, X.; Cheng, C.; Tan, Z.; Li, N.; Tang, M.; Yang, L.; Cao, Y. Emerging roles of lipid metabolism in cancer metastasis. *Mol. Cancer* **2017**, *16*, 76. [CrossRef]
35. McGrath, C.M.; Young, S.P. Lipid and metabolic changes in rheumatoid arthritis. *Curr. Rheumatol. Rep.* **2015**, *17*, 57. [CrossRef]
36. Mennes, E.; Dungan, C.M.; Frendo-Cumbo, S.; Williamson, D.L.; Wright, D.C. Aging-associated reductions in lipolytic and mitochondrial proteins in mouse adipose tissue are not rescued by metformin treatment. *J. Gerontol. Ser. A Biomed. Sci. Med. Sci.* **2014**, *69*, 1060–1068. [CrossRef]
37. Camell, C.D.; Sander, J.; Spadaro, O.; Lee, A.; Nguyen, K.Y.; Wing, A.; Goldberg, E.L.; Youm, Y.-H.; Brown, C.W.; Elsworth, J. Inflammasome-driven catecholamine catabolism in macrophages blunts lipolysis during ageing. *Nature* **2017**, *550*, 119–123. [CrossRef]
38. Szlejf, C.; Parra-Rodríguez, L.; Rosas-Carrasco, O. Osteosarcopenic obesity: Prevalence and relation with frailty and physical performance in middle-aged and older women. *J. Am. Med. Dir. Assoc.* **2017**, *18*, 733.e731–733.e735. [CrossRef]
39. Gross, D.; Van Den Heuvel, A.; Birnbaum, M. The role of FoxO in the regulation of metabolism. *Oncogene* **2008**, *27*, 2320–2336. [CrossRef]
40. Schreiber, R.; Xie, H.; Schweiger, M. Of mice and men: The physiological role of adipose triglyceride lipase (ATGL). *Biochim. Et Biophys. Acta (BBA)—Mol. Cell Biol. Lipids* **2019**, *1864*, 880–899. [CrossRef] [PubMed]
41. Chakrabarti, P.; Kandror, K.V. FoxO1 controls insulin-dependent adipose triglyceride lipase (ATGL) expression and lipolysis in adipocytes. *J. Biol. Chem.* **2009**, *284*, 13296–13300. [CrossRef]
42. Han, Y.; Hu, Z.; Cui, A.; Liu, Z.; Ma, F.; Xue, Y.; Liu, Y.; Zhang, F.; Zhao, Z.; Yu, Y. Post-translational regulation of lipogenesis via AMPK-dependent phosphorylation of insulin-induced gene. *Nat. Commun.* **2019**, *10*, 623. [CrossRef]
43. Jang, M.; Choi, S.I. Schisandrin C isolated from *Schisandra chinensis* fruits inhibits lipid accumulation by regulating adipogenesis and lipolysis through AMPK signaling in 3T3-L1 adipocytes. *J. Food Biochem.* **2022**, *46*, e14454. [CrossRef]
44. Kwon, J.Y.; Kershaw, J.; Chen, C.-Y.; Komanetsky, S.M.; Zhu, Y.; Guo, X.; Myer, P.R.; Applegate, B.; Kim, K.-H. Piceatannol antagonizes lipolysis by promoting autophagy-lysosome-dependent degradation of lipolytic protein clusters in adipocytes. *J. Nutr. Biochem.* **2022**, *105*, 108998. [CrossRef]
45. Lee, J.H.; Kong, J.; Jang, J.Y.; Han, J.S.; Ji, Y.; Lee, J.; Kim, J.B. Lipid droplet protein LID-1 mediates ATGL-1-dependent lipolysis during fasting in *Caenorhabditis elegans*. *Mol. Cell Biol.* **2014**, *34*, 4165–4176. [CrossRef]

46. Stiernagle, T. Maintenance of *C. elegans*. In *Community Worm Book: Worm Book*; TCeR, Ed.; Beijing Institute of Technology Press: Beijing, China, 2006.
47. OECD. *Report of the OECD Seminar on Risk Reduction through Prevention, Detection and Control of the Illegal International Trade in Agricultural Pesticides*; OECD: Paris, France, 2014. [CrossRef]
48. Gomes, W.F.; França, F.R.M.; Denadai, M.; Andrade, J.K.S.; da Silva Oliveira, E.M.; de Brito, E.S.; Rodrigues, S.; Narain, N. Effect of freeze-and spray-drying on physico-chemical characteristics, phenolic compounds and antioxidant activity of papaya pulp. *J. Food Sci. Technol.* **2018**, *55*, 2095–2102. [CrossRef]

Disclaimer/Publisher's Note: The statements, opinions and data contained in all publications are solely those of the individual author(s) and contributor(s) and not of MDPI and/or the editor(s). MDPI and/or the editor(s) disclaim responsibility for any injury to people or property resulting from any ideas, methods, instructions or products referred to in the content.

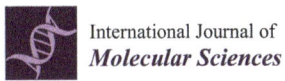

Article

Berberine Protects against High-Energy and Low-Protein Diet-Induced Hepatic Steatosis: Modulation of Gut Microbiota and Bile Acid Metabolism in Laying Hens

Chang Wang, Yitian Yang, Jinyan Chen, Xueyan Dai, Chenghong Xing, Caiying Zhang, Huabin Cao, Xiaoquan Guo, Guoliang Hu * and Yu Zhuang *

Jiangxi Provincial Key Laboratory for Animal Health, Institute of Animal Population Health, College of Animal Science and Technology, Jiangxi Agricultural University, No. 1101 Zhimin Avenue, Economic and Technological Development District, Nanchang 330045, China; 19179147923@163.com (C.W.); yangyitian0810@163.com (Y.Y.); jinyanchen2020@163.com (J.C.); 18722280937@163.com (X.D.); xch20175867@jxau.edu.cn (C.X.); zhangcaiying0916@163.com (C.Z.); chbin20020804@jxau.edu.cn (H.C.); xqguo20720@jxau.edu.cn (X.G.)
* Correspondence: hgljx3818@jxau.edu.cn (G.H.); zhuangyu2019@jxau.edu.cn (Y.Z.); Tel.: +86-138-0708-9905 (G.H.); +86-156-1624-0852 (Y.Z.)

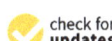

Citation: Wang, C.; Yang, Y.; Chen, J.; Dai, X.; Xing, C.; Zhang, C.; Cao, H.; Guo, X.; Hu, G.; Zhuang, Y. Berberine Protects against High-Energy and Low-Protein Diet-Induced Hepatic Steatosis: Modulation of Gut Microbiota and Bile Acid Metabolism in Laying Hens. *Int. J. Mol. Sci.* **2023**, *24*, 17304. https://doi.org/10.3390/ijms242417304

Academic Editors: Giovanni Tarantino, Marilena Gilca and Adelina Vlad

Received: 7 October 2023
Revised: 3 December 2023
Accepted: 5 December 2023
Published: 9 December 2023

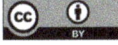

Copyright: © 2023 by the authors. Licensee MDPI, Basel, Switzerland. This article is an open access article distributed under the terms and conditions of the Creative Commons Attribution (CC BY) license (https://creativecommons.org/licenses/by/4.0/).

Abstract: Berberine (BBR) is a natural alkaloid with multiple biotical effects that has potential as a treatment for fatty liver hemorrhagic syndrome (FLHS). However, the mechanism underlying the protective effect of BBR against FLHS remains unclear. The present study aimed to investigate the effect of BBR on FLHS induced by a high-energy, low-protein (HELP) diet and explore the involvement of the gut microbiota and bile acid metabolism in the protective effects. A total of 90 healthy 140-day-old Hy-line laying hens were randomly divided into three groups, including a control group (fed a basic diet), a HELP group (fed a HELP diet), and a HELP+BBR group (high-energy, high-protein diet supplemented with BBR instead of maize). Our results show that BBR supplementation alleviated liver injury and hepatic steatosis in laying hens. Moreover, BBR supplementation could significantly regulate the gut's microbial composition, increasing the abundance of Actinobacteria and Romboutsia. In addition, the BBR supplement altered the profile of bile acid. Furthermore, the gut microbiota participates in bile acid metabolism, especially taurochenodeoxycholic acid and α-muricholic acid. BBR supplementation could regulate the expression of genes and proteins related to glucose metabolism, lipid synthesis (FAS, SREBP-1c), and bile acid synthesis (FXR, CYP27a1). Collectively, our findings demonstrate that BBR might be a potential feed additive for preventing FLHS by regulating the gut microbiota and bile acid metabolism.

Keywords: berberine; high-energy and low-protein diet; fatty liver hemorrhagic syndrome; gut microbiota; bile acids

1. Introduction

Fatty liver hemorrhagic syndrome (FLHS) is a metabolic disease characterized by a lipid metabolism disorder and accompanied by excessively high feed intake, increased body weight, individual obesity, a decreased egg production rate, and engorged, pale combs. Sudden death also occurs, and at necropsy, the syndrome is characterized by an excessive accumulation of fat within the abdominal cavity, a pale and fragile liver sometimes void of structural integrity, multifocal hemorrhages, and large blood clots in the abdominal cavity as a result of liver rupture [1–3]. It is typically brought on by the interaction of genetic and environmental variables, with an excessive intake of foods high in energy and low in protein (HELP) in the diet being a major contributing factor [4,5]. Recently, studies showed that a balanced diet structure and dietary additives can alleviate flora disorders and reduce the development of liver disease [6,7]. High-fat diets alter the gut microbiota ecosystem, resulting in severe liver diseases [8]. Nonalcoholic fatty liver disease (NAFLD), which has been renamed metabolic-associated fatty liver disease (MAFLD) in recent years [9], is a common chronic disease characterized by fatty deposits in hepatic cells and liver steatosis [10]. Liver steatosis is mainly characterized by an imbalance between fat secretion and metabolism after the transportation of fat to the liver [11]. NAFLD is associated with obesity, metabolic syndrome, and certain genetic variations, mainly due to the excessive accumulation of fat in the liver. When compared to healthy people, the gut microbiota of people with NAFLD shows significant structural and compositional abnormalities [12]. Reducing the ratio of Firmicutes to Bacteroidetes (F/B) is a crucial factor in improving NAFLD [13]. Therefore, maintaining a healthy gut microbiome may provide a fundamental strategy for preventing and treating FLHS, leading to a better understanding of the dietary interventions necessary to maintain gut health and minimize liver disease risks.

Gut microbiota plays a critical role in regulating fatty liver illnesses by producing bacterial metabolites, like short-chain fatty acids, secondary bile acids, and trimethylamine [14,15]. Bile acids (BAs), which the liver produces from cholesterol and secretes into the intestine, are metabolites of intestinal micro-organisms and can be effectively utilized by intestinal micro-organisms [16]. Furthermore, they can regulate glucose and lipid metabolism in the liver [17]. An increasing amount of experimental and clinical evidence indicates that BAs hold exceptional potential as a therapeutic approach for fatty liver disease, hypercholesterolemia, and metabolic diseases [18–20]. BA receptors are drawing attention as potential therapeutic targets for liver illnesses because BAs perform their numerous biological actions by attaching to their receptors [21]. More research has revealed that modifications to the gut microbiota affect the host's BA profiles, most notably in the way taurine-conjugated BAs interact with the intestinal farnesol receptor (FXR) [22]. By lowering hepatic and plasma lipid levels, reducing inflammation, and enhancing insulin sensitivity, activation of the FXR may be able to reduce the symptoms of NAFLD [23]. Therefore, BAs can be used as a targeted therapeutic agent for fatty liver diseases.

In recent years, there have been many studies on some natural products as ideal candidates for the treatment of NAFLD, and some of them are about to be approved. Berberine (BBR) is one of them, which has been clearly demonstrated to have significant therapeutic effects on NAFLD in some animal models and clinical studies [24]. However, whether BBR has a positive therapeutic effect on FLHS induced by HELP diets and its mechanism of action is yet to be clarified. BBR is a physiologically active isoquinoline alkaloid extracted mainly from the roots or stems of the herb Coptis chinensis. It possesses various biological effects, including immunomodulatory, antioxidant, and anti-inflammatory effects [25,26]. Recently, studies have revealed that BBR could directly regulate the composition of gut microbiota [27]. The study of Zhu et al. showed that 250 mg/kg BBR added to the feed of 1-day-old yellow-feathered broilers could reduce the Chao 1 and Shannon index, representing the microbial α-diversity and the abundance of the phylum Firmicutes. The genera Lachnospiraceae, Lachnoclostridium, Clostridiales, and Intestinimonas decreased, whereas the abundances of the phylum Bacteroidetes and the genus Bacteroides increased with BBR treatment. These results indicate that BBR improves the growth performance of broilers and reshapes their intestinal flora structure, playing a beneficial role [28]. However, although high doses of berberine can reduce intestinal inflammation in chickens and play a positive role, it can also increase the relative abundance of the family Enterobacteriaceae and decrease the relative abundance of the family Peptostreptococcaceae as well as the protective genera of the Ruminococcaceae and the Lachnospiraceae families, leading to a certain degree of dysbiosis [29]. BBR has also been demonstrated to be connected to the gut microbiota as a lipid-lowering medication by controlling BA turnover and activating subsequent ileal FXR signaling pathways [30]. BBR can reduce body weight, liver fat deposition, and triglyceride content in high-fat diet-induced obesity [31]. Li et al.'s studies have shown that BBR can ameliorate the progression of NAFLD by modulating the gut microbiota and improving the intestinal mucosal barrier function [32]. The protective effects of BBR on the gut microbiota and BA metabolism in FLHS, however, are the subject of few investigations. In the current study, we look at whether BBR can reduce FLHS symptoms caused by HELP in Hy-line brown laying hens. Then, through analyzing the gut microbiota and BA profile, we found that BBR could regulate glucose and lipid metabolism in laying hens by modifying the BA metabolism and gut flora. This research may offer fresh insight into how BBR improves FLHS by controlling the gut flora and BA metabolism.

2. Results

2.1. BBR Alleviated HELP-Induced Blood Lipid Metabolism and Hepatic Lipid Deposition

As shown in Figure 1A, histological observation shows that there is a great deal of lipid-filled vacuoles in the liver cells of the HELP group, and the structure of the hepatic cord and hepatic lobule disappear, while the control group presents normal liver cell structure. The results obtained from transmission electron microscopy indicate that there is an increase in the number of fat vacuoles, and a decrease can be observed in the number of mitochondria within the HELP group (Figure 1B). Furthermore, the biochemical findings indicate that there is a noteworthy elevation in the levels of TG, TC, and LDL-ch ($p < 0.001$) within the HELP group. However, BBR intervention can mitigate pathological changes in liver tissue, alleviate fatty degeneration, and significantly decrease blood lipid levels (Figure 1C–E).

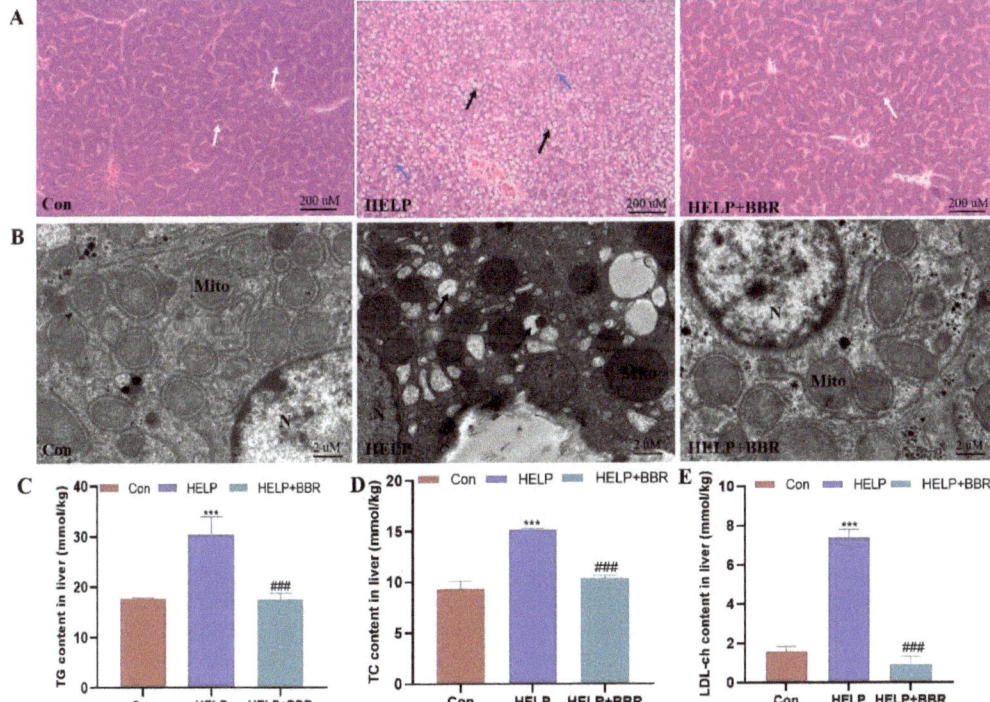

Figure 1. BBR alleviated HELP-induced blood lipid metabolism and hepatic lipid deposition. (**A**) The histological features (magnification: 200×, scale bar = 200 μm) and the frame indicate the location of characteristic lesions. White arrows represent interstitial hepatic cords, black arrows represent cellular steatosis, and blue arrows represent inflammatory cells; (**B**) Ultrastructural features (magnification: 1200×, scale bar = 2 μm), N: nucleus; Mito: mitochondria; (**C**) TG content; (**D**) TC content; (**E**) LDL-ch content. Data were represented as the mean ± SD. *** $p < 0.001$ vs. the Con group; ### $p < 0.001$ vs. the HELP group. Con, control; HELP, high-energy low-protein diet; BBR, berberine. Below is the same.

2.2. BBR Alters the Composition of Gut Microbiota in HELP-Fed Laying Hens

Intestinal flora is a micro-ecosystem in the body, and its diversity is a key indicator of individual health. Therefore, the OTU species of each group were analyzed. There were 295 OTUs in the three groups, among which 136, 222, and 24 OTU species were unique in the Con group, the HELP group, and the BBR + HELP group, respectively (Figure 2A). The alpha diversity index is used to evaluate the richness and uniformity of micro-organisms in samples. As shown in Figure 2B, at the same sequencing depth, ACE and Chao1 were significantly increased in the HELP group and reduced in the HELP+BBR group. To measure the extent of similarity between the microbial communities, beta diversity was calculated using a weighted normalized UniFrac, and PCoA was performed (Figure 2C). The distance between the three groups was obviously separated, and PERMANOVA similarity analysis revealed that the three groups' microbial distributions differed significantly from one another (F = 3.462, p = 0.002).

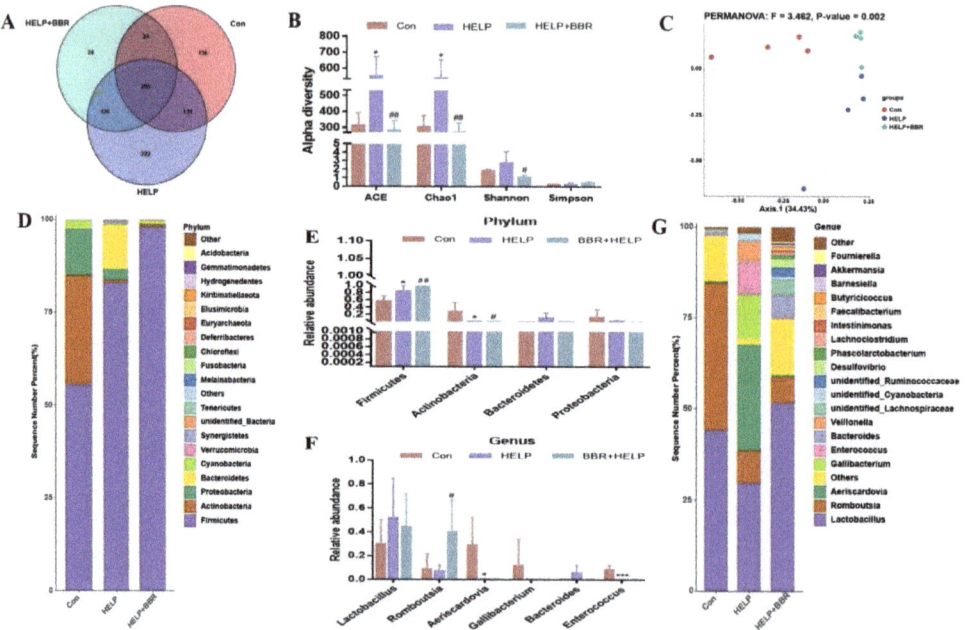

Figure 2. BBR alleviated HELP-induced intestinal microbiota dysbiosis. (**A**) Venn diagram showing the unique and shared OTUs in the diverse groups; (**B**) Alpha diversity; (**C**) Multiple-sample PCoA analysis; (**D**) Relative abundance of gut microbiota at the phylum level; (**E**) Relative abundance of the significantly altered bacteria at the phylum levels from the three groups; (**F**) Relative abundance of the significantly altered bacteria at the genus levels from the three groups; (**G**) Relative abundance of gut microbiota at the genus level. Data are represented as the mean ± SD. * $p < 0.05$ and *** $p < 0.001$ vs. the Con group; # $p < 0.05$ and ## $p < 0.01$ vs. the HELP group.

The flora in each group was examined at the phylum and genus levels to further assess the impact of BBR on intestinal flora. The results at the phylum level are shown in Figure 2D,E. The first four bacterial groups (Firmicutes, Actinobacteria, Bacteroidetes, and Proteobacteria) in the intestine of each group account for more than 90% of total phylum levels. Firmicute abundance was significantly upregulated, Actinobacterium and Proteobacterium abundances were significantly downregulated, and Bacteroidota abundance was raised in the HELP group. Compared to the HELP group, the addition of BBR in the HELP diet can further improve Firmicute abundance and reduce the abundance of Actinobacteria, Proteobacteria and Bacteroidetes. At the genus level, 21 species of bacteria, such as *Lactobacillus* and *Romboutsia*, were detected, among which *Lactobacillus* was the dominant bacteria with a relatively high abundance (Figure 2G,F). After BBR intervention, the abundance of *Lactobacillus* in the HELP group showed an increase by approximately 25% compared to the HELP group. Conversely, the abundance of *Lactobacillus* experienced a reduction of about 10% post-BBR intervention. *Bacteroides* were elevated in the HELP group, and bacterial abundance tended to be normal after BBR intervention. In addition, the abundance of *Romboutsia* flora showed a downward trend in the HELP group, but after the addition of BBR intervention, the abundance of flora increased significantly. The abundance of *Aeriscardovia*, *Gallibacterium*, and *Enterococcus* bacteria significantly decreased in the HELP group but did not improve after BBR intervention.

2.3. Regulation of BBR on Bile Acid Metabolism Disorder in Chicken Feces

In the case of FLHS, the change in intestinal flora structure can lead to the abnormal metabolism of bile acid, and the intestinal immune balance and the stability of the intestinal barrier can be destroyed. BBR can further affect the metabolism of bile acid molecules by modifying the makeup of the intestinal flora. In Figure 3A, the control group and the HELP group can be observed to have different bile acid distributions. Specifically, the bile acid reaches the maximum distance in both groups but is congregated in two distinct quadrants for each group. However, when BBR is added to the HELP diet, the bile acid metabolism in the feces of FLHS laying hens changes. In addition, 15 bile acids in the intestinal contents of FLHS laying hens were accurately quantified and analyzed by the partial least-squares method. Ten free bile acids, five conjugated bile acids, eight primary bile acids, and five secondary bile acids were detected. Compared to the control group, the content of chenodeoxycholic acid declined, and the content of Taurochenodeoxycholic_acid, Taurocholic_acid, Cholic_acid, and Allocholic_acid increased in the HELP group (Figure 3B–D). However, bile acid content continued to decrease with the addition of BBR, indicating that BBR plays an important regulatory role in the bile acid metabolism of FLHS laying hens induced by HELP.

Finally, this study analyzed the correlation between bile acid molecules and intestinal microflora at the phylum and genus levels, respectively. The results showed that bile acid was closely related to intestinal flora. At the phylum level (Figure 4A), the bacterial abundance of ileal *Actinobacteria* was significantly positively correlated with Chenodeoxycholic_acid, Taurolithocholic_acid, and Allocholic_acid. In addition, the content of *Fusobacteria* was positively correlated with 7_ketodeoxycholic_acid, 3_dehydrocholic_acid, and 12_dehydrocholic_acid. *Melainabacteria* and *Synergistetes* were positively correlated with 3_dehydrocholic_acid and taurochenodeoxycholic_acid, respectively. *Firmicuteria* was negatively correlated with Chenodeoxycholic_acid. At the genus level (Figure 4B), the bacterial abundance of *Aeriscardovia*, *Enterococcus*, and *Veillonella* were positively correlated with taurolithocholic_acid, and significantly negatively correlated with taurochenodeoxycholic_acid. *Campylobacter* and *Romboutsia* were negatively correlated with allocholic_acid, and *gallibacterium* and *lawsonia* were significantly negatively correlated with 7_ketodeoxycholic_acid.

2.4. BBR Alleviated HELP-Induced Abnormal Bile Acid Biosynthesis

As shown in Figure 5A,B,G,H, compared to the control group, FXR receptor-related genes *ASBT*, *FGF19* (ileum), and *FGF19* (liver) mRNA levels declined ($p < 0.001$) in the HELP group. The FXR gene and protein were significantly increased in the HELP group. ($p < 0.001$; $p < 0.01$); bile acid synthesis genes *CYP7a1* and *ABCB11* mRNA levels were downregulated in the HELP group compared to the control group ($p < 0.001$; $p < 0.05$). Among them, *CYP8b1* and *CYP27a1* mRNA levels were upregulated in the HELP group compared to the control group ($p < 0.001$; $p < 0.05$). However, added BBR can significantly increase the expression of *ASBT*, *FGF19* (ileum), *FGF19* (liver), *CYP27a1*, and *ABCB11* mRNA levels ($p < 0.001$). The results of CYP27a1 protein were consistent with the results of gene expression.

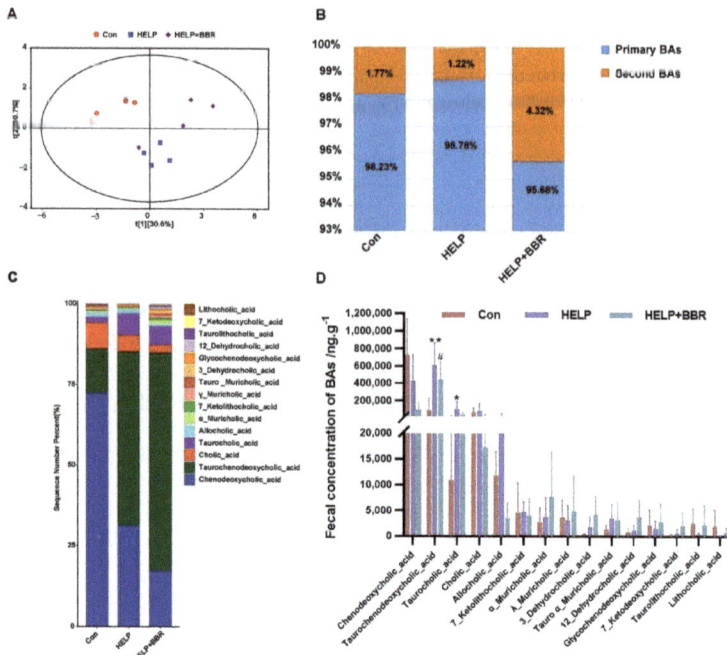

Figure 3. Regulation of BBR on bile acid metabolism disorder in chicken feces. (**A**) PLS-DA score plots for discriminating the fecal BA profiles from three groups; (**B**) Ratio of primary bile acid to secondary bile acid; (**C**) Composition of bile acid pool in feces; (**D**) Relative abundance of the significantly changed BAs from different groups. Data are represented as the mean ± SD. * $p < 0.05$ and ** $p < 0.01$ vs. the Con group; # $p < 0.05$ vs. the HELP group.

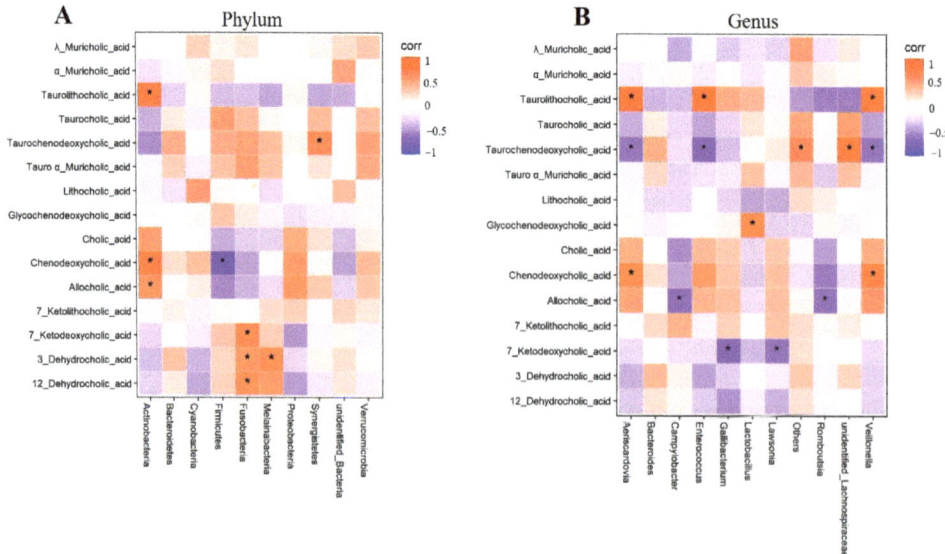

Figure 4. Heatmap analysis of the Spearman correlation of fecal BAs and gut microbiota. (**A**) Spearman correlation of fecal BA and gut microbiota at the phylum level; (**B**) Spearman correlation of

fecal BA and gut microbiota at the genus level. Squares in red with an asterisk refer to a significant positive correlation, and squares in blue with an asterisk indicate a significant negative correlation. Data are represented as the mean ± SD. * $p < 0.05$ vs. the Con group.

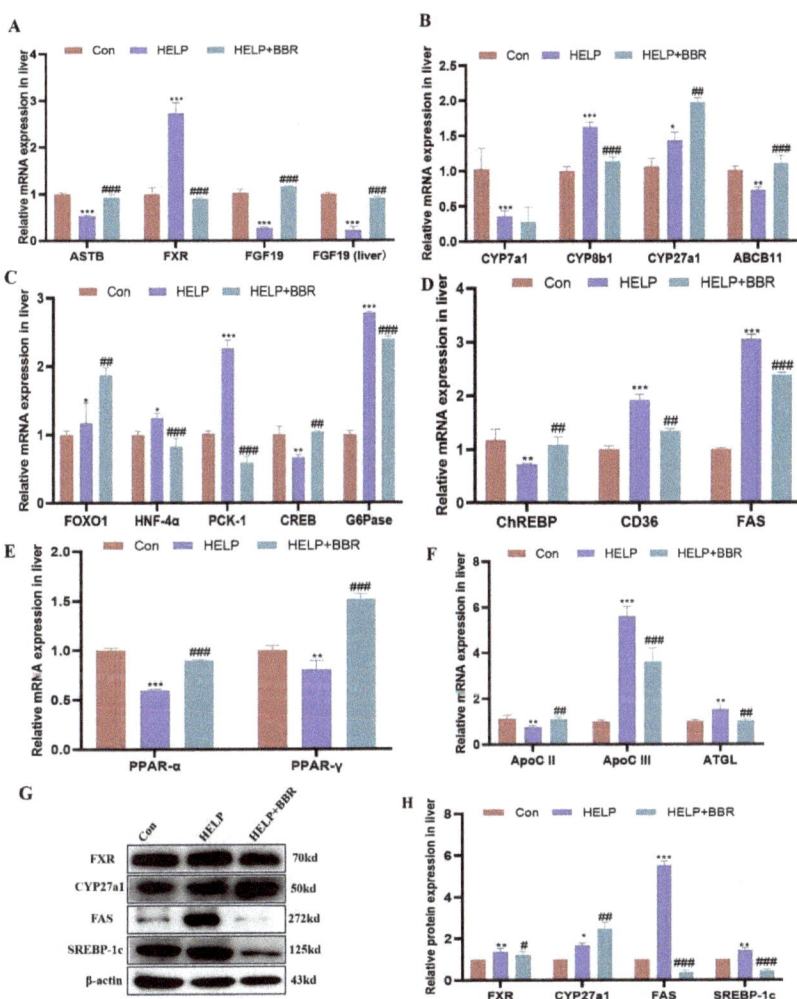

Figure 5. BBR alleviated HELP-induced lipid metabolism. (**A**) Bile acid biosynthesis-related mRNA expression level; (**B**) FXR receptor-related mRNA expression level; (**C**) Gluconeogenesis-related mRNA expression level; (**D**) lipid synthesis-related mRNA expression level; (**E**) lipid oxidation-related mRNA expression level; (**F**) Triglyceride hydrolysis-related mRNA expression level; (**G**) protein bands; (**H**) The results of gray-value analysis of protein bands. Data are represented as the mean ± SD. * $p < 0.05$, ** $p < 0.01$ and *** $p < 0.001$ vs. the Con group; # $p < 0.05$, ## $p < 0.01$ and ### $p < 0.001$ vs. the HELP group.

2.5. BBR Alleviated HELP-Induced Abnormal Glucose and Lipid Metabolism

As shown in Figure 5C–F, compared to the control group involved in glucose metabolism genes, *FOXO1*, *HNF-4α*, *PCK-1*, and *G6Pase* mRNA levels increased ($p < 0.001$), but *CREB* mRNA level declined ($p < 0.01$) in the HELP group. For the added BBR in the HELP diet, the mRNA levels of *FOXO1*, *HNF-4α*, *PCK-1*, and *G6Pase* significantly declined ($p < 0.01$ or $p < 0.001$). Meanwhile, compared to the control group, lipid metabolism genes *chREBP*, *PPARα*, and *PPAR-γ* mRNA levels were reduced ($p < 0.05$), but *CD36* and *FAS* mRNA levels were upregulated ($p < 0.01$; $p < 0.001$) in the HELP group. Added BBR can significantly upregulate *chREBP*, *PPARα*, and *PPAR-γ* mRNA levels ($p < 0.01$ or $p < 0.001$) in the BBR+HELP group. At the same time, the expression of lipid synthesis proteins FAS and SREBP-1c in the HELP group significantly increased ($p < 0.01$; $p < 0.001$), and the addition of BBR could reduce the expression of proteins ($p < 0.001$) (Figure 5G,H). Additionally, compared to the control group, ApoC II mRNA levels were reduced ($p < 0.01$), but *ApoC III* and *ATGL* mRNA levels were upregulated ($p < 0.01$ or $p < 0.001$) in the HELP group. For added BBR in the HELP diet, the mRNA levels of *ApoC III* and *ATGL* were significantly reduced ($p < 0.01$), and *ApoC II* mRNA level was upregulated ($p < 0.05$).

3. Discussion

FLHS is a prevalent nutritional metabolic disease that affects laying hens, causing liver injury and a sudden decline in egg production during the peak laying period. However, a complete understanding of the underlying mechanisms concerning the development and advancement of FLHS remains to be fully elucidated. Recently, mounting evidence has suggested that the participation of the gastrointestinal–hepatic axis plays a crucial role in the emergence and advancement of NAFLD [33,34]. The gut microbiota, a fundamental component of the gut–liver axis, has been extensively recognized for its pivotal role in rewiring the energy metabolism of the host. In the present study, we successfully induced liver fat deposition in laying hens through a HELP diet (3100 kcal/kg, 12% crude protein), thus corroborating our previous study [5]. Furthermore, BBR has a direct impact on the microbiota in the intestine and controls the metabolism of bile acid through the regulation of the FXR signaling pathway. As a result, it enhances liver lipid metabolism in laying hens.

The gastrointestinal–hepatic axis plays a key role in the development of NAFLD [35]. The expression of fatty acid synthase (FAS) and sterol regulatory element binding protein-1c (SREBP-1c) in the liver has been demonstrated to be inhibited by gut microbiota-derived metabolites derived from tryptophan metabolism. These metabolites control lipid metabolism by activating the hepatic aromatic hydrocarbon receptor (AHR) [36]. Accumulating evidence indicates the potential therapeutic effects of fecal microbiota transplantation in mitigating high-fat diet-induced steatohepatitis in murine models [37]. This effect may be due to an increase in beneficial gut microbiota, which improves the integrity of intestinal tight junctions and reduces the levels of lipopolysaccharides (LPS) [38]. In the present study, the intestinal microbiota structure in laying hens promotes hepatic lipid deposition, as demonstrated by alterations in intestinal microbiota α-diversity and β-diversity. Additionally, the supplementation of BBR has the potential to modulate the intestinal microbiota.

Recent research has indicated that BBR may directly improve the function of the intestinal barrier, reduce inflammation, control the bile acid signal pathway, and regulate the axis of bacteria–gut–brain [39]. In both normal-chow-diet (NCD) and high-fat-diet (HFD) conditions, BBR had a significant impact on the makeup of the gut microbiota [40]. In particular, within the order Clostridiales, families Streptococcaceae, Clostridiaceae, and Prevotellaceae, as well as genera *Streptococcus* and *Prevotella*, BBR has shown a particular capacity to diminish the relative abundance of bacteria involved in the formation of branched-chain amino acids (BCAAs) [41]. In our results, according to the PCoA score plots, all three groups were significantly separated compared with themselves, indicating changes in bacterial communities. At the phylum level, the HELP group showed an increase in Firmicutes and Bacteroidetes. Firmicutes, as opposed to Bacteroidetes, digest sugar more effectively and favor energy resorption, the process by which surplus energy is converted to fat and stored in liver tissue when it is not used [42]. At the genus level, we found that the *Romboutsia* significantly increases in the BBR group compared with the HELP group.

Romboutsia was dramatically reduced in obese individuals [43]. Other studies have connected *Romboutsia* to glycerophospholipids, which have been connected to obesity-related fatty liver disease [44,45]. Therefore, we speculate that BBR may improve lipid metabolism in HELP laying hens by regulating changes in the abundance of *Romboutsia*.

The field of metabolomics has recently gained popularity in biomedical research, although identifying many metabolites in untargeted metabolomics remains challenging. However, in nonalcoholic fatty liver disease, BA metabolism emerges as a desirable therapeutic target [46]. Therefore, in the current investigation, BA-targeted metabolomics was used to identify the alterations to BA in FLHS following BBR administration. A total of 15 bile acid metabolites were identified, among which the HELP group's primary BA-to-secondary-BA ratio was higher than that of the Con group. After BBR treatment, the ratio of primary BA to secondary BA changed, manifested in Tauro chenodeoxycholic acid (TDCA) and Taurocholic acid (TCA). TUDCA, a derivative of Ursodeoxycholic acid (UDCA), was used for the treatment of liver dysfunction and increased HFD-induced obesity in a rat model [47,48]. Simultaneously, Cholic acid was converted into taurocholic acid, which could affect the metabolism of lipids and lipoproteins, glycolysis and gluconeogenesis, and fatty acid production [49]. These findings align with our experimental results that suggest that when FLHS occurs in laying hens, the body can relieve liver damage by secreting UDCA and TCA. However, additional supplementation of BBR can exogenously reduce damage and reduce the secretion of UDCA and TCA. Furthermore, by regulating the intestinal transit of bile acids, the gut microbiota can maintain bile acid homeostasis and regulate bile acid metabolism. According to earlier studies, gut microbes deconjugate primary bile acids generated from the host using bile salt hydrolases found in Actinobacteria [50]. At the phylum level, our analysis also revealed a substantial positive correlation between Actinobacteria and Chenodeoxycholic acid, Taurolithocholic acid, and Allocholic acid. Likewise, Aeriscardoviay was inversely connected with Taurochenodeoxychlic acid at the genus level but had a positive correlation with Chenodeoxycholic acid and Taurolithocholic acid.

By activating FXR and TGR5, BAs function as signal molecules that regulate not only their biosynthesis but also vital metabolic processes [51,52]. Therefore, we investigated whether the FXR signaling pathway is involved in the effects on BA production of the enhanced intestinal microbiota caused by BBR. Our findings in the current study showed that BBR stimulated liver FXR signaling to affect hepatic BA problems, and downstream bile acid synthesis-related genes (*CYP27a1* and *ABCB11* ($p < 0.01$)) are markedly upregulated in the BBR group, indicating that BBR can promote bile acid metabolism. Recent investigations have highlighted the significance of FXR as a critical therapeutic target in NAFLD, with encouraging findings showcasing the substantial amelioration of pathological manifestations in patients with NASH upon treatment with FXR agonists [53]. *Penthorum chinense* Pursh extract promotes bile acid biosynthesis and further reduces NAFLD in mice that are fed a high-cholesterol diet by promoting the production of the enzymes *CYP7a1* and *CYP8b1* and activating the liver's FXR receptor [54]. By contrast, in our results, we found that BBR can reduce the expression of *CYP7a1* and *CYP8b1* and inhibit the activation of *FXR*. Moreover, based on Chao Yang et al., 28 weeks of FLA treatment substantially decreases the development of NASH in NAFL-model mice fed an HFD. These advantageous effects can be attributed to the regulation and enhancement of gut flora- and microbiota-related BAs, which in turn activate the intestinal FXR-FGF15 and TGR5-NF-κB pathways [55]. Additionally, Triglyceride and fatty acid metabolism are regulated by FXR. Haczeyni et al. demonstrated that Obeticholic acid reduced SREBP-1c expression and increased PPARα expression through the hepatic FXR signaling pathway in the liver of HFD mice [56]. Moreover, PPARγ and SREBP-1c expression are suppressed, and PPARα expression is increased by FXR, which is one strategy for preventing fat accumulation [57]. In the present study, BBR downregulated the glucose metabolism genes (*FOXO1*, *HNF-4α*, *PCK-1*, and *G6Pase* ($p < 0.001$)) and downstream lipogenic genes (*FAS* and *CD36* ($p < 0.001$)), as well as upregulating the expression of *PPARα*, *PPARγ*, and downregulating downstream triglyceride hydrolysis genes (*ApoC III* and *ATGL* ($p < 0.01$)). Thus, from our results that detect the genes and proteins of glucose and lipid metabolism downstream of the FXR signaling pathway, it is also shown that BBR has a positive therapeutic effect on liver lipid deposition caused by HELP.

4. Materials and Methods

4.1. Animals and Experimental Design

This study was approved by the Committee for the Care and Use of Experimental Animals at Jiangxi Agricultural University (No: JXAULL-202218). All experimental procedures adhered to the standards established by Jiangxi Agricultural University's Experimental Animal Care and Use Committee. A total of 90 Hy-line laying hens, aged 140 days and in good health, were randomly distributed among three groups: control (Con), high-energy low-protein (HELP), and berberine (BBR)+ HELP. The diets provided to the laying hens in these groups comprised the basal diet, HELP diet, and HELP diet enriched with 100 mg/kg BBR, respectively. The experiment lasted for 140 days, during which all groups of hens received sufficient food and water. The nutritional requirements for the hens' baseline diet were formulated in accordance with the standard guidelines specified by the National Research Council (1998). The HELP diet differed only in its energy and protein standards. The composition of both the basal and HELP diets can be found in Table 1.

Table 1. Composition and nutrient levels of diets (air-dry basis) %.

Composition of Diet %	Control Group	HELP Group
Corn	64.00	70.00
Wheat Bran	2.00	1.20
Soybean Meal	24.00	14.58
Fat-Soybean Oil	0	4.22
Calcium	8.00	8.00
* Premix	2.00	2.00
Total	100.00	100.00
Nutrient level		
Crude Protein CP	15.86	12.00
Available Phosphorus (AP)	0.51	0.46
Arginine	1.03	0.74
Methionine	0.37	0.32
Valine	0.77	0.58
Metabolic Energy (kcal/kg)	2678.99	3100.00
Met + Cys	0.67	0.56

* The ingredient of premix: The ingredient of premix: multiple vitamins, 30 mg; cupric sulfate, 4.6 mg; ferrous sulfate, 28.4 mg; manganous sulfate, 35.46 mg; zinc sulfate, 76 mg; zeolite powder, 6 mg; sodium selenite, 5 mg; anti-oxidizing quinolone, 50 mg; choline, 90 mg; bacitracin zinc, 26.7 mg; bran, 350 mg; methionine, 100 mg.

After the 140-day experiment, each of the hens underwent anesthesia induced by an intravenous injection of sodium pentobarbital, administered at a dosage of 50 mg/kg following a 12-hour fast. Subsequently, samples of liver, distal ileum tissue, and ileal feces were carefully preserved at temperatures of $-20\ °C$ or $-80\ °C$. Additionally, a segment of the liver tissue was preserved in a solution containing 4% paraformaldehyde to facilitate the examination of the corresponding indicators.

4.2. Histopathological Examination

The specific experimental method is consistent with Gao et al. [58]. The liver tissue specimens were washed with normal saline and then fixed in a 4% paraformaldehyde solution. After one week, the samples were routinely embedded and sliced (5 μm) and stained with hematoxylin and eosin (H&E). Afterward, pathological sections were observed using an optical microscope, and photographs were taken.

4.3. Determination of Liver Biochemical Indexes

We assessed the levels of triglyceride (TG), total cholesterol (TC), and low-density lipoprotein cholesterol (LDL-ch). In short, an appropriate amount of liver tissue (tissue weight: homogenate medium = 1:9) was weighed to prepare tissue homogenate. The homogenate was then centrifuged at 2500 rpm for 10 min to obtain the supernatant for testing, following the instructions provided by the manufacturer, the Nanjing Jiancheng Bioengineering Institute (based in Nanjing, China).

4.4. Sequencing of 16S rDNA

The total microbial genomic DNA from the hen's ileum feces was extracted and sent to BIOTREE (Shanghai, China). The DNA concentration and purity were assessed. A total of 1 ng/μL DNA concentration was selected as the template to amplify the V3–V4 fragment and the 16S rDNA gene using forward primer (5-CCTACGGGNGGCWGCAG-3) and reverse primer (5-GACTACHVGGG TATCTAATCC-3), and specific primers and high-fidelity enzymes were selected for PCR amplification [59]. The PCR amplification of the 16S rDNA gene was performed as follows: initial denaturation at 95 °C for 3 min, followed by 27 cycles of denaturing at 95 °C for 30 s, annealing at 55 °C for 30 s, and extension at 72 °C for 45 s, and single extension at 72 °C for 10 min, and ending at 4 °C. The PCR mixtures contained 5 × Trans Start Fast Pfu buffer 4 μL, 2.5 mM dNTPs 2 μL, forward primer (5 μM) 0.8 μL, reverse primer (5 μM) 0.8 μL, Trans Start Fast Pfu DNA Polymerase 0.4 μL, template DNA 10 ng, and ddH$_2$O up to 20 μL. PCR reactions were performed in triplicate. The PCR product was extracted from 2% agarose gel and purified using the AxyPrep DNA Gel Extraction Kit (Axygen Biosciences, Union City, CA, USA) according to the manufacturer's instructions and quantified using Quantus™ Fluorometer (Promega, WI, USA). Purified amplicons were pooled in equimolar, and paired-end sequenced (2 × 300) on an Illumina MiSeq platform (Illumina, San Diego, CA, USA). The 16S rDNA gene sequencing reads were demultiplexed, quality-filtered by Trimmomatic, and merged by FLASH with the following criteria: (i) 300 bp reads were truncated at any site receiving an average quality score of <20 over a 50 bp sliding window, and truncated reads shorter than 50 bp were discarded. Reads containing ambiguous characters were also discarded; (ii) only overlapping sequences longer than 10 bp were assembled according to their overlapped sequence. The maximum mismatch ratio of the overlap region was 0.2. Reads that could not be assembled were discarded; (iii) samples were distinguished according to the barcode and primers, and the sequence direction was adjusted for exact barcode matching and 2 nucleotide mismatches in primer matching.

Operational taxonomic units (OTUs) with 97% similarity cutoff were clustered using UPARSE (version 7.1, http://drive5.com/uparse/, 6 August 2022), and chimeric sequences were identified and removed. The taxonomy of each OTU representative sequence was analyzed by the RDP Classifier (http://rdp.cme.msu.edu/, 6 August 2022) against the 16S rDNA database (e.g., Silva 132/16s_bacteria) using a confidence threshold of 0.7.

4.5. Quantitative Analysis of BA Profile in Ileal Feces

The concentration of BA in the samples was determined using UPLC–TQMS, a method developed in a previous study [60,61]. In short, 1000 μL of formic acid extract containing 0.1% formic acid was added to 25 mg of fecal samples, vortexed, and mixed under ice-water bath conditions, ground ultrasonically, left to stand at −40 °C, and centrifuged. Finally, the supernatant was extracted for UPLC–TQMS analysis.

4.6. Quantitative Real-Time PCR Analysis

Total RNA was extracted from liver tissues using the Trizol reagent (Takara, Dalian, China), as directed by the manufacturer. The RNA was then dissolved in 40 μL of clean, diethyl pyrocarbonate-treated water and stored at −80 °C. A biophotometer (Eppendorf, Germany) and agarose gel electrophoresis were used to evaluate the quantity and quality of the RNA. A One-Step gDNA Removal and cDNA Synthesis SuperMix kit from TransGen,

Beijing, China, was used for the reverse-transcription (RT) procedure. The Anchored Oligo (dT)18 Primer, 10 µL of 2XES Reaction Mix, 1 µL of RT Enzyme Mix, 1 µL of gDNA Remover, and 7 µL of RNase-free ddH$_2$O and cDNA made up the 20 µL of RT reactions. The reaction was carried out at 42 °C for 15 min, followed by 85 °C for 5 s, and finally, 4 °C indefinitely. The resulting cDNA was stored at −20 °C for real-time PCR.

The acquired chicken gene sequences and NCBI GenBank accession numbers are shown in Table 2. Shanghai Bioengineering Co., Ltd. was tasked with creating the primers for the housekeeping gene actin using the Primer Express 3.0 program. The ABI Quant Studio 7 Flex PCR apparatus was used to carry out the experiment. The reaction process was carried out in the following steps: predenaturation at 95 °C for 30 s, denaturation at 95 °C for 5 s, and annealing at 60 °C for 34 s. A total of 40 cycles were carried out. The $2^{-\Delta\Delta ct}$ approach was used to determine the relative mRNA levels.

Table 2. Gene primer sequence and their GenBank accession number.

Gene Name	Accession Number	Primer Sequences (5′ to 3′)
FXR	AF49249.7	Forward: CTCTCGCAAAATGGGGCAGT Reverse: CGCGGGAATTCGATTGGC
ASBT	AB970773.1	Forward: ACCATGAAATTGAAACAAGAGTGAA Reverse: TGGGATAACTTTAGCCTGTCCA
FGF19	NM_204674.3	Forward: GCCAGAGGTCTACTCATCGC Reverse: ACCTGCAACATTCTGCGGTA
CYP7a1	NM_001001753.2	Forward: GCTCCGCATGTTCCTGAATG Reverse: ATGGTGTTAGCTTGCGAGGC
CYP8b1	NM_001389480.2	Forward: TACCAAGGGACAGGGAACAAGGAG Reverse: GGAGGCAACACGGCATAGGC
ABCB11	XM_046921923.1	Forward: ATCTTGGCCATCCAGCAAGG Reverse: ACTGGCTCTTGCTCAACAACACC
G6Pase	BM439740.1	Forward: TCCAGCACATCCACTCCATCTACC Reverse: TCAACACCAAGCATCCGCAGAAG
CREB	CAJNRD030001119.1	Forward: ACCTGCCATTGCCACTGTTACG Reverse: CTCCATCCGTGCCGTTGTTAGAC
FOXO1	NM_204328.2	Forward: ACACAGTGAACCCCATGTCA Reverse: AGGGGCATACGGGTTCATAG
HNF-4α	AY700581.1	Forward: AGGATGTCTTGCTGCTAGGG Reverse: GCAGGCGTATTCATTGTCGT
FAS	AB495724.1	Forward: ACTGTGGGCTCCAAATCTTCA Reverse: CAAGGAGCCATCGTGTAAAGC
ATGL	EU240627.2	Forward: GCTGATCCAGGCCTGTGTCT Reverse: TGGAGGTATCTGCCCACAGTAGA
PPAR-γ	AB045597.1	Forward: CACTGCAGGAACAGAACAAAGAA Reverse: TCCACAGAGCGAAACTGACATC
CD36	NM_001030731.1	Forward: CTGGGAAGGTTACTGCGATT Reverse: GCGAGGAACTGTGAAACGATA
ChREBP	EU152408.1	Forward: GATGAGCACCGCAAACCAGAGG Reverse: TCGGAGCCGCTTCTTGTAGTAGG
PPAR-α	AF163809.1	Forward: GACACCCTTTCACCAGCATC Reverse: CCCTTACAACCTTCACAAGCA
ApoC II	CM040951.1	Forward: CCTCCCAGCTCACCCAATT Reverse: CAGGATCCCGGTGTAAGTCA
ApoC III	NM_001302127.2	Forward: AAGGTGCAGGAGTACGTCAA Reverse: GCGTTGTCTGACAGCCATTT
CYP27a1	XM_040676620.2	Forward: CTTCCCCAAGAACACCCTCT Reverse: AAGGGATGGAGCTGAAAGGG
PCK-1	NM_205471.2	Forward: TCAACACCAGATTCCCAGGC Reverse: CCTCATGCTAGCCACCACAT
β-actin	L08165.1	Forward: ATTGCTGCGCTCGTTGTT Reverse: CTTTTGCTCTGGGCTTCA

4.7. Western Blot Analysis

An appropriate amount of liver tissue was taken and homogenized by adding lysate tissue. The tissue homogenate was then centrifuged at 4 °C at 15,000 rpm for 10 min. The total protein content of the liver samples was determined using the BCA protein detection kit (Solarbio, Beijing, China). The primary antibodies of FXR (1:1000) (Cat No. TD12402S) and CYP27a1 (1:1000) (Cat No. T58677S) were procured from ABMART. SREBP-1c (Cat No. 14088-1-AP), FAS (1:1000) (Cat No. 60196-1-lg), and β-actin (1:5000) (Cat No. 81115-1-RR) were procured from Proteinates. The Bio-Rad ChemiDoc Touch imager (Bio-Rad ChemiDoc Touch, California, USA) captured the signal. Finally, the gray cost of the corresponding protein was analyzed using ImageJ software V1.8.0 (ImageJ, RRID:SCR_003070).

4.8. Statistical Analysis

The data were presented as mean ± standard deviation (SD). GraphPad Prism 9.0 (GraphPad Inc., La Jolla, CA, USA), Microsoft Excel 2019, and SPSS version 26.0 (SPSS Inc., Chicago, IL, USA) were utilized for data analysis. One-way analysis of variance (ANOVA) and post hoc testing, known as the least significant difference (LSD), was employed in the data analysis. Statistical significance was set at a p-value of less than 0.05 ($p < 0.05$). Correlation analysis between fecal BA-related bacteria was performed using Spearman's rank correlation, with a coefficient of $> |0.5|$, as well as a p-value < 0.05.

5. Conclusions

In summary, our study suggests that BBR has a potential therapeutic effect on FLHS, potentially through modulating the gut microbiota and regulating lipid metabolism. This novel finding provides important insights into the pathogenesis of FLHS and may contribute to the development of new treatments for FLHS.

Author Contributions: Conceptualization, C.X. and C.Z.; Data curation, Y.Y.; Formal analysis, H.C. and X.G.; Funding acquisition, G.H.; Methodology, J.C.; Project administration, Y.Z.; Resources, G.H.; Supervision, X.D.; Writing—original draft, C.W.; Writing—review and editing, Y.Z. All authors have read and agreed to the published version of the manuscript.

Funding: This project was supported by the National Natural Science Foundation of China (No. 32060819; Beijing, China), Jiangxi Province introduces and trains high-level talents of innovation and entrepreneurship "Thousand Talents Plan" (No. jxsq2023201060, Jiangxi, China) and Graduate Innovative Special Fund Projects of Jiangxi Province (No. YC2022-B100 and YC2022-s387 Jiangxi, China). The APC was funded by [No. 32060819; Beijing, China]. All authors thank all members of the clinical veterinary medicine laboratory in the College of Animal Science and Technology, Jiangxi Agricultural University, for help in the experimental process.

Institutional Review Board Statement: This experiment was approved by the Committee for the Care and Use of Experimental Animals at Jiangxi Agricultural University No: JXAULL-202218).

Informed Consent Statement: Animal care and experimental procedures were approved by the Animal Care Committee of Jiangxi Agricultural University (Nanchang, China) and adhered to the university's guidelines for animal research.

Data Availability Statement: The datasets analyzed during the current study are available from the corresponding author upon reasonable request.

Conflicts of Interest: The authors declare no conflict of interest.

References

1. Chen, W.; Shi, Y.; Li, G.; Huang, C.; Zhuang, Y.; Shu, B.; Cao, X.; Li, Z.; Hu, G.; Liu, P.; et al. Preparation of the peroxisome proliferator-activated receptor alpha polyclonal antibody: Its application in fatty liver hemorrhagic syndrome. *Int. J. Biol. Macromol.* **2021**, *182*, 179–186. [CrossRef] [PubMed]
2. Grimes, J.L.; Maurice, D.V.; Lightsey, S.F.; Bridges, W.J. Research note: Relationship of comb color to liver appearance and fat content in Single Comb White Leghorn laying hens. *Poult. Sci.* **1991**, *70*, 2544–2546. [CrossRef] [PubMed]
3. Rozenboim, I.; Mahato, J.; Cohen, N.A.; Tirosh, O. Low protein and high-energy diet: A possible natural cause of fatty liver hemorrhagic syndrome in caged White Leghorn laying hens. *Poult. Sci.* **2016**, *95*, 612–621. [CrossRef] [PubMed]

4. Diaz, G.J.; Squires, F.J.; Julian, R.J. The use of selected plasma enzyme activities for the diagnosis of fatty liver-hemorrhagic syndrome in laying hens. *Avian Dis.* **1999**, *43*, 768–773. [CrossRef]
5. Zhuang, Y.; Xing, C.; Cao, H.; Zhang, C.; Luo, J.; Guo, X.; Hu, G. Insulin resistance and metabonomics analysis of fatty liver haemorrhagic syndrome in laying hens induced by a high-energy low-protein diet. *Sci. Rep.* **2019**, *9*, 10141. [CrossRef] [PubMed]
6. Ma, S.; Sun, Y.; Zheng, X.; Yang, Y. Gastrodin attenuates perfluorooctanoic acid-induced liver injury by regulating gut microbiota composition in mice. *Bioengineered* **2021**, *12*, 11546–11556. [CrossRef] [PubMed]
7. Han, K.H.; Ohashi, S.; Sasaki, K.; Nagata, R.; Pelpolage, S.; Fukuma, N.; Reed, J.D.; Shimada, K.I.; Kadoya, N.; Fukushima, M. Dietary adzuki bean paste dose-dependently reduces visceral fat accumulation in rats fed a normal diet. *Food Res. Int.* **2020**, *130*, 108890. [CrossRef] [PubMed]
8. Yu, J.; Marsh, S.; Hu, J.; Feng, W.; Wu, C. The pathogenesis of nonalcoholic fatty liver disease: Interplay between diet, gut microbiota, and genetic background. *Gastroenterol. Res. Pract.* **2016**, *2016*, 2862173. [CrossRef]
9. Eslam, M.; Sanyal, A.J.; George, J. MAFLD: A consensus-driven proposed nomenclature for metabolic associated fatty liver disease. *Gastroenterology* **2020**, *158*, 1999–2014. [CrossRef]
10. Marchesini, G.; Brizi, M.; Bianchi, G.; Tomassetti, S.; Bugianesi, E.; Lenzi, M.; McCullough, A.J.; Natale, S.; Forlani, G.; Melchionda, N. Nonalcoholic fatty liver disease: A feature of the metabolic syndrome. *Diabetes* **2001**, *50*, 1844–1850. [CrossRef]
11. Vuppalanchi, R.; Chalasani, N. Nonalcoholic fatty liver disease and nonalcoholic steatohepatitis: Selected practical issues in their evaluation and management. *Hepatology* **2009**, *49*, 306–317. [CrossRef] [PubMed]
12. Long, X.; Liu, D.; Gao, Q.; Ni, J.; Qian, L.; Ni, Y.; Fang, Q.; Jia, W.; Li, H. Bifidobacterium adolescents alleviates liver steatosis and steatohepatitis by increasing fibroblast growth factor 21 sensitivity. *Front. Endocrinol.* **2021**, *12*, 773340. [CrossRef] [PubMed]
13. Wang, B.; Jiang, X.; Cao, M.; Ge, J.; Bao, Q.; Tang, L.; Chen, Y.; Li, L. Altered fecal microbiota correlates with liver biochemistry in nonobese patients with Non-alcoholic fatty liver disease. *Sci. Rep.* **2016**, *6*, 32002. [CrossRef] [PubMed]
14. Abilos, A.; de Gottardi, A.; Rescigno, M. The gut-liver axis in liver disease: Pathophysiological basis for therapy. *J. Hepatol.* **2020**, *72*, 558–577. [CrossRef]
15. Juarez-Hernandez, E.; Chavez-Tapia, N.C.; Uribe, M.; Barbero-Becerra, V.J. Role of bioactive fatty acids in nonalcoholic fatty liver disease. *Nutr. J.* **2016**, *15*, 72. [CrossRef] [PubMed]
16. Presides, G.A.; Keaton, M.A.; Campeau, P.M.; Bessard, B.C.; Conner, M.E.; Hotez, P.J. The undernourished neonatal mouse metabolome reveals evidence of liver and biliary dysfunction, inflammation, and oxidative stress. *J. Nutr.* **2014**, *144*, 273–281. [CrossRef]
17. Ichimura-Shimizu, M.; Watanabe, S.; Kashirajima, Y.; Nagatomo, A.; Wada, H.; Tsuneyama, K.; Omagari, K. Dietary cholic acid exacerbates liver fibrosis in NASH model of sprague-dawley rats Fed a high-fat and high-cholesterol diet. *Int. J. Mol. Sci.* **2022**, *23*, 9268. [CrossRef]
18. Huang, W.; Ma, K.; Zhang, J.; Qatan ani, M.; Cuvillier, J.; Liu, J.; Dong, B.; Huang, X.; Moore, D.D. Nuclear receptor-dependent bile acid signaling is required for normal liver regeneration. *Science* **2006**, *312*, 233–236. [CrossRef] [PubMed]
19. Safari, H.; Kaczorowski, N.; Felder, M.L.; Brannon, E.R.; Varghese, M.; Singer, K.; Eniola-Adefeso, O. Biodegradable, bile salt microparticles for localized fat dissolution. *Sci. Adv.* **2020**, *6*, eabd8019. [CrossRef]
20. Sinal, C.J.; Tohkin, M.; Miyata, M.; Ward, J.M.; Lambert, G.; Gonzalez, F.J. Targeted disruption of the nuclear receptor FXR/BAR impairs bile acid and lipid homeostasis. *Cell* **2000**, *102*, 731–744. [CrossRef]
21. Li, R.; Palmiotti, A.; de Vries, H.D.; Hovingh, M.V.; Koehorst, M.; Mulder, N.L.; Zhang, Y.; Kats, K.; Bloks, V.W.; Fu, J.; et al. Low production of 12alpha-hydroxylated bile acids prevents hepatic steatosis in Cyp2c70(-/-) mice by reducing fat absorption. *J. Lipid. Res.* **2021**, *62*, 100134. [CrossRef]
22. Park, M.Y.; Kim, S.J.; Ko, E.K.; Ahn, S.H.; Seo, H.; Sung, M.K. Gut microbiota-associated bile acid deconjugation accelerates hepatic steatosis in ob/ob mice. *J. Appl. Microbiol.* **2016**, *121*, 800–810. [CrossRef]
23. Yao, J.; Zhou, C.S.; Ma, X.; Fu, B.Q.; Tao, L.S.; Chen, M.; Xu, Y.P. FXR agonist GW4064 alleviates endotoxin-induced hepatic inflammation by repressing macrophage activation. *World J. Gastroenterol.* **2014**, *20*, 14430–14441. [CrossRef]
24. Tarantino, G.; Balsano, C.; Santini, S.J.; Brienza, G.; Clemente, I.; Cosimini, B.; Sinatti, G. It is high time physicians thought of natural products for alleviating NAFLD. Is there sufficient evidence to use them? *Int. J. Mol. Sci.* **2021**, *22*, 13424. [CrossRef]
25. Pirillo, A.; Catapano, A.L. Berberine, a plant alkaloid with lipid- and glucose-lowering properties: From in vitro evidence to clinical studies. *Atherosclerosis* **2015**, *243*, 449–461. [CrossRef] [PubMed]
26. Song, D.; Hao, J.; Fan, D. Biological properties and clinical applications of berberine. *Front. Med.* **2020**, *14*, 564–582. [CrossRef] [PubMed]
27. Habtemariam, S. Berberine pharmacology and the gut microbiota: A hidden therapeutic link. *Pharmacol. Res.* **2020**, *155*, 104722. [CrossRef] [PubMed]
28. Zhu, C.; Huang, K.; Bai, Y.; Feng, X.; Gong, L.; Wei, C.; Huang, H.; Zhang, H. Dietary supplementation with berberine improves growth performance and modulates the composition and function of cecal microbiota in yellow-feathered broilers. *Poult. Sci.* **2021**, *100*, 1034–1048. [CrossRef] [PubMed]
29. Dehau, T.; Cherlet, M.; Croubels, S.; van Immerseel, F.; Goossens, E. A high dose of dietary berberine improves gut wall morphology, despite an expansion of Enterobacteriaceae and a reduction in beneficial microbiota in broiler chickens. *mSystems* **2023**, *8*, e0123922. [CrossRef] [PubMed]

30. Sun, R.; Yang, N.; Kong, B.; Cao, B.; Feng, D.; Yu, X.; Ge, C.; Huang, J.; Shen, J.; Wang, P.; et al. Orally administered berberine modulates hepatic lipid metabolism by altering microbial bile acid metabolism and the intestinal FXR signaling pathway. *Mol. Pharmacol.* **2017**, *91*, 110–122. [CrossRef] [PubMed]
31. Noh, J.W.; Jun, M.S.; Yang, H.K.; Lee, B.C. Cellular and molecular mechanisms and effects of berberine on obesity-induced inflammation. *Biomedicines* **2022**, *10*, 1739. [CrossRef]
32. Li, D.; Zheng, J.; Hu, Y.; Hou, H.; Hao, S.; Liu, N.; Wang, Y. Amelioration of intestinal barrier dysfunction by berberine in the treatment of nonalcoholic fatty liver disease in rats. *Pharmacogn. Mag.* **2017**, *13*, 677–682. [CrossRef] [PubMed]
33. Zhu, L.; Baker, S.S.; Gill, C.; Liu, W.; Alkhouri, R.; Baker, R.D.; Gill, S.R. Characterization of gut microbiomes in nonalcoholic steatohepatitis (NASH) patients: A connection between endogenous alcohol and NASH. *Hepatology* **2013**, *57*, 601–609. [CrossRef] [PubMed]
34. Jiang, D.; Zhang, J.; Lin, S.; Wang, Y.; Chen, Y.; Fan, J. Prolyl endopeptidase gene disruption improves gut dysbiosis and non-alcoholic fatty liver disease in mice induced by a high-fat diet. *Front. Cell Dev. Biol.* **2021**, *9*, 628143. [CrossRef] [PubMed]
35. Aron-Wisnewsky, J.; Vigliotti, C.; Witjes, J.; Le, P.; Holleboom, A.G.; Verheij, J.; Nieuwdorp, M.; Clement, K. Gut microbiota and human NAFLD: Disentangling microbial signatures from metabolic disorders. *Nat. Rev. Gastroenterol. Hepatol.* **2020**, *17*, 279–297. [CrossRef]
36. Krishnan, S.; Ding, Y.; Saedi, N.; Choi, M.; Sridharan, G.V.; Sherr, D.H.; Yarmush, M.L.; Alaniz, R.C.; Jayaraman, A.; Lee, K. Gut microbiota-derived tryptophan metabolites modulate inflammatory response in hepatocytes and macrophages. *Cell Rep.* **2018**, *23*, 1099–1111. [CrossRef]
37. Zhou, D.; Pan, Q.; Shen, F.; Cao, H.X.; Ding, W.J.; Chen, Y.W.; Fan, J.G. Total fecal microbiota transplantation alleviates high-fat diet-induced steatohepatitis in mice via beneficial regulation of gut microbiota. *Sci. Rep.* **2017**, *7*, 1529. [CrossRef]
38. Li, J.; Li, Y.; Feng, S.; He, K.; Guo, L.; Chen, W.; Wang, M.; Zhong, L.; Wu, C.; Peng, X.; et al. Differential effects of dietary white meat and red meat on NAFLD progression by modulating gut microbiota and metabolites in rats. *Oxidative Med. Cell. Longev.* **2022**, *2022*, 6908934. [CrossRef]
39. Wang, H.; Zhang, H.; Gao, Z.; Zhang, Q.; Gu, C. The mechanism of berberine alleviating metabolic disorder based on gut microbiome. *Front. Cell. Infect. Microbiol.* **2022**, *12*, 854885. [CrossRef]
40. Yu, M.; Alimujiang, M.; Hu, L.; Liu, F.; Bao, Y.; Yin, J. Berberine alleviates lipid metabolism disorders via inhibition of mitochondrial complex I in gut and liver. *Int. J. Biol. Sci.* **2021**, *17*, 1693–1707. [CrossRef]
41. Yue, S.J.; Liu, J.; Wang, A.T.; Meng, X.T.; Yang, Z.R.; Peng, C.; Guan, H.S.; Wang, C.Y.; Yan, D. Berberine alleviates insulin resistance by reducing peripheral branched-chain amino acids. *Am. J. Physiol.-Endocrinol. Metab.* **2019**, *316*, E73–E85. [CrossRef] [PubMed]
42. Wu, G.; Sun, X.; Cheng, H.; Xu, S.; Li, D.; Xie, Z. Large yellow tea extract ameliorates metabolic syndrome by suppressing lipogenesis through SIRT6/SREBP1 pathway and modulating microbiota in leptin receptor knockout rats. *Foods* **2022**, *11*, 1638. [CrossRef] [PubMed]
43. Martinez-Cuesta, M.C.; Del, C.R.; Garriga-Garcia, M.; Pelaez, C.; Requena, T. Taxonomic characterization and short-chain fatty acids production of the obese microbiota. *Front. Cell. Infect. Microbiol.* **2021**, *11*, 598093. [CrossRef]
44. Zeng, Q.; Li, D.; He, Y.; Li, Y.; Yang, Z.; Zhao, X.; Liu, Y.; Wang, Y.; Sun, J.; Feng, X.; et al. Discrepant gut microbiota markers for the classification of obesity-related metabolic abnormalities. *Sci. Rep.* **2019**, *9*, 13424. [CrossRef] [PubMed]
45. Vazquez-Moreno, M.; Perez-Herrera, A.; Locia-Morales, D.; Dizzel, S.; Meyre, D.; Stearns, J.C.; Cruz, M. Association of gut microbiome with fasting triglycerides, fasting insulin and obesity status in Mexican children. *Pediatr. Obes.* **2021**, *16*, e12748. [CrossRef] [PubMed]
46. Zhao, W.W.; Xiao, M.; Wu, X.; Li, X.W.; Li, X.X.; Zhao, T.; Yu, L.; Chen, X.Q. Ilexsaponin A (1) ameliorates diet-induced nonalcoholic fatty liver disease by regulating bile acid metabolism in mice. *Front. Pharmacol.* **2021**, *12*, 771976. [CrossRef] [PubMed]
47. Jiang, C.; Xie, C.; Lv, Y.; Li, J.; Krausz, K.W.; Shi, J.; Brocker, C.N.; Desai, D.; Amin, S.G.; Bisson, W.H.; et al. Intestine-selective farnesoid X receptor inhibition improves obesity-related metabolic dysfunction. *Nat. Commun.* **2015**, *6*, 10166. [CrossRef] [PubMed]
48. Lin, H.; An, Y.; Tang, H.; Wang, Y. Alterations of bile acids and gut microbiota in obesity induced by high fat diet in rat model. *J. Agric. Food. Chem.* **2019**, *67*, 3624–3632. [CrossRef]
49. Zhu, K.; Nie, S.; Gong, D.; Xie, M. Effect of polysaccharide from Ganoderma atrum on the serum metabolites of type 2 diabetic rats. *Food Hydrocoll.* **2016**, *53*, 31–36. [CrossRef]
50. He, Z.; Ma, Y.; Yang, S.; Zhang, S.; Liu, S.; Xiao, J.; Wang, Y.; Wang, W.; Yang, H.; Li, S.; et al. Gut microbiota-derived ursodeoxycholic acid from neonatal dairy calves improves intestinal homeostasis and colitis to attenuate extended-spectrum beta-lactamase-producing enteroaggregative Escherichia coli infection. *Microbiome* **2022**, *10*, 79. [CrossRef]
51. Sirvent, A.; Claudel, T.; Martin, G.; Brozek, J.; Kosykh, V.; Darteil, R.; Hum, D.W.; Fruchart, J.C.; Staels, B. The farnesoid X receptor induces very low-density lipoprotein receptor gene expression. *FEBS Lett.* **2004**, *566*, 173–177. [CrossRef]
52. Staels, B.; Fonseca, V.A. Bile acids and metabolic regulation: Mechanisms and clinical responses to bile acid sequestration. *Diabetes Care* **2009**, *32* (Suppl. S2), S237–S245. [CrossRef] [PubMed]
53. Neuschwander-Tetri, B.A.; Loomba, R.; Sanyal, A.J.; Lavine, J.E.; Van Natta, M.L.; Abdelmalek, M.F.; Chalasani, N.; Dasarathy, S.; Diehl, A.M.; Hameed, B.; et al. Farnesoid X nuclear receptor ligand obeticholic acid for non-cirrhotic, non-alcoholic steatohepatitis (FLINT): A multicentre, randomised, placebo-controlled trial. *Lancet* **2015**, *385*, 956–965. [CrossRef] [PubMed]

54. Li, X.; Zhao, W.; Xiao, M.; Yu, L.; Chen, Q.; Hu, X.; Zhao, Y.; Xiong, L.; Chen, X.; Wang, X.; et al. Penthorum chinense Pursh. extract attenuates non-alcholic fatty liver disease by regulating gut microbiota and bile acid metabolism in mice. *J. Ethnopharmacol.* **2022**, *294*, 115333. [CrossRef] [PubMed]
55. Yang, C.; Wan, M.; Xu, D.; Pan, D.; Xia, H.; Yang, L.; Sun, G. Flaxseed powder attenuates non-alcoholic steatohepatitis via modulation of gut microbiota and bile acid metabolism through gut-liver axis. *Int. J. Mol. Sci.* **2021**, *22*, 10858. [CrossRef] [PubMed]
56. Haczeyni, F.; Poekes, L.; Wang, H.; Mridha, A.R.; Barn, V.; Geoffrey, H.W.; Ioannou, G.N.; Yeh, M.M.; Leclercq, I.A.; Teoh, N.C.; et al. Obeticholic acid improves adipose morphometry and inflammation and reduces steatosis in dietary but not metabolic obesity in mice. *Obesity* **2017**, *25*, 155–165. [CrossRef] [PubMed]
57. Hassan, H.M.; Guo, H.; Yousef, B.A.; Guerram, M.; Hamdi, A.M.; Zhang, L.; Jiang, Z. Role of inflammatory and oxidative stress, cytochrome P450 2E1, and bile acid disturbance in rat liver injury induced by isoniazid and lipopolysaccharide cotreatment. *Antimicrob. Agents. Chemother.* **2016**, *60*, 5285–5293. [CrossRef]
58. Gao, X.; Liu, P.; Wu, C.; Wang, T.; Liu, G.; Cao, H.; Zhang, C.; Hu, G.; Guo, X. Effects of fatty liver hemorrhagic syndrome on the AMP-activated protein kinase signaling pathway in laying hens. *Poult. Sci.* **2019**, *98*, 2201–2210. [CrossRef]
59. Huang, F.; Zheng, X.; Ma, X.; Jiang, R.; Zhou, W.; Zhou, S.; Zhang, Y.; Lei, S.; Wang, S.; Kuang, J.; et al. Theabrownin from Pu-erh tea attenuates hypercholesterolemia via modulation of gut microbiota and bile acid metabolism. *Nat. Commun.* **2019**, *10*, 4971. [CrossRef] [PubMed]
60. Zheng, X.; Huang, F.; Zhao, A.; Lei, S.; Zhang, Y.; Xie, G.; Chen, T.; Qu, C.; Rajani, C.; Dong, B.; et al. Bile acid is a significant host factor shaping the gut microbiome of diet-induced obese mice. *BMC Biol.* **2017**, *15*, 120. [CrossRef]
61. Xie, G.; Wang, Y.; Wang, X.; Zhao, A.; Chen, T.; Ni, Y.; Wong, L.; Zhang, H.; Zhang, J.; Liu, C.; et al. Profiling of serum bile acids in a healthy Chinese population using UPLC-MS/MS. *J. Proteome Res.* **2015**, *14*, 850–859. [CrossRef] [PubMed]

Disclaimer/Publisher's Note: The statements, opinions and data contained in all publications are solely those of the individual author(s) and contributor(s) and not of MDPI and/or the editor(s). MDPI and/or the editor(s) disclaim responsibility for any injury to people or property resulting from any ideas, methods, instructions or products referred to in the content.

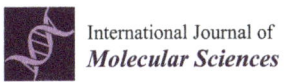

Review

Therapeutic Applications of Ginseng Natural Compounds for Health Management

Syed Sayeed Ahmad [1,2], Khurshid Ahmad [1,2], Ye Chan Hwang [1], Eun Ju Lee [1,2] and Inho Choi [1,2,*]

1. Department of Medical Biotechnology, Yeungnam University, Gyeongsan 38541, Republic of Korea; sayeedahmad4@gmail.com (S.S.A.); ahmadkhursheed2008@gmail.com (K.A.); 1230hyc@naver.com (Y.C.H.); gorapadoc0315@hanmail.net (E.J.L.)
2. Research Institute of Cell Culture, Yeungnam University, Gyeongsan 38541, Republic of Korea
* Correspondence: inhochoi@ynu.ac.kr; Tel.: +82-01-3264-9392

Abstract: Ginseng is usually consumed as a daily food supplement to improve health and has been shown to benefit skeletal muscle, improve glucose metabolism, and ameliorate muscle-wasting conditions, cardiovascular diseases, stroke, and the effects of aging and cancers. Ginseng has also been reported to help maintain bone strength and liver (digestion, metabolism, detoxification, and protein synthesis) and kidney functions. In addition, ginseng is often used to treat age-associated neurodegenerative disorders, and ginseng and ginseng-derived natural products are popular natural remedies for diseases such as diabetes, obesity, oxidative stress, and inflammation, as well as fungal, bacterial, and viral infections. Ginseng is a well-known herbal medication, known to alleviate the actions of several cytokines. The article concludes with future directions and significant application of ginseng compounds for researchers in understanding the promising role of ginseng in the treatment of several diseases. Overall, this study was undertaken to highlight the broad-spectrum therapeutic applications of ginseng compounds for health management.

Keywords: ginseng; compounds; treatment; disease; mechanism

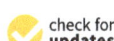

Citation: Ahmad, S.S.; Ahmad, K.; Hwang, Y.C.; Lee, E.J.; Choi, I. Therapeutic Applications of Ginseng Natural Compounds for Health Management. *Int. J. Mol. Sci.* **2023**, *24*, 17290. https://doi.org/10.3390/ijms242417290

Academic Editors: Marilena Gilca and Adelina Vlad

Received: 15 November 2023
Revised: 6 December 2023
Accepted: 7 December 2023
Published: 9 December 2023

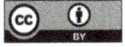

Copyright: © 2023 by the authors. Licensee MDPI, Basel, Switzerland. This article is an open access article distributed under the terms and conditions of the Creative Commons Attribution (CC BY) license (https://creativecommons.org/licenses/by/4.0/).

1. Introduction

Natural products are viewed as a primary source of therapeutic agents and have been identified in plants, microorganisms, animals, insects, and marine organisms [1]. Natural products have diverse pharmacological properties and play important roles in drug discovery and development by serving as novel lead templates. Aspirin (from willow tree bark), digoxin (from the flower; *Digitalis lanata*), morphine (from opium), artemisinin, camptothecin, lovastatin, maytansine, reserpine, and silibinin are just a few examples of drugs directly or indirectly derived from natural products [2]. Some semi-synthetic therapeutic agents (hybrids of natural and synthetic sources), such as penicillin [3] and paclitaxel (an anti-cancer drug derived from the Pacific yew, *Taxus brevifolia*) [4], are typically produced by chemically transforming natural products [5]. The chemical, functional, and structural diversities of small molecule natural products have been explored [2]. The interactions between biological macromolecules (mainly proteins) and natural products explain the therapeutic efficacies of natural products. Furthermore, natural products do not cause as many adverse effects as synthetic compounds and combinatorial libraries [2].

The use of Chinese medicine has risen in popularity after the 2015 Nobel Prize was awarded for the discovery that artemisinin is an effective treatment for malaria [6]. Ginseng (a medicinal herb) and its derived natural products are amongst the most popular natural remedies and are used to treat various diseases and conditions such as diabetes [7], anti-oxidative [8], inflammation [9], cancers [10], fungal, bacterial, viral, stress [11], and neurodegenerative diseases (ND) [12], as well as brain ischemia [13], hypertension [14], obesity [15], cardiovascular diseases and stroke [16], sarcopenia [17], muscle-wasting conditions [18–20], muscle aging, and cancer cachexia [21–23]. Known side effects of ginseng include headaches, diarrhea, blood pressure changes, skin irritations, and vaginal bleeding [24]. Overall, ginseng has been reported to be a useful management option for many diseases, as is suggested by its name—Panax is derived from the Greek pan akheia, meaning "cures all diseases" [25]. A summary of known ginseng compounds is provided in Table 1.

Table 1. List of several known compounds of ginseng along with their molecular formula and weight. The compounds known in the different parts of the ginseng plant, such as root and flower bud, having higher molecular weight as compared to other parts of the ginseng plant.

Part of Ginseng	Compounds Name	PubChem ID	Molecular Formula	Molecular Weight (g/mol)
Hydrolysis	Protopanaxadiol (PPD)	9920281	$C_{30}H_{52}O_3$	460.7
	Protopanaxatriol (PPT)	9847853	$C_{30}H_{52}O_4$	476.7
	Panaxadiol	73498	$C_{30}H_{52}O_3$	460.7
	Panaxatriol	73599	$C_{30}H_{52}O_4$	476.7
Leaves	Ginsenoside F1	9809542	$C_{36}H_{62}O_9$	638.9
	Ginsenoside F2	9918692	$C_{42}H_{72}O_{13}$	785.0
	Ginsenoside F3	46887678	$C_{41}H_{70}O_{13}$	771.0
	Ginsenoside F4	102004835	$C_{42}H_{70}O_{12}$	767.0
	Ginsenoside Ki	102294899	$C_{37}H_{64}O_{10}$	668.9
	Ginsenoside Km	102294900	$C_{37}H_{64}O_{10}$	668.9
	Ginsenoside Rh6	131752646	$C_{36}H_{62}O_{11}$	670.9
	Ginsenoside Rh7	101096472	$C_{36}H_{60}O_9$	636.9
	Ginsenoside Rh8	85245726	$C_{36}H_{60}O_9$	636.9
Roots	Ginsenoside Ra1	100941542	$C_{58}H_{98}O_{26}$	1211.4
	Ginsenoside Ra2	100941543	$C_{58}H_{98}O_{26}$	1211.4
	Ginsenoside Ra3	73157064	$C_{59}H_{100}O_{27}$	1241.4
	Ginsenoside Rb1	9898279	$C_{54}H_{92}O_{23}$	1109.3
	Malonylginsenoside Rb1	118987129	$C_{57}H_{94}O_{26}$	1195.3
	Ginsenoside Rb2	6917976	$C_{53}H_{90}O_{22}$	1079.3
	Ginsenoside Rb3	12912363	$C_{53}H_{90}O_{22}$	1079.3
	Ginsenoside Rc	12855889	$C_{53}H_{90}O_{22}$	1079.3
	Ginsenoside Rd	11679800	$C_{48}H_{82}O_{18}$	947.2
	Ginsenoside Rf	441922	$C_{42}H_{72}O_{14}$	801.0
	20-Glucoginsenoside Rf	3052077	$C_{48}H_{82}O_{19}$	963.2
	Ginsenoside Rg1	441923	$C_{42}H_{72}O_{14}$	801.0
	Ginsenoside Rg2	21599924	$C_{42}H_{72}O_{13}$	785.0
	Ginsenoside Ro	11815492	$C_{48}H_{76}O_{19}$	957.1
	Ginsenoside Rs1	85044013	$C_{55}H_{92}O_{23}$	1121.3
	Ginsenoside Rs2	162343294	$C_{55}H_{92}O_{23}$	1121.3

Table 1. Cont.

Part of Ginseng	Compounds Name	PubChem ID	Molecular Formula	Molecular Weight (g/mol)
Steamed roots	Ginsenoside Rg3	9918693	$C_{42}H_{72}O_{13}$	785.0
	Ginsenoside Rg5	11550001	$C_{42}H_{70}O_{12}$	767.0
	Ginsenoside Rg6	91895489	$C_{42}H_{70}O_{12}$	767.0
	Ginsenoside Rh1	12855920	$C_{36}H_{62}O_9$	638.9
	Ginsenoside Rh2	119307	$C_{36}H_{62}O_8$	622.9
	Ginsenoside Rh3	20839223	$C_{36}H_{60}O_7$	604.9
	Ginsenoside Rh4	21599928	$C_{36}H_{60}O_8$	620.9
	Ginsenoside Rh5	10699455	$C_{37}H_{64}O_9$	652.9
	Ginsenoside Rk1	11499198	$C_{42}H_{70}O_{12}$	767.0
	Ginsenoside Rk2	90472238	$C_{36}H_{60}O_7$	604.9
	Ginsenoside Rk3	75412555	$C_{36}H_{60}O_8$	620.9
	Ginsenoside Rs3	100937823	$C_{44}H_{74}O_{14}$	827.0
	Ginsenoside Rs5	102021585	$C_{44}H_{72}O_{13}$	809.0
Flower buds	Floralginsenoside A	16655581	$C_{42}H_{72}O_{16}$	833.0
	Floralginsenoside B	101423532	$C_{50}H_{84}O_{21}$	1021.2
	Floralginsenoside C	16655212	$C_{42}H_{72}O_{15}$	817.0
	Floralginsenoside D	16655213	$C_{42}H_{72}O_{15}$	817.0
	Floralginsenoside E	101423533	$C_{41}H_{70}O_{15}$	803.0
	Floralginsenoside F	101423534	$C_{48}H_{82}O_{20}$	979.2
	Floralginsenoside G	101423535	$C_{48}H_{82}O_{21}$	995.2
	Floralginsenoside H	101423536	$C_{53}H_{90}O_{25}$	1127.3
	Floralginsenoside I	16655580	$C_{42}H_{72}O_{16}$	833.0
	Floralginsenoside J	101423537	$C_{41}H_{70}O_{15}$	803.0
	Floralginsenoside K	101423538	$C_{50}H_{84}O_{21}$	1021.2
	Floralginsenoside Lb	102512867	$C_{48}H_{82}O_{19}$	963.2
	Floralginsenoside M	101423540	$C_{48}H_{82}O_{19}$	963.2
	Floralginsenoside N	101423541	$C_{53}H_{90}O_{22}$	1079.3
	Floralginsenoside O	101423542	$C_{53}H_{90}O_{22}$	1079.3
	Floralginsenoside P	101423543	$C_{53}H_{90}O_{23}$	1095.3
	Floralginsenoside Ta	46224641	$C_{36}H_{60}O_{10}$	652.9
	Floralginsenoside Tb	46224642	$C_{35}H_{62}O_{11}$	658.9
	Floralginsenoside Tc	46224643	$C_{53}H_{90}O_{25}$	1127.3
	Floralginsenoside Td	46224646	$C_{53}H_{90}O_{25}$	1127.3
	Ginsenoside I	102050355	$C_{48}H_{82}O_{20}$	979.2
	Ginsenoside II	101717751	$C_{48}H_{82}O_{19}$	963.2
Fruits	25-Hydroxyprotopanaxadiol	158501	$C_{30}H_{54}O_4$	478.7
Seeds	Panaxadione	25233029	$C_{30}H_{48}O_5$	488.7

Seventeen Panax species are now recognized, but commercial *P. ginseng* cultivars are largely found in South Korea and China [26]. The two most well-known are *Panax ginseng* and *Panax quinquefolius* [27]. The world's major ginseng producers are China,

South Korea, Canada, and the United States [27], and South Korea is the largest ginseng distributor [27]. *P. ginseng* and its ginsenoside components are non-toxic and used to treat chemotherapy-induced side effects such as nephrotoxicity, hepatotoxicity, cardiotoxicity, immunotoxicity, and hematopoietic suppression [28]. Here, we report the broad-spectrum therapeutic applications of known ginseng compounds. The strategy used to identify the articles include performing thorough searches in reputable academic databases such as PubMed, Scopus, SciFinder, Science Direct, Google Scholar, and the Scientific Information Database. The study focused on English language papers with particular keywords related to ginseng plants, natural compounds, biological investigations, and activities. The aim of this review was to explore ginseng-related natural compounds with potential use for the management of human health.

2. Protopanaxadiol (PPD) and Protopanaxatriol (PPT)

Protopanaxadiol (PPD) and protopanaxatriol (PPT) are active compounds found in members of the *Panax* genus, mainly in the roots, stems, leaves, and flowers. PPD is used to treat endometriosis and has been shown to significantly upregulate endometrial receptivity-related molecules, such as interleukin 6 family cytokine, insulin-like growth factor-binding protein 1, and collagens, to restrict the pelvic macrophage inflammatory response and to recover fertility in mice with endometriosis. Thus, the literature shows that PPD prevents and is a promising treatment for endometriosis [29]. On the other hand, PPT ginsenosides have pharmacological effects on the central nervous and cardiovascular systems [30], and PPT reportedly acts as a PPARγ antagonist [31]; thus, targeting PPARγ is considered a promising treatment option for obesity.

3. Ginsenoside F1 (GF1)

GF1 is a ginseng saponin isolated from a traditional Chinese medicine used to treat ischemic stroke. GF1 activates the IGF-1/IGF1R pathway [32] to promote angiogenesis, which reduces cerebral ischemia. In addition, GF1 may improve cerebrovascular function and accelerate recovery from ischemic stroke. In zebrafish, GF1 repaired vascular defects caused by axitinib [33], and in vivo and in vitro studies revealed that GF1 protects against Aβ accumulation. At 2.5 µM, GF1 reduced Aβ-induced cytotoxicity by reducing Aβ accumulation in mouse neuroblastoma neuro-2a (N2a) and human neuroblastoma SH-SY5Y neuronal cell lines. Additionally, GF1 reduced Aβ plaques in the hippocampus of (APP/PS1) double-transgenic AD mice [34,35]. Collectively, studies have shown GF1 is a highly active component in *P. ginseng* that can cross the BBB and has therapeutic potential for treating ND. Furthermore, GF1 reduces eosinophilic inflammation in chronic rhinosinusitis by enhancing NK cell activity [36].

4. Ginsenoside F2 (GF2)

GF2 is a minor component in *P. ginseng* with therapeutic applications in inflammatory diseases [37]. GF2 treatment attenuated liver damage in C57BL/6J WT mice (a model of alcoholic liver injury) [37] and suppressed the expression of TGF-β2 (a pro-apoptotic factor) to reduce hair loss in a dihydrotestosterone-induced mouse model [38]. It has been well established that excessive alcohol consumption can result in vitamin/mineral shortages (possibly due to liver damage) and subsequent hair loss because appropriate nourishment is required to maintain hair quality. In addition, alcohol suppresses nutrient breakdown and the body's capacity to absorb nutrients. Currently, hair loss is a major issue among young men. We suggest that the effects of GF2 on known targets of hair loss should be investigated to manage this condition.

5. Ginsenoside F3 (GF3)

GF3 was isolated from the leaves of *P. ginseng* [39]. At concentrations ranging from 0.1 to 100 µmol/L, GF3 not only stimulated murine spleen cell proliferation but also raised the production of IL-2 and IFN-γ. It improved immunity by modulating the synthesis and gene expression of type 1 and 2 cytokines in murine spleen cells [40].

6. Ginsenoside F4 (GF4)

GF4 considerably enhanced the hyperglycemic state of db/db mice, alleviated dyslipidemia, and helped in SM glucose uptake. Protein tyrosine phosphatase 1B (PTP1B) is a major negative regulator of the insulin signaling pathway. The inhibition of this enzyme by GF4 resulted in increased insulin receptor and insulin receptor substrate 1 tyrosine phosphorylation and enhanced insulin sensitivity. Overall, GF4 activates the insulin signaling pathway by inhibiting PTP1B [41]. Further, GF4 has an inhibitory effect on human lymphocytoma Jurkat (JK) cell by inducing apoptosis [42].

7. Ginsenoside Ra1 (GRa1)

GRa1 is a key active ingredient in ginseng with immune regulatory, anti-inflammatory, and anti-oxidant properties [43]. Little is known about the effects of GRa1 on human health compared to other known ginseng compounds. GRa1 can affect the cardiovascular system, immune regulation, and nervous system [44]. It is present in both red ginseng powder and red ginseng concentrate samples [45]. GRa1 has been reported as a significant inhibitor of protein tyrosine kinase activation induced by in vitro hypoxia/reoxygenation in cultured human umbilical vein endothelial cells [46]. However, GRa1 has been shown to have anti-inflammatory and anti-oxidant properties, and thus it might be effective for the management of cancers and other inflammation-related diseases such as autoimmune diseases (rheumatoid arthritis), cardiovascular diseases (high blood pressure and heart disease), and gastrointestinal disorders (inflammatory bowel disease).

8. Ginsenoside Rb1 (GRb1)

In vitro and in vivo studies have demonstrated GRb1 to have diverse pharmacological applications in metabolic disorders due to its anti-apoptotic effects and ability to regulate oxidative stress, inflammatory responses, and autophagy. In addition, GRb1 suppresses obesity, hyperglycemia, and diabetes by regulating glycolipid metabolism and improving insulin and leptin sensitivities [47]. GRb1 may increase insulin sensitivity by downregulating 11β-hydroxysteroid dehydrogenase type 1 in T2D [48]. The administration of GRb1 (60 mg/kg of body mass intraperitoneally (i.p.)) daily for 12 days decreased adipose tissue and leptin levels in KK-Ay DM mice [49]. Furthermore, GRb1 (20 mg/kg of body mass, daily) reduced hepatic fat formation and enhanced insulin sensitivity in obese diabetic db/db mice; these effects were confirmed by reductions in liver weight and hepatic triglyceride contents [50]. GRb1 at 10 mg/kg of body mass (i.p.) daily considerably reduced body weight gain, improved glucose tolerance, and increased fasting plasma insulin levels in high-fat diet-induced obese mice and rats [51,52]. In addition, GRb1 increased GLUT4 translocation in C2C12 myotubes and 3T3-L1 cells by activating the adiponectin signaling pathway [53]. Notably, GRb1 is a major component of ginseng [53], which is frequently used as a natural medication in diabetic patients. Altogether, GRb1 has the potential to be used as an anti-obesity, anti-hyperglycemic, and anti-diabetic drug that affects multiple targets.

9. Ginsenoside Rb2 (GRb2)

It is a PPD-type saponin abundant in the stems and leaves of ginseng [54]. GRb2 significantly enhanced the viability of HT22 murine hippocampal neuronal cells [55] and inhibited the growth, migration, and invasion of colorectal cancer cells (HT29 and SW620 cell lines) [56]. GRb2 has been used to manage atherosclerosis [57], insulin resistance and obesity [58], endothelial cell senescence [59], and suppression of glutamate-induced neurotoxicity [55]. Thus, GRb2 appears to have potential for treating diabetes, obesity, tumors, viral infections, and cardiovascular conditions.

10. Ginsenoside Rb3 (GRb3)

GRb3 is a ginseng-derived natural product with cardioprotective properties [60] that can reduce the risk of myocardial infarction by inhibiting oxidative stress and suppressing inflammation [61]. It was found in an in vivo study to reduce the levels of the inflammatory markers NF-κB and CD45 and enhance the activities of crucial proteins of the contraction unit (cardiac troponin protein I (cTnI) and α-actinin) to recover cardiac function [62]. Furthermore, in vivo and in vitro studies have shown GRb3 mitigates oxidative stress by triggering the anti-oxidation signaling of PERK/Nrf2/HMOX1 [63]. Studies indicate that GRb3 may be helpful for treating heart-related disorders.

11. Ginsenoside Rc (GRc)

GRc has been reported to enhance bone development in ovariectomy-induced osteoporotic mice and to stimulate osteogenic differentiation in vitro through the Wnt/β-catenin signaling pathway [64]. Additionally, an in vivo study demonstrated that GRc administration significantly attenuated acetaminophen-induced hepatotoxicity, repaired liver damage, and improved survival [65]. In addition, in a dose-dependent manner, GRc reduced the proliferation and viability of 3T3L1 preadipocytes, adipocyte numbers, and lipid accumulation in maturing 3T3L1 preadipocytes, indicating it inhibited lipogenesis [66]. Collectively, it would appear that GRc has potential utility for managing several diseases.

12. Ginsenoside Rd (GRd)

The leading causes of muscle wasting are aging and cancer, and there are no effective cures for these conditions. However, GRd has been shown to alleviate muscle wasting. In mice, GRd administration suppressed age- and cancer-induced muscle atrophy and improved grip strength, hanging times, muscle mass, and muscle tissue cross-sectional areas; at the molecular level, GRd inhibited STAT3 phosphorylation and suppressed atrogin-1, muscle RING-finger protein-1 (MuRF-1), and myostatin levels [67]. Myostatin is a well-known inhibitor of muscle development [68]. MuRF1 is a key factor in the SM atrophy process that occurs during catabolic conditions, making MuRF1 a promising target for pharmaceutical therapies for muscle-wasting conditions [69]. SM improvement is necessary for healthy life [70,71]. Furthermore, GRd improved ischemic stroke-induced damage by suppressing oxidative stress and inflammation, prolonging neural cell survival by upregulating the endogenous anti-oxidant system and phosphoinositide-3-kinase/AKT signaling [72]. Thus, GRd may be an innovative natural product for treating muscle-wasting conditions, act as an anti-diabetic therapy by improving muscle health, and have anti-inflammatory, neuroprotective, and cardioprotective properties.

13. Ginsenoside Rf (GRf)

GRf is a constituent of Korean ginseng and upregulates markers of myoblast differentiation and mitochondrial biogenesis. GRf improves exercise tolerance in mice, possibly by enhancing mitochondrial biogenesis and myoblast differentiation via AMPK and p38 MAPK signaling pathways, suggesting that GRf boosts energy production to meet the increased demands of working muscle cells [73]. In addition, GRf has been reported to have neuroprotective and anti-inflammatory effects under hypoxic conditions. The binding of GRf at the active site of PPARγ suggests that it binds at the position used by known agonists [74]. In 3T3L1 adipocytes, GRf treatment downregulated PPARγ and perilipin (lipid droplet-associated protein) levels and reduced lipid accumulation [75]. These observations suggest GRf might be useful for treating obesity.

14. Ginsenoside Rg2 (GRg2)

GRg2 promotes porcine mesenchymal stem cell (pMSC) proliferation, prevents D-galactose-induced oxidative stress and senescence, and increases autophagic activity through the AMPK signaling pathway. Furthermore, long-term culture with GRg2 promoted pMSC proliferation, prevented replicative senescence, and preserved stemness [76].

In addition, the ability of GRg2 to exert its anti-atherosclerotic effects at the cellular and animal levels supports ginseng's role as a functional dietary regulator [77]. Additionally, GRg2 was found to decrease mRNA levels of the inflammatory factors TNF, IL-6, and IL-8, and at 20 µM, it considerably suppressed IL-6, IL-8, and IL-1 [77]. These findings suggest a strategy for muscle regeneration based on the in vitro expansion of pMSCs.

15. Ginsenoside Rg3 (GRg3)

Acute pancreatitis (AP) is a systemic inflammatory response syndrome. In a study performed using a cerulein-induced murine model of AP to investigate the effect of GRg3, cerulein increased serum amylase, TNFα, IL-6, IL-1β, ROS, and Fe^{2+} levels, and GRg3 co-treatment decreased cerulein-induced ROS buildup and cell death in pancreatic tissues [78]. Due to the lack of an effective delivery approach, it is difficult to deliver GRg3 to body organs due to its hydrophobic nature. However, the intramyocardial injection of GRg3-loaded PEG-b-PPS nanoparticles in a rat ischemia–reperfusion model improved cardiac functions and reduced infarct sizes [79].

16. Ginsenoside Rg5 (GRg5)

GRg5 was administered to nude mice bearing A549/T tumors to combat multidrug resistance. Treatment with GRg5 and docetaxel considerably suppressed the growth of drug-resistant tumors without increasing toxicity compared to docetaxel alone at the same dose [80]. In another study, GRg5 remarkably suppressed breast cancer cell propagation by inducing mitochondria-mediated apoptosis and autophagic cell death. It was also found that GRg5 decreased the phosphorylation of PI3K, Akt, and mTOR and attenuated PI3K/Akt signaling in breast cancer [81]. Thus, GRg5 has therapeutic potential as a breast cancer treatment. Furthermore, GRg5 [82] and GRh1 [83] can both alleviate cisplatin-induced nephrotoxicity [82], presumably due to their anti-oxidant, anti-apoptotic, and anti-inflammatory effects.

17. Ginsenoside Rh1 (GRh1)

GRh1 is obtained from red ginseng and used to improve physical fitness. In a cisplatin-induced injury model, GRh1 enhanced the vitality of HK-2 cells and inhibited ROS production and apoptosis [83], which suggested that GRh1 has potential use for alleviating cisplatin-induced nephrotoxicity in cancer patients. In addition, GRh1 was found to have an anti-cancer effect on breast cancer by inhibiting the ROS-mediated PI3K/Akt pathway and causing cell cycle arrest, apoptosis, and autophagy [84]. An in vitro study reported that GRh1 (at 100 µM) significantly inhibited cell migration and invasion and effectively inhibited colorectal cancer development [85]. Currently, GRh1 is mostly being used as an anticancer agent and could be further explored for its use against various other cancers.

18. Ginsenoside Rh2 (GRh2)

GRh2 is obtained from the roots of *P. ginseng* and has been reported to have anti-tumor effects by immunomodulating the tumor microenvironment (TME) [86], regulating HMGB1/NF-κB signaling, and improving the oxygen–glucose deprived environment of cardiomyocytes [87]. However, the in vivo effects of GRh2 have not yet been well explored, and its therapeutic effects are unknown.

19. Ginsenoside Rh3 (GRh3)

Lung cancer is the second most common cause of cancer-related death after breast cancer [88]. In vitro, GRh3 (at 50 µM) inhibited the proliferation of A549 and PC9 cells, and in another in vitro study, GRh3 inhibited tumor growth by causing cell arrest in the G1 phase. In vivo, GRh3 at 50 and 100 mg/kg significantly inhibited lung cancer metastasis [89]. GRh3 also inhibited HCT116 (colon cancer) cell proliferation, invasion, migration, and arrested cells in the G1 phase by downregulating genes related to DNA replication [90]. In addition, GRh3 significantly ameliorated myocardial necrosis and caspase 3 levels in male Sprague Dawley rat myocardial tissues by hindering the p38 MAPK pathway [91].

20. Ginsenoside Rh4 (GRh4)

GRh4 significantly inhibited the production of pro-inflammatory cytokines (TNF-α, IL-6, and IL-1β) in RAW264.7 cells (macrophages). JAK-STAT, TNF, NF-κB, and PI3K-Akt were identified as the main pathways used by GRh4 to reduce inflammation [92]. It has also been reported that GRh4 protects kidneys from cisplatin-induced oxidative injury [93]. GRh4 has been shown to have a high anti-lung adenocarcinoma efficacy in vitro and in vivo. Lung adenocarcinoma is a typical cellular breakdown in the lungs with a high harm that desperately should be treated [94]. Further, it is reported that GRh4 inhibits colorectal cancer cell proliferation [95], breast cancer growth [96], and delays SM aging through the SIRT1 pathway [97].

21. Ginsenoside Rh7 (GRh7)

GRh7 has been reported to inhibit H1299 (a lymph node-derived human non-small cell lung cancer cell line) growth (by 83%) and proliferation. In the same study, A549 (also an NSCLC cell line) and H1299 cells were used to study the time-dependent effects of GRh7 on cell growth. After treatment with 25 μM GRh7 for 4 days, A549 growth was inhibited by 72% and H1299 growth by 75% compared to non-treated controls [98]. These results suggest GRh7 has anti-cancerous properties that warrant further investigation.

22. Ginsenoside Rk1 (GRk1)

GRk1 is produced by thermally dehydrating GRg3, a saponin present in *Panax ginseng* Meyer. GRk1 effectively inhibited N-methyl-D-aspartate receptors in cultured hippocampal neurons [99] and protected human melanocytes from H_2O_2-induced death. PIG1 melanocytes were pretreated with GRk1 at 0, 0.1, 0.2, or 0.4 mM for 2 h and then exposed to H_2O_2 under cytotoxic conditions (at 1.0 mM for 24 h). GRk1 pretreatment at 0.2 or 0.4 mM for 2 h considerably improved cell viability and decreased cell shrinkage versus H_2O_2 treatment controls [100]. In another study, GRk1 treatment reversed cisplatin-induced increases in the protein levels of Bax, cleaved caspase 3 and 9, and Bcl-2 [101]. GRk1 was also reported to have anti-tumor activity against lung squamous cell carcinoma [102], and at 30 mg/kg, GRk1 injections markedly inhibited tumor xenograft growth [103].

23. Ginsenoside Rk3 (GRk3)

GRk3 is a key bioactive constituent in ginseng and has robust anti-oxidant properties. GRk3 was found to enhance neuronal apoptosis, decrease intracellular ROS production, and restore mitochondrial membrane potentials in PC12 and primary neuronal cells. GRk3 also improved spatial learning and reduced memory deficits in an amyloid precursor protein (APP)/presenilin 1 (PS1) double transgenic mouse model of Alzheimer's disease (AD) [104]. AD has devastating effects on society with a limited number of approaches for its treatment [105]. AD is caused by mutations in one of the genes that codes for APP and presenilins 1 and 2. The majority of these gene mutations boost Aβ42 production [106]. Parkinson's disease (PD) is the second most common ND without any proper cure [107] and is categorized as a movement disorder. Natural products for the management of PD have also been reported [108]. Additionally, several other natural products have been reported for the management of AD and other NDs [109,110]. The anti-cancer effects of GRk3 were also checked in Eca109 and KYSE150 cell lines (both esophageal squamous carcinoma cell lines), and it was observed that GRk3 suppressed proliferation and colony formation for both cell types. This inhibition was ascribed to blocking of the PI3K/Akt/mTOR pathway and consequent activation of apoptosis and autophagy [111]. GRk3 might be an effective anti-tumor agent for esophageal cancer and for the treatment of renal dysfunctions caused by cisplatin-induced oxidative injury [93]. Furthermore, GRk3 improved hematopoietic function in myelosuppressed mice [112] and inhibited the proliferation, migration, and invasion associated with the extramedullary infiltration of leukemia [113].

24. Ginsenoside Ro (GRo)

GRo is a primary saponin in *P. ginseng* C.A. Meyer with several biological actions. In B16F10 tumor-bearing mice, GRo significantly inhibited tumor growth [114], LPS-induced lung damage, and TNF, IL-6, and IL-1 transcript levels in tumor tissues. Furthermore, in a dose-dependent manner, GRo suppressed the phosphorylation of NF-κB and MAPKs and the nuclear translocation of the p65 subunit. These findings imply that GRo targets inflammation by directly inhibiting the TLR4 signaling pathway [115]. The anti-inflammatory effects of GRo have been linked to a significant decrease in levels of pro-inflammatory cytokines generated by lipopolysaccharides. In a dose-dependent manner, GRo enhances cell survival while lowering reactive oxygen species (ROS) and nitric oxide generation produced by lipopolysaccharides [116]. Further, GRo improves obesity and insulin resistance in mice [117].

25. Floralginsenoside A (FGA)

Melanin provides UV protection and removes ROS from the skin. However, excessive melanin production and its accumulation in the skin can result in pigmentation disorders (e.g., solar lentigo, melasma, and freckles) [118]. Melan-a cells, an immortalized C57BL/6 mouse melanocyte cell line containing high levels of melanin, were used to investigate the melanin-inhibitory activity of FGA. At a concentration of 160 μM, FGA inhibited melanin activity by 23.9% without causing cytotoxicity. Tyrosinase is a key player in the biosynthesis of melanin, and the main mechanism underlying the anti-melanogenesis effects of inhibitory agents involves the downregulation of MITF (microphthalmia-related transcription factor) due to the ERK-induced phosphorylation of MITF at serine-73, which triggers the ubiquitination of MITF and its subsequent degradation. The phosphorylation of MITF at serine 29 activates Akt signaling and inhibits melanin production. FGA can block MITF–tyrosinase signaling and/or activate ERK–Akt signaling, which are both involved in melanogenesis. In addition, FGA treatment dose-dependently decreases the expressions of tyrosinase and MITF. Furthermore, FGA (at 160 μM) significantly and dose-dependently augmented phospho-ERK and Akt signaling pathways [119]. Tyrosinase activity and melanin content inhibition may result in skin whitening. However, the potential carcinogenic side effects of the agent currently used (kojic acid) to whiten skin [120] necessitates the development of new, safer, more effective depigmenting agents, and natural products feature prominently in these studies. Makeup/cosmetic production is expanding, especially in South Korea. Thus, the identification of natural makeup agents is likely to result in commercially attractive health and skin care products.

26. Future Perspectives

This study was performed to summarize what is known about the influence of ginseng and its derived natural products on diseases. It is well known that synthetic drugs are associated with adverse effects and that herbal remedies have been used for millennia and are relatively free of side effects. As a result, perceptions are changing in favor of natural therapies and traditional medicines. In particular, ginseng has been administered as an herbal medicine for thousands of years and is now commercially available in pill and tea forms. Intriguingly, one clinical study reported that patients who took ginseng after curative surgery had a 38% higher overall survival rate and a 35% higher 5-year disease-free rate [19,121].

The roles and functions of a number of ginseng compounds are listed in Table 2. Several of the natural products isolated from ginseng are therapeutically beneficial. Natural products have been thoroughly investigated in vitro and in vivo, and we suggest in silico studies be undertaken to aid in the primary screening of ginseng natural products. It has been reported that in silico-screened compounds produce better results during subsequent in vitro or in vivo testing [122–124]. Most of the natural products mentioned have anti-diabetic, anti-neuroprotective, anti-cancer, anti-oxidant, and anti-inflammatory effects. We suggest that the repurposing of these compounds be attempted to improve their therapeutic effects.

Table 2. Therapeutic application of different ginseng compounds in disease management.

Compound Name	Function	Model/Object/Experiments	Reference
Protopanaxadiol	recovery from endometriosis	mice	[29]
Ginsenoside F2	alcoholic liver damage improvement	C57BL/6J WT or IL-10 knockout mice	[37]
Ginsenoside F1	repair the vascular defects caused by axitinib in zebrafish	in vivo tests in zebrafish	[33]
	reduce Aβ-induced cytotoxicity	neuroblastoma neuro-2a (mouse) and neuroblastoma SH-SY5Y (human)	[34]
Ginsenoside Rh7	anticancerous properties	A549 and H1299 cell line	[98]
Ginsenoside Rb1	decrease adipose tissue and leptin levels	KK-Ay DM mice	[49]
	reduce hepatic fat formation	obese diabetic db/db mice	[50]
	reduce body weight gain	HFD-induced obese mice	[51]
	increase GLUT4 translocation	C2C12 and 3T3-L1 cells	[53]
Ginsenoside Rb2	improve cell viability	HT22 murine hippocampal neuronal cells	[55]
	inhibit the growth of colorectal cancer cells	HT29 and SW620 cell lines	[56]
Ginsenoside Rc	enhance bone development	ovariectomy-induced osteoporosis mice	[64]
	reduce the proliferation and viability process	3T3L1	[66]
Ginsenoside Rd	enhance hypertrophy	aged mice	[67]
Ginsenoside Rg2	encourage pMSC proliferation	MTT assay	[76]
Ginsenoside Ro	inhibit tumor growth	B16F10 tumor-bearing mice	[114]
Ginsenoside Rg3	decrease ROS buildup	mice	[78]
Ginsenoside Rh2	improve the oxygen–glucose deprivation environment of cardiomyocytes	regulate the HMGB1/NF-κB signaling	[87]
Ginsenoside Rh1	anticancer effect on breast cancer cells	inhibition of the ROS-mediated PI3K/Akt pathway	[84]
Ginsenoside Rh3	inhibit proliferation	A549 and PC9 cells	[89]
Ginsenoside Rk3	improve neuronal apoptosis	PC12 and primary neuronal cells	[104]
Floralginsenoside A	melanin inhibitory activity	C57BL/6 mouse melanocyte cell line	[119]

27. Conclusions

Ginseng and ginseng-derived natural products are attractive candidates for the treatment of several disease. Furthermore, this study showed that ginseng and its derived natural products are powerful therapeutic agents/supplements that improve health and increase energy. Therefore, we suggest that clinical trials be performed to confirm the therapeutic efficacies of ginsenosides in cancer, stroke, obesity, aging, and NDs.

Author Contributions: S.S.A., K.A. and Y.C.H.: conceptualization; writing—original draft preparation; S.S.A. and K.A. data curation, E.J.L. and I.C.: supervision, writing—reviewing and editing. All authors have read and agreed to the published version of the manuscript.

Funding: This research was supported by the Basic Science Research Program of the National Research Foundation of Korea (NRF), funded by the Ministry of Education (2020R1A6A1A03044512), the National Research Foundation of Korea (NRF), and the Korean government (NRF-2021R1A2C2004177). In addition, the study was supported by the Forestry (IPET) through High Value-added Food Technology Development Program of the Korea Institute of Planning and Evaluation for Technology in Food and Agriculture, funded by the Ministry of Agriculture, Food, and Rural Affairs (MAFRA) (Grant nos. 322008-5).

Institutional Review Board Statement: Not applicable.

Informed Consent Statement: Not applicable.

Data Availability Statement: Not applicable.

Conflicts of Interest: The author declares no conflict of interest.

References

1. Ji, H.F.; Li, X.J.; Zhang, H.Y. Natural products and drug discovery. Can thousands of years of ancient medical knowledge lead us to new and powerful drug combinations in the fight against cancer and dementia? *EMBO Rep.* **2009**, *10*, 194–200. [CrossRef] [PubMed]
2. Mathur, S.; Hoskins, C. Drug development: Lessons from nature. *Biomed. Rep.* **2017**, *6*, 612–614. [CrossRef]
3. Oshiro, B.T. The semisynthetic penicillins. *Prim. Care Update OB/GYNS* **1999**, *6*, 56–60. [CrossRef]
4. Lahlou, M. The success of natural products in drug discovery. *Pharmacol. Pharmacy* **2013**, *4*, 17–31. [CrossRef]
5. Cragg, G.M.; Newman, D.J. Natural products: A continuing source of novel drug leads. *Biochim. Biophys. Acta* **2013**, *1830*, 3670–3695. [CrossRef] [PubMed]
6. Tu, Y. Artemisinin-A Gift from Traditional Chinese Medicine to the World (Nobel Lecture). *Angew. Chem. Int. Ed. Engl.* **2016**, *55*, 10210–10226. [CrossRef]
7. Bai, L.; Gao, J.; Wei, F.; Zhao, J.; Wang, D.; Wei, J. Therapeutic Potential of Ginsenosides as an Adjuvant Treatment for Diabetes. *Front. Pharmacol.* **2018**, *9*, 423. [CrossRef]
8. He, N.W.; Zhao, Y.; Guo, L.; Shang, J.; Yang, X.B. Antioxidant, antiproliferative, and pro-apoptotic activities of a saponin extract derived from the roots of *Panax notoginseng* (Burk.) F.H. Chen. *J. Med. Food* **2012**, *15*, 350–359. [CrossRef] [PubMed]
9. Lee, I.S.; Uh, I.; Kim, K.S.; Kim, K.H.; Park, J.; Kim, Y.; Jung, J.H.; Jung, H.J.; Jang, H.J. Anti-Inflammatory Effects of Ginsenoside Rg3 via NF-κB Pathway in A549 Cells and Human Asthmatic Lung Tissue. *J. Immunol. Res.* **2016**, *2016*, 7521601. [CrossRef]
10. Lu, M.; Fei, Z.; Zhang, G. Synergistic anticancer activity of 20(S)-Ginsenoside Rg3 and Sorafenib in hepatocellular carcinoma by modulating PTEN/Akt signaling pathway. *Biomed. Pharmacother.* **2018**, *97*, 1282–1288. [CrossRef]
11. Lee, M.H.; Lee, B.H.; Jung, J.Y.; Cheon, D.S.; Kim, K.T.; Choi, C. Antiviral effect of Korean red ginseng extract and ginsenosides on murine norovirus and feline calicivirus as surrogates for human norovirus. *J. Ginseng Res.* **2011**, *35*, 429–435. [CrossRef]
12. Wang, Y.; Yang, G.; Gong, J.; Lu, F.; Diao, Q.; Sun, J.; Zhang, K.; Tian, J.; Liu, J. Ginseng for Alzheimer's Disease: A Systematic Review and Meta-Analysis of Randomized Controlled Trials. *Curr. Top. Med. Chem.* **2016**, *16*, 529–536. [CrossRef]
13. Kim, K.H.; Lee, D.; Lee, H.L.; Kim, C.E.; Jung, K.; Kang, K.S. Beneficial effects of *Panax ginseng* for the treatment and prevention of neurodegenerative diseases: Past findings and future directions. *J. Ginseng Res.* **2018**, *42*, 239–247. [CrossRef]
14. Park, S.H.; Chung, S.; Chung, M.Y.; Choi, H.K.; Hwang, J.T.; Park, J.H. Effects of *Panax ginseng* on hyperglycemia, hypertension, and hyperlipidemia: A systematic review and meta-analysis. *J. Ginseng Res.* **2022**, *46*, 188–205. [CrossRef]
15. Li, Z.; Ji, G.E. Ginseng and obesity. *J. Ginseng Res.* **2018**, *42*, 1–8. [CrossRef]
16. Lee, C.H.; Kim, J.H. A review on the medicinal potentials of ginseng and ginsenosides on cardiovascular diseases. *J. Ginseng Res.* **2014**, *38*, 161–166. [CrossRef] [PubMed]
17. Cho, D.E.; Choi, G.M.; Lee, Y.S.; Hong, J.P.; Yeom, M.; Lee, B.; Hahm, D.H. Long-term administration of red ginseng non-saponin fraction rescues the loss of skeletal muscle mass and strength associated with aging in mice. *J. Ginseng Res.* **2022**, *46*, 657–665. [CrossRef] [PubMed]
18. Kim, T.J.; Pyun, D.H.; Kim, M.J.; Jeong, J.H.; Abd El-Aty, A.M.; Jung, T.W. Ginsenoside compound K ameliorates palmitate-induced atrophy in C2C12 myotubes via promyogenic effects and AMPK/autophagy-mediated suppression of endoplasmic reticulum stress. *J. Ginseng Res.* **2022**, *46*, 444–453. [CrossRef] [PubMed]
19. Ahmad, S.S.; Chun, H.J.; Ahmad, K.; Choi, I. Therapeutic applications of ginseng for skeletal muscle-related disorder management. *J. Ginseng Res.* **2023**; in press. [CrossRef]
20. Ahmad, K.; Shaikh, S.; Ahmad, S.S.; Lee, E.J.; Choi, I. Cross-Talk Between Extracellular Matrix and Skeletal Muscle: Implications for Myopathies. *Front. Pharmacol.* **2020**, *11*, 142. [CrossRef]
21. Kim, R.; Kim, J.W.; Lee, S.J.; Bae, G.U. Ginsenoside Rg3 protects glucocorticoid-induced muscle atrophy in vitro through improving mitochondrial biogenesis and myotube growth. *Mol. Med. Rep.* **2022**, *25*, 94. [CrossRef]
22. Ahmad, S.S.; Ahmad, K.; Shaikh, S.; You, H.J.; Lee, E.Y.; Ali, S.; Lee, E.J.; Choi, I. Molecular Mechanisms and Current Treatment Options for Cancer Cachexia. *Cancers* **2022**, *14*, 2107. [CrossRef]

23. Lee, E.J.; Ahmad, S.S.; Lim, J.H.; Ahmad, K.; Shaikh, S.; Lee, Y.S.; Park, S.J.; Jin, J.O.; Lee, Y.H.; Choi, I. Interaction of Fibromodulin and Myostatin to Regulate Skeletal Muscle Aging: An Opposite Regulation in Muscle Aging, Diabetes, and Intracellular Lipid Accumulation. *Cells* **2021**, *10*, 2083. [CrossRef]
24. Ginseng. *Drugs and Lactation Database (LactMed®)*; Bethesda: Rockville, MD, USA, 2006.
25. Yun, T.K. Brief introduction of *Panax ginseng* C.A. Meyer. *J. Korean Med. Sci.* **2001**, *16*, 63–65. [CrossRef] [PubMed]
26. Zhang, H.; Abid, S.; Ahn, J.C.; Mathiyalagan, R.; Kim, Y.J.; Yang, D.C.; Wang, Y. Characteristics of *Panax ginseng* Cultivars in Korea and China. *Molecules* **2020**, *25*, 2635. [CrossRef] [PubMed]
27. Baeg, I.H.; So, S.H. The world ginseng market and the ginseng (Korea). *J. Ginseng Res.* **2013**, *37*, 1–7. [CrossRef] [PubMed]
28. Wan, Y.; Wang, J.; Xu, J.F.; Tang, F.; Chen, L.; Tan, Y.Z.; Rao, C.L.; Ao, H.; Peng, C. *Panax ginseng* and its ginsenosides: Potential candidates for the prevention and treatment of chemotherapy-induced side effects. *J. Ginseng Res.* **2021**, *45*, 617–630. [CrossRef]
29. Lai, Z.Z.; Yang, H.L.; Shi, J.W.; Shen, H.H.; Wang, Y.; Chang, K.K.; Zhang, T.; Ye, J.F.; Sun, J.S.; Qiu, X.M.; et al. Protopanaxadiol improves endometriosis associated infertility and miscarriage in sex hormones receptors-dependent and independent manners. *Int. J. Biol. Sci.* **2021**, *17*, 1878–1894. [CrossRef]
30. Zhou, C.; Gong, T.; Chen, J.; Chen, T.; Yang, J.; Zhu, P. Production of a Novel Protopanaxatriol-Type Ginsenoside by Yeast Cell Factories. *Bioengineering* **2023**, *10*, 463. [CrossRef]
31. Zhang, Y.; Yu, L.; Cai, W.; Fan, S.; Feng, L.; Ji, G.; Huang, C. Protopanaxatriol, a novel PPARgamma antagonist from *Panax ginseng*, alleviates steatosis in mice. *Sci. Rep.* **2014**, *4*, 7375. [CrossRef]
32. Ahmad, S.S.; Ahmad, K.; Lee, E.J.; Lee, Y.H.; Choi, I. Implications of Insulin-like Growth Factor-1 in Skeletal Muscle and Various Diseases. *Cells* **2020**, *9*, 1773. [CrossRef]
33. Zhang, J.; Liu, M.; Huang, M.; Chen, M.; Zhang, D.; Luo, L.; Ye, G.; Deng, L.; Peng, Y.; Wu, X.; et al. Ginsenoside F1 promotes angiogenesis by activating the IGF-1/IGF1R pathway. *Pharmacol. Res.* **2019**, *144*, 292–305. [CrossRef]
34. Yun, Y.J.; Park, B.H.; Hou, J.; Oh, J.P.; Han, J.H.; Kim, S.C. Ginsenoside F1 Protects the Brain against Amyloid Beta-Induced Toxicity by Regulating IDE and NEP. *Life* **2022**, *12*, 58. [CrossRef] [PubMed]
35. Han, J.; Oh, J.P.; Yoo, M.; Cui, C.H.; Jeon, B.M.; Kim, S.C.; Han, J.H. Minor ginsenoside F1 improves memory in APP/PS1 mice. *Mol. Brain* **2019**, *12*, 77. [CrossRef]
36. Kim, S.J.; Lee, J.; Choi, W.S.; Kim, H.J.; Kim, M.Y.; Kim, S.C.; Kim, H.S. Ginsenoside F1 Attenuates Eosinophilic Inflammation in Chronic Rhinosinusitis by Promoting NK Cell Function. *J. Ginseng Res.* **2021**, *45*, 695–705. [CrossRef] [PubMed]
37. Kim, M.H.; Kim, H.H.; Jeong, J.M.; Shim, Y.R.; Lee, J.H.; Kim, Y.E.; Ryu, T.; Yang, K.; Kim, K.R.; Jeon, B.M.; et al. Ginsenoside F2 attenuates chronic-binge ethanol-induced liver injury by increasing regulatory T cells and decreasing Th17 cells. *J. Ginseng Res.* **2020**, *44*, 815–822. [CrossRef] [PubMed]
38. Shin, H.S.; Park, S.Y.; Hwang, E.S.; Lee, D.G.; Mavlonov, G.T.; Yi, T.H. Ginsenoside F2 reduces hair loss by controlling apoptosis through the sterol regulatory element-binding protein cleavage activating protein and transforming growth factor-beta pathways in a dihydrotestosterone-induced mouse model. *Biol. Pharm. Bull.* **2014**, *37*, 755–763. [CrossRef] [PubMed]
39. Yoshizaki, K.; Yahara, S. New triterpenoid saponins from leaves of *Panax japonicus* (3). Saponins of the specimens collected in Miyazaki prefecture. *Nat. Prod. Commun.* **2012**, *7*, 491–493. [CrossRef] [PubMed]
40. Yu, J.L.; Dou, D.Q.; Chen, X.H.; Yang, H.Z.; Guo, N.; Cheng, G.F. Immunoenhancing activity of protopanaxatriol-type ginsenoside-F3 in murine spleen cells. *Acta Pharmacol. Sin.* **2004**, *25*, 1671–1676.
41. Zhao, Y.; Liu, Y.; Deng, J.; Zhu, C.; Ma, X.; Jiang, M.; Fan, D. Ginsenoside F4 Alleviates Skeletal Muscle Insulin Resistance by Regulating PTP1B in Type II Diabetes Mellitus. *J. Agric. Food Chem.* **2023**, *71*, 14263–14275. [CrossRef]
42. Chen, B.; Shen, Y.P.; Zhang, D.F.; Cheng, J.; Jia, X.B. The apoptosis-inducing effect of ginsenoside F4 from steamed notoginseng on human lymphocytoma JK cells. *Nat. Prod. Res.* **2013**, *27*, 2351–2354. [CrossRef] [PubMed]
43. Liu, J.; Nile, S.H.; Xu, G.; Wang, Y.; Kai, G. Systematic exploration of *Astragalus membranaceus* and *Panax ginseng* as immune regulators: Insights from the comparative biological and computational analysis. *Phytomedicine* **2021**, *86*, 153077. [CrossRef] [PubMed]
44. Sim, U.; Sung, J.; Lee, H.; Heo, H.; Jeong, H.S.; Lee, J. Effect of calcium chloride and sucrose on the composition of bioactive compounds and antioxidant activities in buckwheat sprouts. *Food Chem.* **2020**, *312*, 126075. [CrossRef]
45. Park, H.W.; In, G.; Han, S.T.; Lee, M.W.; Kim, S.Y.; Kim, K.T.; Cho, B.G.; Han, G.H.; Chang, I.M. Simultaneous determination of 30 ginsenosides in *Panax ginseng* preparations using ultra performance liquid chromatography. *J. Ginseng Res.* **2013**, *37*, 457–467. [CrossRef]
46. Dou, D.Q.; Zhang, Y.W.; Zhang, L.; Chen, Y.J.; Yao, X.S. The inhibitory effects of ginsenosides on protein tyrosine kinase activated by hypoxia/reoxygenation in cultured human umbilical vein endothelial cells. *Planta Med.* **2001**, *67*, 19–23. [CrossRef]
47. Zhou, P.; Xie, W.; He, S.; Sun, Y.; Meng, X.; Sun, G.; Sun, X. Ginsenoside Rb1 as an Anti-Diabetic Agent and Its Underlying Mechanism Analysis. *Cells* **2019**, *8*, 204. [CrossRef] [PubMed]
48. Song, B.; Ding, L.; Zhang, H.; Chu, Y.; Chang, Z.; Yu, Y.; Guo, D.; Zhang, S.; Liu, X. Ginsenoside Rb1 increases insulin sensitivity through suppressing 11beta-hydroxysteroid dehydrogenase type I. *Am. J. Transl. Res.* **2017**, *9*, 1049–1057. [PubMed]
49. Zhong, Z.D.; Wang, C.M.; Wang, W.; Shen, L.; Chen, Z.H. Major hypoglycemic ingredients of *Panax notoginseng* saponins for treating diabetes. *Sichuan Da Xue Xue Bao Yi Xue Ban.* **2014**, *45*, 235–239.
50. Yu, X.; Ye, L.; Zhang, H.; Zhao, W.; Wang, G.; Guo, C.; Shang, W. Ginsenoside Rb1 ameliorates liver fat accumulation by upregulating perilipin expression in adipose tissue of db/db obese mice. *J. Ginseng Res.* **2015**, *39*, 199–205. [CrossRef] [PubMed]

51. Wu, Y.; Yu, Y.; Szabo, A.; Han, M.; Huang, X.F. Central inflammation and leptin resistance are attenuated by ginsenoside Rb1 treatment in obese mice fed a high-fat diet. *PLoS ONE* **2014**, *9*, e92618. [CrossRef]
52. Xiong, Y.; Shen, L.; Liu, K.J.; Tso, P.; Xiong, Y.; Wang, G.; Woods, S.C.; Liu, M. Antiobesity and antihyperglycemic effects of ginsenoside Rb1 in rats. *Diabetes* **2010**, *59*, 2505–2512. [CrossRef]
53. Tabandeh, M.R.; Jafari, H.; Hosseini, S.A.; Hashemitabar, M. Ginsenoside Rb1 stimulates adiponectin signaling in C2C12 muscle cells through up-regulation of AdipoR1 and AdipoR2 proteins. *Pharm. Biol.* **2015**, *53*, 125–132. [CrossRef] [PubMed]
54. Miao, L.; Yang, Y.; Li, Z.; Fang, Z.; Zhang, Y.; Han, C.C. Ginsenoside Rb2: A review of pharmacokinetics and pharmacological effects. *J. Ginseng Res.* **2022**, *46*, 206–213. [CrossRef] [PubMed]
55. Kim, D.H.; Kim, D.W.; Jung, B.H.; Lee, J.H.; Lee, H.; Hwang, G.S.; Kang, K.S.; Lee, J.W. Ginsenoside Rb2 suppresses the glutamate-mediated oxidative stress and neuronal cell death in HT22 cells. *J. Ginseng Res.* **2019**, *43*, 326–334. [CrossRef] [PubMed]
56. Phi, L.T.H.; Wijaya, Y.T.; Sari, I.N.; Yang, Y.G.; Lee, Y.K.; Kwon, H.Y. The anti-metastatic effect of ginsenoside Rb2 in colorectal cancer in an EGFR/SOX2-dependent manner. *Cancer Med.* **2018**, *7*, 5621–5631. [CrossRef]
57. Wang, S.; Yang, S.; Chen, Y.; Chen, Y.; Li, R.; Han, S.; Kamili, A.; Wu, Y.; Zhang, W. Ginsenoside Rb2 Alleviated Atherosclerosis by Inhibiting M1 Macrophages Polarization Induced by MicroRNA-216a. *Front. Pharmacol.* **2021**, *12*, 764130. [CrossRef] [PubMed]
58. Lin, Y.; Hu, Y.; Hu, X.; Yang, L.; Chen, X.; Li, Q.; Gu, X. Ginsenoside Rb2 improves insulin resistance by inhibiting adipocyte pyroptosis. *Adipocyte* **2020**, *9*, 302–312. [CrossRef] [PubMed]
59. Chen, Y.; Wang, S.; Yang, S.; Li, R.; Yang, Y.; Chen, Y.; Zhang, W. Inhibitory role of ginsenoside Rb2 in endothelial senescence and inflammation mediated by microRNA-216a. *Mol. Med. Rep.* **2021**, *23*, 1–11. [CrossRef]
60. Heras, G.; Namuduri, A.V.; Traini, L.; Shevchenko, G.; Falk, A.; Bergstrom Lind, S.; Jia, M.; Tian, G.; Gastaldello, S. Muscle RING-finger protein-1 (MuRF1) functions and cellular localization are regulated by SUMO1 post-translational modification. *J. Mol. Cell Biol.* **2019**, *11*, 356–370. [CrossRef]
61. Chen, X.; Liu, T.; Wang, Q.; Wang, H.; Xue, S.; Jiang, Q.; Li, J.; Li, C.; Wang, W.; Wang, Y. Synergistic Effects of Ginsenoside Rb3 and Ferruginol in Ischemia-Induced Myocardial Infarction. *Int. J. Mol. Sci.* **2022**, *23*, 15935. [CrossRef]
62. Shao, M.; Gao, P.; Cheng, W.; Ma, L.; Yang, Y.; Lu, L.; Li, C.; Wang, W.; Wang, Y. Ginsenoside Rb3 upregulates sarcoplasmic reticulum Ca^{2+}-ATPase expression and improves the contractility of cardiomyocytes by inhibiting the NF-κB pathway. *Biomed. Pharmacother.* **2022**, *154*, 113661. [CrossRef]
63. Sun, J.; Yu, X.; Huangpu, H.; Yao, F. Ginsenoside Rb3 protects cardiomyocytes against hypoxia/reoxygenation injury via activating the antioxidation signaling pathway of PERK/Nrf2/HMOX1. *Biomed. Pharmacother.* **2019**, *109*, 254–261. [CrossRef] [PubMed]
64. Yang, N.; Zhang, X.; Li, L.; Xu, T.; Li, M.; Zhao, Q.; Yu, J.; Wang, J.; Liu, Z. Ginsenoside Rc Promotes Bone Formation in Ovariectomy-Induced Osteoporosis In Vivo and Osteogenic Differentiation In Vitro. *Int. J. Mol. Sci.* **2022**, *23*, 6187. [CrossRef] [PubMed]
65. Zhong, Y.; Chen, Y.; Pan, Z.; Tang, K.; Zhong, G.; Guo, J.; Cui, T.; Li, T.; Duan, S.; Yang, X.; et al. Ginsenoside Rc, as an FXR activator, alleviates acetaminophen-induced hepatotoxicity via relieving inflammation and oxidative stress. *Front. Pharmacol.* **2022**, *13*, 1027731. [CrossRef] [PubMed]
66. Yang, J.W.; Kim, S.S. Ginsenoside Rc promotes anti-adipogenic activity on 3T3-L1 adipocytes by down-regulating C/EBPalpha and PPARgamma. *Molecules* **2015**, *20*, 1293–1303. [CrossRef] [PubMed]
67. Wijaya, Y.T.; Setiawan, T.; Sari, I.N.; Park, K.; Lee, C.H.; Cho, K.W.; Lee, Y.K.; Lim, J.Y.; Yoon, J.K.; Lee, S.H.; et al. Ginsenoside Rd ameliorates muscle wasting by suppressing the signal transducer and activator of transcription 3 pathway. *J. Cachexia Sarcopenia Muscle* **2022**, *13*, 3149–3162. [CrossRef] [PubMed]
68. Baig, M.H.; Ahmad, K.; Moon, J.S.; Park, S.Y.; Ho Lim, J.; Chun, H.J.; Qadri, A.F.; Hwang, Y.C.; Jan, A.T.; Ahmad, S.S.; et al. Myostatin and its Regulation: A Comprehensive Review of Myostatin Inhibiting Strategies. *Front. Physiol.* **2022**, *13*, 876078. [CrossRef]
69. Peris-Moreno, D.; Taillandier, D.; Polge, C. MuRF1/TRIM63, Master Regulator of Muscle Mass. *Int. J. Mol. Sci.* **2020**, *21*, 6663. [CrossRef]
70. Ahmad, K.; Shaikh, S.; Lim, J.H.; Ahmad, S.S.; Chun, H.J.; Lee, E.J.; Choi, I. Therapeutic application of natural compounds for skeletal muscle-associated metabolic disorders: A review on diabetes perspective. *Biomed. Pharmacother.* **2023**, *168*, 115642. [CrossRef] [PubMed]
71. Ahmad, K.; Shaikh, S.; Chun, H.J.; Ali, S.; Lim, J.H.; Ahmad, S.S.; Lee, E.J.; Choi, I. Extracellular matrix: The critical contributor to skeletal muscle regeneration-a comprehensive review. *Inflamm. Regen.* **2023**, *43*, 58. [CrossRef]
72. Nabavi, S.F.; Sureda, A.; Habtemariam, S.; Nabavi, S.M. Ginsenoside Rd and ischemic stroke; a short review of literatures. *J. Ginseng Res.* **2015**, *39*, 299–303. [CrossRef] [PubMed]
73. Lim, W.C.; Shin, E.J.; Lim, T.G.; Choi, J.W.; Song, N.E.; Hong, H.D.; Cho, C.W.; Rhee, Y.K. Ginsenoside Rf Enhances Exercise Endurance by Stimulating Myoblast Differentiation and Mitochondrial Biogenesis in C2C12 Myotubes and ICR Mice. *Foods* **2022**, *11*, 1709. [CrossRef] [PubMed]
74. Song, H.; Park, J.; Choi, K.; Lee, J.; Chen, J.; Park, H.J.; Yu, B.I.; Iida, M.; Rhyu, M.R.; Lee, Y. Ginsenoside Rf inhibits cyclooxygenase-2 induction via peroxisome proliferator-activated receptor gamma in A549 cells. *J. Ginseng Res.* **2019**, *43*, 319–325. [CrossRef] [PubMed]
75. Siraj, F.M.; Natarajan, S.; Huq, M.A.; Kim, Y.J.; Yang, D.C. Structural investigation of ginsenoside Rf with PPARgamma major transcriptional factor of adipogenesis and its impact on adipocyte. *J. Ginseng Res.* **2015**, *39*, 141–147. [CrossRef]

76. Che, L.; Zhu, C.; Huang, L.; Xu, H.; Ma, X.; Luo, X.; He, H.; Zhang, T.; Wang, N. Ginsenoside Rg2 Promotes the Proliferation and Stemness Maintenance of Porcine Mesenchymal Stem Cells through Autophagy Induction. *Foods* **2023**, *12*, 1075. [CrossRef]
77. Xue, Q.; Yu, T.; Wang, Z.; Fu, X.; Li, X.; Zou, L.; Li, M.; Cho, J.Y.; Yang, Y. Protective effect and mechanism of ginsenoside Rg2 on atherosclerosis. *J. Ginseng Res.* **2023**, *47*, 237–245. [CrossRef] [PubMed]
78. Shan, Y.; Li, J.; Zhu, A.; Kong, W.; Ying, R.; Zhu, W. Ginsenoside Rg3 ameliorates acute pancreatitis by activating the NRF2/HO-1 mediated ferroptosis pathway. *Int. J. Mol. Med.* **2022**, *50*, 89. [CrossRef]
79. Li, L.; Wang, Y.; Guo, R.; Li, S.; Ni, J.; Gao, S.; Gao, X.; Mao, J.; Zhu, Y.; Wu, P.; et al. Ginsenoside Rg3-loaded, reactive oxygen species-responsive polymeric nanoparticles for alleviating myocardial ischemia-reperfusion injury. *J. Control Release* **2020**, *317*, 259–272. [CrossRef] [PubMed]
80. Feng, S.L.; Luo, H.B.; Cai, L.; Zhang, J.; Wang, D.; Chen, Y.J.; Zhan, H.X.; Jiang, Z.H.; Xie, Y. Ginsenoside Rg5 overcomes chemotherapeutic multidrug resistance mediated by ABCB1 transporter: In vitro and in vivo study. *J. Ginseng Res.* **2020**, *44*, 247–257. [CrossRef]
81. Liu, Y.; Fan, D. The Preparation of Ginsenoside Rg5, Its Antitumor Activity against Breast Cancer Cells and Its Targeting of PI3K. *Nutrients* **2020**, *12*, 246. [CrossRef] [PubMed]
82. Li, W.; Yan, M.H.; Liu, Y.; Liu, Z.; Wang, Z.; Chen, C.; Zhang, J.; Sun, Y.S. Ginsenoside Rg5 Ameliorates Cisplatin-Induced Nephrotoxicity in Mice through Inhibition of Inflammation, Oxidative Stress, and Apoptosis. *Nutrients* **2016**, *8*, 566. [CrossRef]
83. Yang, Q.; Qian, L.; Zhang, S. Ginsenoside Rh1 Alleviates HK-2 Apoptosis by Inhibiting ROS and the JNK/p53 Pathways. *Evid. Based Complement. Alternat Med.* **2020**, *2020*, 3401067. [CrossRef] [PubMed]
84. Huynh, D.T.N.; Jin, Y.; Myung, C.S.; Heo, K.S. Ginsenoside Rh1 Induces MCF-7 Cell Apoptosis and Autophagic Cell Death through ROS-Mediated Akt Signaling. *Cancers* **2021**, *13*, 1892. [CrossRef] [PubMed]
85. Lyu, X.; Xu, X.; Song, A.; Guo, J.; Zhang, Y.; Zhang, Y. Ginsenoside Rh1 inhibits colorectal cancer cell migration and invasion in vitro and tumor growth in vivo. *Oncol. Lett.* **2019**, *18*, 4160–4166. [CrossRef] [PubMed]
86. Xiaodan, S.; Ying, C. Role of ginsenoside Rh2 in tumor therapy and tumor microenvironment immunomodulation. *Biomed. Pharmacother.* **2022**, *156*, 113912. [CrossRef] [PubMed]
87. Qi, Z.; Yan, Z.; Wang, Y.; Ji, N.; Yang, X.; Zhang, A.; Li, M.; Xu, F.; Zhang, J. Ginsenoside Rh2 Inhibits NLRP3 Inflammasome Activation and Improves Exosomes to Alleviate Hypoxia-Induced Myocardial Injury. *Front. Immunol.* **2022**, *13*, 883946. [CrossRef] [PubMed]
88. Thandra, K.C.; Barsouk, A.; Saginala, K.; Aluru, J.S.; Barsouk, A. Epidemiology of lung cancer. *Contemp. Oncol.* **2021**, *25*, 45–52. [CrossRef]
89. Xue, X.; Liu, Y.; Qu, L.; Fan, C.; Ma, X.; Ouyang, P.; Fan, D. Ginsenoside Rh3 Inhibits Lung Cancer Metastasis by Targeting Extracellular Signal-Regulated Kinase: A Network Pharmacology Study. *Pharmaceuticals* **2022**, *15*, 758. [CrossRef]
90. Teng, S.; Lei, X.; Zhang, X.; Shen, D.; Liu, Q.; Sun, Y.; Wang, Y.; Cong, Z. Transcriptome Analysis of the Anti-Proliferative Effects of Ginsenoside Rh3 on HCT116 Colorectal Cancer Cells. *Molecules* **2022**, *27*, 5002. [CrossRef] [PubMed]
91. Cao, L.; Gao, Y.; Zhu, J.; Zhang, J.; Dong, M.; Mao, Y. Protective action of the ginsenoside Rh3 in a rat myocardial ischemia-reperfusion injury model by inhibition of apoptosis induced via p38 mitogen-activated protein kinase/caspase-3 signaling. *J. Int. Med. Res.* **2020**, *48*, 300060520969090. [CrossRef]
92. To, K.I.; Zhu, Z.X.; Wang, Y.N.; Li, G.A.; Sun, Y.M.; Li, Y.; Jin, Y.H. Integrative network pharmacology and experimental verification to reveal the anti-inflammatory mechanism of ginsenoside Rh4. *Front. Pharmacol.* **2022**, *13*, 953871. [CrossRef] [PubMed]
93. Baek, S.H.; Shin, B.K.; Kim, N.J.; Chang, S.Y.; Park, J.H. Protective effect of ginsenosides Rk3 and Rh4 on cisplatin-induced acute kidney injury in vitro and in vivo. *J. Ginseng Res.* **2017**, *41*, 233–239. [CrossRef] [PubMed]
94. Zhang, Y.; Ma, P.; Duan, Z.; Liu, Y.; Mi, Y.; Fan, D. Ginsenoside Rh4 Suppressed Metastasis of Lung Adenocarcinoma via Inhibiting JAK2/STAT3 Signaling. *Int. J. Mol. Sci.* **2022**, *23*, 2018. [CrossRef] [PubMed]
95. Wu, Y.; Pi, D.; Chen, Y.; Zuo, Q.; Zhou, S.; Ouyang, M. Ginsenoside Rh4 Inhibits Colorectal Cancer Cell Proliferation by Inducing Ferroptosis via Autophagy Activation. *Evid. Based Complement. Alternat Med.* **2022**, *2022*, 6177553. [CrossRef]
96. Dong, F.; Qu, L.; Duan, Z.; He, Y.; Ma, X.; Fan, D. Ginsenoside Rh4 inhibits breast cancer growth through targeting histone deacetylase 2 to regulate immune microenvironment and apoptosis. *Bioorg. Chem.* **2023**, *135*, 106537. [CrossRef]
97. Zhu, A.; Duan, Z.; Chen, Y.; Zhu, C.; Fan, D. Ginsenoside Rh4 delays skeletal muscle aging through SIRT1 pathway. *Phytomedicine* **2023**, *118*, 154906. [CrossRef]
98. Chen, X.; Liu, W.; Liu, B. Ginsenoside Rh7 Suppresses Proliferation, Migration and Invasion of NSCLC Cells through Targeting ILF3-AS1 Mediated miR-212/SMAD1 Axis. *Front. Oncol.* **2021**, *11*, 656132. [CrossRef] [PubMed]
99. Ryoo, N.; Rahman, M.A.; Hwang, H.; Ko, S.K.; Nah, S.Y.; Kim, H.C.; Rhim, H. Ginsenoside Rk1 is a novel inhibitor of NMDA receptors in cultured rat hippocampal neurons. *J. Ginseng Res.* **2020**, *44*, 490–495. [CrossRef]
100. Xiong, J.; Yang, J.; Yan, K.; Guo, J. Ginsenoside Rk1 protects human melanocytes from H_2O_2-induced oxidative injury via regulation of the PI3K/AKT/Nrf2/HO-1 pathway. *Mol. Med. Rep.* **2021**, *24*, 1–9. [CrossRef]
101. Hu, J.N.; Xu, X.Y.; Jiang, S.; Liu, Y.; Liu, Z.; Wang, Y.P.; Gong, X.J.; Li, K.K.; Ren, S.; Li, W. Protective effect of ginsenoside Rk1, a major rare saponin from black ginseng, on cisplatin-induced nephrotoxicity in HEK-293 cells. *Kaohsiung J. Med. Sci.* **2020**, *36*, 732–740. [CrossRef]
102. An, X.; Fu, R.; Ma, P.; Ma, X.; Fan, D. Ginsenoside Rk1 inhibits cell proliferation and promotes apoptosis in lung squamous cell carcinoma by calcium signaling pathway. *RSC Adv.* **2019**, *9*, 25107–25118. [CrossRef]

103. Oh, J.M.; Lee, J.; Im, W.T.; Chun, S. Ginsenoside Rk1 Induces Apoptosis in Neuroblastoma Cells through Loss of Mitochondrial Membrane Potential and Activation of Caspases. *Int. J. Mol. Sci.* **2019**, *20*, 1213. [CrossRef]
104. She, L.; Xiong, L.; Li, L.; Zhang, J.; Sun, J.; Wu, H.; Ren, J.; Wang, W.; Zhao, X.; Liang, G. Ginsenoside Rk3 ameliorates Abeta-induced neurotoxicity in APP/PS1 model mice via AMPK signaling pathway. *Biomed. Pharmacother.* **2023**, *158*, 114192. [CrossRef]
105. Ahmad, S.S.; Khalid, M.; Kamal, M.A.; Younis, K. Study of Nutraceuticals and Phytochemicals for the Management of Alzheimer's Disease: A Review. *Curr. Neuropharmacol.* **2021**, *19*, 1884–1895. [CrossRef] [PubMed]
106. Ahmad, S.S.; Kamal, M.A. Current Updates on the Regulation of Beta-Secretase Movement as a Potential Restorative Focus for Management of Alzheimer's Disease. *Protein Pept. Lett.* **2019**, *26*, 579–587. [CrossRef] [PubMed]
107. Corona, J.C. Natural Compounds for the Management of Parkinson's Disease and Attention-Deficit/Hyperactivity Disorder. *Biomed. Res. Int.* **2018**, *2018*, 4067597. [CrossRef] [PubMed]
108. Zhong, Z.; He, X.; Ge, J.; Zhu, J.; Yao, C.; Cai, H.; Ye, X.Y.; Xie, T.; Bai, R. Discovery of small-molecule compounds and natural products against Parkinson's disease: Pathological mechanism and structural modification. *Eur. J. Med. Chem.* **2022**, *237*, 114378. [CrossRef] [PubMed]
109. Ahmad, S.S.; Khatoon, A.; Khan, M.S.; Khalid, M.; Alharbi, A.M.; Siddiqui, M.H. Evaluation of vincamine against acetylcholinesterase enzyme. *Cell. Mol. Biol.* **2022**, *68*, 14–21. [CrossRef] [PubMed]
110. Abitbol, A.; Mallard, B.; Tiralongo, E.; Tiralongo, J. Mushroom Natural Products in Neurodegenerative Disease Drug Discovery. *Cells* **2022**, *11*, 3938. [CrossRef]
111. Liu, H.; Zhao, J.; Fu, R.; Zhu, C.; Fan, D. The ginsenoside Rk3 exerts anti-esophageal cancer activity in vitro and in vivo by mediating apoptosis and autophagy through regulation of the PI3K/Akt/mTOR pathway. *PLoS ONE* **2019**, *14*, e0216759. [CrossRef]
112. Han, J.; Xia, J.; Zhang, L.; Cai, E.; Zhao, Y.; Fei, X.; Jia, X.; Yang, H.; Liu, S. Studies of the effects and mechanisms of ginsenoside Re and Rk(3) on myelosuppression induced by cyclophosphamide. *J. Ginseng Res.* **2019**, *43*, 618–624. [CrossRef] [PubMed]
113. Ma, S.; Huang, Q.; Hu, Q.; Gao, R.; Lan, J.; Yu, X.; Zhao, Y.; Shen, F.; Mi, A.; Wang, B. Ginsenoside Rk3 Inhibits the Extramedullary Infiltration of Acute Monocytic Leukemia Cell via miR-3677-5p/CXCL12 Axis. *Evid. Based Complement. Alternat Med.* **2022**, *2022*, 3065464. [CrossRef]
114. Zheng, S.W.; Xiao, S.Y.; Wang, J.; Hou, W.; Wang, Y.P. Inhibitory Effects of Ginsenoside Ro on the Growth of B16F10 Melanoma via Its Metabolites. *Molecules* **2019**, *24*, 2985. [CrossRef] [PubMed]
115. Xu, H.L.; Chen, G.H.; Wu, Y.T.; Xie, L.P.; Tan, Z.B.; Liu, B.; Fan, H.J.; Chen, H.M.; Huang, G.Q.; Liu, M.; et al. Corrigendum to "Ginsenoside Ro, an oleanolic saponin of *Panax ginseng*, exerts anti-inflammatory effect by direct inhibiting toll like receptor 4 signaling pathway" [J Ginseng Res 46 (2022) 156–166]. *J. Ginseng Res.* **2022**, *46*, 315–319. [CrossRef] [PubMed]
116. Kim, S.; Oh, M.H.; Kim, B.S.; Kim, W.I.; Cho, H.S.; Park, B.Y.; Park, C.; Shin, G.W.; Kwon, J. Upregulation of heme oxygenase-1 by ginsenoside Ro attenuates lipopolysaccharide-induced inflammation in macrophage cells. *J. Ginseng Res.* **2015**, *39*, 365–370. [CrossRef]
117. Jiang, L.S.; Li, W.; Zhuang, T.X.; Yu, J.J.; Sun, S.; Ju, Z.C.; Wang, Z.T.; Ding, L.L.; Yang, L. Ginsenoside Ro Ameliorates High-Fat Diet-Induced Obesity and Insulin Resistance in Mice via Activation of the G Protein-Coupled Bile Acid Receptor 5 Pathway. *J. Pharmacol. Exp. Ther.* **2021**, *377*, 441–451. [CrossRef]
118. Chiang, H.M.; Chien, Y.C.; Wu, C.H.; Kuo, Y.H.; Wu, W.C.; Pan, Y.Y.; Su, Y.H.; Wen, K.C. Hydroalcoholic extract of *Rhodiola rosea* L. (Crassulaceae) and its hydrolysate inhibit melanogenesis in B16F0 cells by regulating the CREB/MITF/tyrosinase pathway. *Food Chem. Toxicol.* **2014**, *65*, 129–139. [CrossRef]
119. Lee, D.Y.; Lee, J.; Jeong, Y.T.; Byun, G.H.; Kim, J.H. Melanogenesis inhibition activity of floralginsenoside A from *Panax ginseng* berry. *J. Ginseng Res.* **2017**, *41*, 602–607. [CrossRef]
120. Kim, S.; Jung, S.H.; Cho, C.W. Physicochemical studies of a newly synthesized molecule, 6-methyl-3-phenethyl-3,4-dihydro-1H-quinazoline-2-thione (JSH18) for topical formulations. *Arch. Pharm. Res.* **2008**, *31*, 1363–1368. [CrossRef]
121. Zhang, S.; Chen, C.; Lu, W.; Wei, L. Phytochemistry, pharmacology, and clinical use of *Panax notoginseng* flowers buds. *Phytother. Res.* **2018**, *32*, 2155–2163. [CrossRef]
122. Ahmad, S.S.; Ahmad, K.; Lee, E.J.; Shaikh, S.; Choi, I. Computational Identification of Dithymoquinone as a Potential Inhibitor of Myostatin and Regulator of Muscle Mass. *Molecules* **2021**, *26*, 5407. [CrossRef] [PubMed]
123. Shaikh, S.; Ali, S.; Lim, J.H.; Chun, H.J.; Ahmad, K.; Ahmad, S.S.; Hwang, Y.C.; Han, K.S.; Kim, N.R.; Lee, E.J.; et al. Dipeptidyl peptidase-4 inhibitory potentials of *Glycyrrhiza uralensis* and its bioactive compounds licochalcone A and licochalcone B: An in silico and in vitro study. *Front. Mol. Biosci.* **2022**, *9*, 1024764. [CrossRef] [PubMed]
124. Lee, E.J.; Shaikh, S.; Baig, M.H.; Park, S.Y.; Lim, J.H.; Ahmad, S.S.; Ali, S.; Ahmad, K.; Choi, I. MIF1 and MIF2 Myostatin Peptide Inhibitors as Potent Muscle Mass Regulators. *Int. J. Mol. Sci.* **2022**, *23*, 4222. [CrossRef] [PubMed]

Disclaimer/Publisher's Note: The statements, opinions and data contained in all publications are solely those of the individual author(s) and contributor(s) and not of MDPI and/or the editor(s). MDPI and/or the editor(s) disclaim responsibility for any injury to people or property resulting from any ideas, methods, instructions or products referred to in the content.

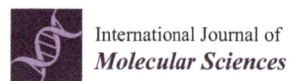

Article

Ellagic Acid from Hull Blackberries: Extraction, Purification, and Potential Anticancer Activity

Jialuan Wang [1,†], Fengyi Zhao [1,†], Wenlong Wu [1], Lianfei Lyu [1], Weilin Li [2,*] and Chunhong Zhang [1,*]

[1] Jiangsu Key Laboratory for the Research and Utilization of Plant Resources, Institute of Botany, Jiangsu Province and Chinese Academy of Sciences (Nanjing Botanical Garden Mem. Sun Yat-Sen), Qian Hu Hou Cun No. 1, Nanjing 210014, China; wjl163youxiang@163.com (J.W.); zhaofengyi92@163.com (F.Z.); 1964wwl@163.com (W.W.); njbglq@163.com (L.L.)

[2] Co-Innovation Center for Sustainable Forestry in Southern China, College of Forestry, Nanjing Forestry University, 159 Longpan Road, Nanjing 210037, China

* Correspondence: wlli@njfu.edu.cn (W.L.); chzhang@cnbg.net (C.Z.)

† These authors contributed equally to this work.

Abstract: Ellagic acid (EA) is present at relatively high concentrations in many berries and has many beneficial health effects, including anticancer properties. To improve the development and utilization of blackberry fruit nutrients, we divided Hull blackberry fruits into five growth periods according to color and determined the EA content in the fruits in each period. The EA content in the green fruit stage was the highest at 5.67 mg/g FW. Single-factor tests and response surface methodology were used to optimize the extraction process, while macroporous resin adsorption and alkali dissolution, acid precipitation, and solvent recrystallization were used for purification. The highest purity of the final EA powder was 90%. The anticancer assessment results determined by MTT assay showed that EA inhibited HeLa cells with an IC_{50} of 35 μg/mL, and the apoptosis rate of the cells increased in a dose-dependent manner, with the highest rate of about 67%. We evaluated the changes in the mRNA levels of genes related to the EA-mediated inhibition of cancer cell growth and initially verified the PI3K/PTEN/AKT/mTOR pathway as the pathway by which EA inhibits HeLa cell growth. We hope to provide a theoretical basis for the deep exploration and utilization of this functional food.

Keywords: blackberry; ellagic acid; extraction; purification; anticancer activity

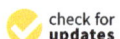

Citation: Wang, J.; Zhao, F.; Wu, W.; Lyu, L.; Li, W.; Zhang, C. Ellagic Acid from Hull Blackberries: Extraction, Purification, and Potential Anticancer Activity. *Int. J. Mol. Sci.* **2023**, *24*, 15228. https://doi.org/10.3390/ijms242015228

Academic Editors: Marilena Gilca and Adelina Vlad

Received: 28 September 2023
Revised: 11 October 2023
Accepted: 12 October 2023
Published: 16 October 2023

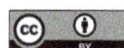

Copyright: © 2023 by the authors. Licensee MDPI, Basel, Switzerland. This article is an open access article distributed under the terms and conditions of the Creative Commons Attribution (CC BY) license (https://creativecommons.org/licenses/by/4.0/).

1. Introduction

Blackberries (*Rubus* spp.) are fruits of interest owing to their high content of anthocyanins and ellagitannins as well as other phenolic compounds that contribute to their good biological activities [1], including antioxidant [2], anticancer [3], anti-inflammatory [4], antibacterial [5] and others. This fruit is composed of an aggregate of droplets 1–3 cm in diameter that change color from green to red to black as it ripens [6]. However, the majority of blackberry varieties have a sour taste when fresh and are not easy to store, which is detrimental to the development and utilization of blackberries. Consequently, studying the functional components of blackberries by optimizing the extraction and utilization process is important.

Reportedly, the highest concentrations of ellagic acid (EA) are found in fruits of plants of the genus Rubus [7]. In plants, EA is a biologically active polyphenolic compound that occurs naturally as a secondary metabolite in many plants, where it is produced mainly by hydrolyzing ellagitannins [8]. Structurally, EA is considered a dimeric gallic acid derivative because it constitutes a dilactone of hexahydroxy-diphenic acid (HHDP) (Figure 1) [9]. In recent decades, EA has attracted increasing attention due to its pronounced antioxidant [10,11], anticancer [12–14], anti-inflammatory [15,16], and antimutagenic properties [17,18]. Many studies have shown that EA can regulate a range of cell signaling pathways to prevent, mitigate or slow the progression of chronic diseases such as cardiovascular disease [19] and neurodegenerative diseases [20], diabetes [21], and cancer [13,14,22].

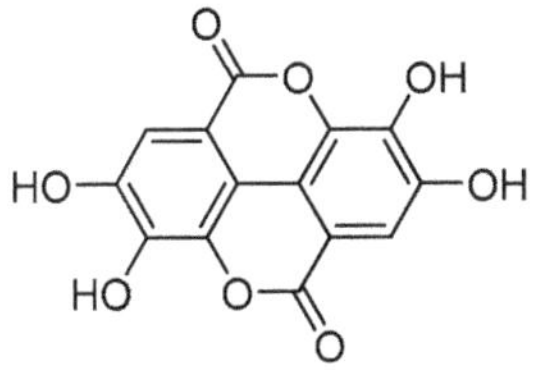

Figure 1. Chemical structure of ellagic acid.

The evidence from epidemiologic and clinical studies suggests that a daily intake of 400–800 g of vegetables and fruits may prevent 20% or more of cancer cases. Studies in vitro, animal, and clinical studies have demonstrated the potential role of berry phenolic compounds in reducing cancer risk [23]. EA has a significant inhibitory effect on chemical-induced carcinogenesis and many other types of carcinogenesis, such as liver, lung, colon, breast, and cervical cancer [24–29]. Cervical cancer is the fourth leading cause of cancer death in women [27]. Long-term infection with human papillomavirus (HPV) is one of the causes of cervical cancer, and approximately 91% of cervical cancer patients are infected with high-risk HPV [30]. Studies have found that 16/18 are the two most prevalent HPV subtypes in patients with cervical cancer. Several studies have shown that the E6/E7 gene is the most abundant viral transcript in biopsies and HPV-positive cells from HPV-positive cervical cancer patients. E6/E7 plays a key role in the process of viral replication and carcinogenesis. The open reading frames of E6/E7 sequences are directly involved in regulating the growth and proliferation of cervical cancer cells and are closely related to apoptosis [31–35]. In this paper, apoptosis-related pathways and E6/E7 genes were selected. Changes in the mRNA levels of the related pathway genes were determined by qPCR, which initially revealed the related pathway of EA to inhibit the growth of HeLa cells. This provides part of the theoretical basis for the further development of EA in blackberry fruit.

EA has special physicochemical properties and low solubility in many solvents, so improving its extraction efficiency is significant for its utilization and research. In this study, the different growth stages of Hull were divided into five periods according to color, including green fruiting (S1), green to red (S2), red fruiting (S3), red to purple (S4), and ripening (S5). We determined the EA content as well as other antioxidants in fresh fruits at each stage. After determination and analysis, we selected the S1 period fruits for extraction and purification. After finally obtaining 90% pure EA powder, we further investigated the in vitro anticancer activity of EA and its possible pathway to inhibit cancer cells. It is hoped that this work will provide a theoretical basis for exploring the effective utilization value of blackberries and developing more functional foods.

2. Results

2.1. Determination of EA

The important morphological indicators and EA content in Hull fruits were measured at each ripening stage. Fifteen fruits were randomly selected to measure their weights and diameters, as shown in Figure 2b. The EA content showed a decreasing trend with fruit growth and development. Among the five stages, the highest EA content was found at the S1 stage at 5.67 mg/g (Figure 2c), while the lowest EA content was found at the S5 stage at 0.77 mg/g. Others were S2 with 1.54 mg/g, S3 with 0.89 mg/g, and S4 with 0.99 mg/g.

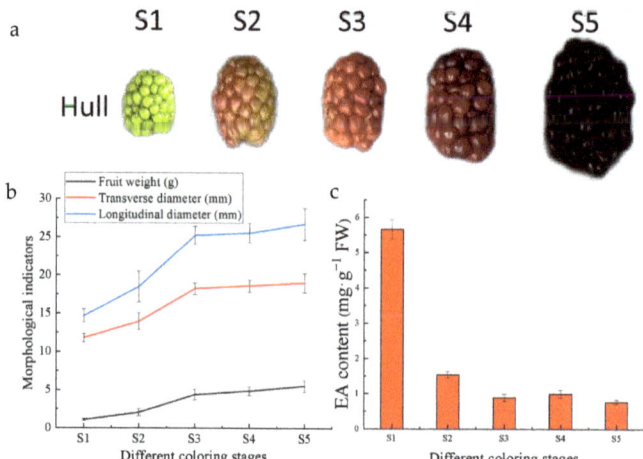

Figure 2. Hull fruit indicators: (**a**) Hull fruit appearance at each stage; (**b**) morphological indicators of Hull fruits at different coloring stages; (**c**) EA content in Hull fruits at different coloring stages.

2.2. Measurement of Fruit Quality Indexes

The antioxidant capacity and antioxidant substances as well as the content of saccharides in the fruits of Hull at different coloring stages were determined, which showed that the antioxidant substances and antioxidant capacity declined gradually with fruit growth and development (Figure 3). Among them, vitamin C decreased and then increased during fruit development, and the content was the highest in the S1 stage, while anthocyanin, which is related to fruit color, gradually accumulated with fruit growth and development. The total antioxidant capacity of fruits in Hull was 857.90 U·mgprot^{-1} FW in S1 period, DPPH scavenging capacity was higher at 340.07 mg Trolox·g^{-1} FW, and the highest content of anthocyanin was 0.91 mg·g^{-1} FW in S5 stage.

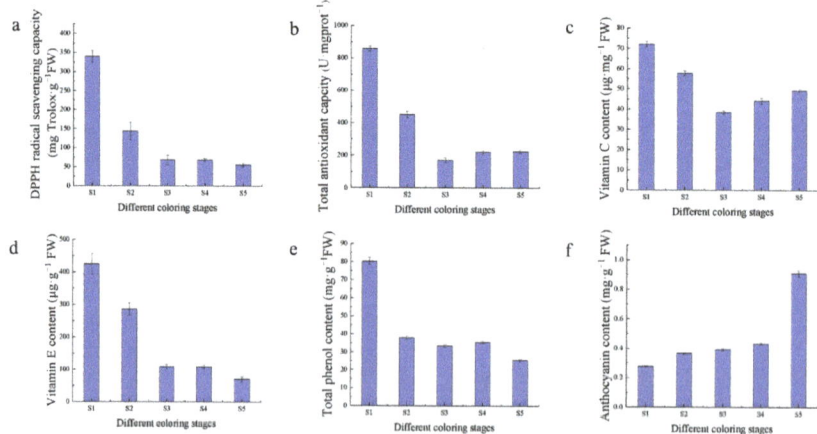

Figure 3. Antioxidant indicators: (**a**) DPPH radical scavenging capacity; (**b**) total antioxidant capacity; (**c**) vitamin C content; (**d**) vitamin E content; (**e**) total phenol content; (**f**) anthocyanin content.

Sugars are one of the important evaluation indexes of fruit flavor, which gradually accumulated with fruit growth and development, and reached the highest in the S5 period. The soluble sugar content increased linearly during fruit development, with the highest content of 61.78 mg/g in the S5 period, while the fructose content decreased gradually in the

S1–S3 period, with the lowest content of 12.71 mg/g in the S3 period. The fructose content increased linearly in the middle and late stages of fruit development, with the highest content of 56.65 mg/g in the S5 period (Figure 4). EA synthesis pathway is the mangiferolic acid pathway, the starting material is phosphoenolpyruvic acid, EA can combine with sugar to form glycosides, which leads to a decrease in free EA content. The high content of antioxidants and the low content of sugars in the S1 period during fruit growth and development make it suitable as a sample for EA extraction.

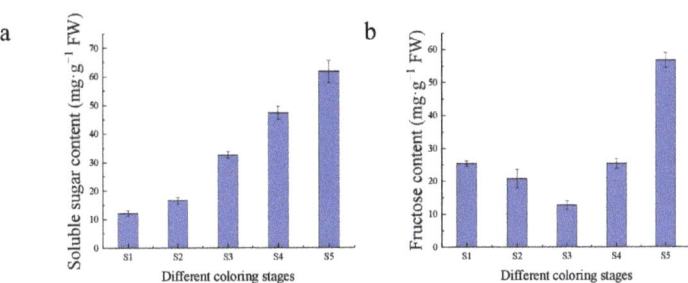

Figure 4. Sugars content. (**a**) Soluble sugar content; (**b**) fructose content.

2.3. Single-Factor Tests for EA Extraction

EA lyophilized powder was made from S1 fruits with the highest EA content. Four factors, including ethanol concentration, solid–liquid ratio, extraction time, and extraction temperature, were used to analyze the extraction process. The EA extracted under different conditions was determined and the optimal extraction conditions were studied. The results of the single-factor experiment showed that the optimal extraction conditions were a solid–liquid ratio of 1:20, an ethanol concentration of 40%, an extraction time of 20 min, and an extraction temperature of 80 °C.

The extraction efficiency of EA increased gradually with the increase in ethanol volume fraction and reached a peak extraction of 47.39 mg/g when the ethanol concentration reached 40%. However, the extraction efficiency decreased gradually when the ethanol concentration exceeded 40%. Therefore, the optimum concentration of ethanol is 40% (Figure 5a).

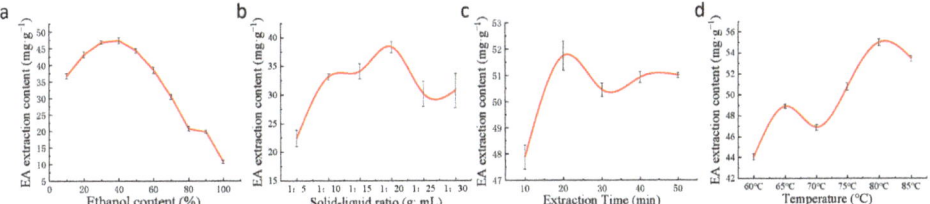

Figure 5. The effect of each single factor on the extraction efficiency of EA. (**a**) Ethanol concentration; (**b**) solid–liquid ratio; (**c**) ultrasonication time; (**d**) ultrasonication temperature.

The solid–liquid ratio has a strong influence on the extraction efficiency of EA. The smaller the solid–liquid ratio is, the more incomplete the extraction is and the lower the extraction efficiency is; the larger the solid–liquid ratio is, the more unnecessary waste will be produced, which also reduces the extraction efficiency. When the solid–liquid ratio was 1:20, the EA had been fully precipitated, and the EA content was 38.33 mg/g. Finally, 1:20 was chosen as the optimal solid–liquid ratio (Figure 5b).

Ultrasound can destroy the cell wall and make the cell contents more soluble in the extraction solvent. As the extraction time increased, the extraction rate of EA gradually increased, but a too-prolonged extraction time would consume a lot of time and cause problems such as EA aging, so the best extraction time was 20 min (Figure 5c). When the ultrasonic extraction time was 20 min, the maximum amount of EA extracted was 51.75 mg/g.

EA is not sensitive to high temperatures and is not highly soluble in many solvents. The extraction rate and solubility increased with increasing extraction temperature. When the temperature reached 80 °C, the EA content also reached the highest value of 53.46 mg/g. However, prolonged extraction at high temperatures will lead to the aging of EA and reduce its activity. Hence, 80 °C was chosen as the optimal extraction temperature. The best extraction conditions derived from the single-factor test were solid–liquid ratio of 1:20, ethanol concentration of 40%, ultrasonic extraction temperature of 80 °C, and time of 20 min. Under these conditions, the content of the extracted EA lyophilized powder was 55.20 mg/g (Figure 5d).

Solvent extraction is the earliest and most classical method. And ultrasonic waves have the advantages of penetration and cavitation, which can make the liquid molecules collide and interact with each other, thus rapidly rupturing the plant cell wall and releasing phenolic compounds. Ultrasonic extraction is easier to operate, with lower instrument costs, and is more efficient than other techniques [36,37]. Because of its similar polarity to EA, acetone is difficult to react with hydrolyzed tannins compared to other solvents. Li and colleagues used acetone as an extraction solvent and determined that an 80% acetone solution (containing HCl and vitamins) with a solid–liquid ratio of 1:12 (g/mL) was the most effective for EA extraction (323 µg/g) at 80 °C and reflux extraction for 90 min [38]. Ethanol is recognized as a low-toxicity organic reagent. Wang and coworkers used anhydrous ethanol as a solvent to extract EA from raspberries by ultrasound-assisted extraction. The best extraction conditions were as follows: solid–liquid ratio of 1:14 (g/mL), ultrasonic extraction for 20 min, and extraction temperature at 80 °C, and 670.28 µg/g of EA was obtained [39].

2.4. Response Surface Methodology to Optimize EA Extraction

According to the results of the single-factor experiments, the best three values were selected, and the above four critical factors were optimized using the experimental design software Design-Expert 8.0.6.1 (Stat-Ease, Minneapolis, MN, USA) and the Box–Behnken design method; the related process mathematical models were established and verified. The results of EA extraction were determined according to the experimental conditions shown in Tables 1 and 2.

Table 1. Response surface design experimental setup and results.

Number	A (°C)	B (min)	C (mL/g)	D/%	Ellagic Acid Content (mg/g)
1	1	0	1	0	48.28
2	0	0	0	0	54.84
3	1	1	0	0	51.24
4	0	−1	1	0	46.26
5	0	0	−1	1	48.12
6	−1	0	−1	0	50.21
7	0	1	1	0	49.06
8	−1	0	1	0	48.73
9	0	−1	−1	0	47.22
10	0	1	0	1	48.82
11	0	1	−1	0	50.83
12	1	0	0	−1	50.75
13	0	0	0	0	54.86
14	−1	−1	0	0	48.62
15	1	0	0	1	49.51
16	0	−1	0	1	46.36

Table 1. Cont.

Number	A (°C)	B (min)	C (mL/g)	D/%	Ellagic Acid Content (mg/g)
17	0	0	1	1	47.11
18	0	0	1	−1	47.95
19	−1	0	0	1	49.70
20	1	0	−1	0	50.10
21	−1	1	0	0	52.04
22	0	0	0	0	55.55
23	0	1	0	−1	52.18
24	−1	0	0	−1	52.50
25	1	−1	0	0	47.52
26	0	0	0	0	55.72
27	0	−1	0	−1	46.87
28	0	0	−1	−1	50.95
29	0	0	0	0	54.71

Table 2. Analysis of variance (ANOVA) of the fitted quadratic polynomial model.

Source	Sum of Squares	DF	Mean Square	F Value	p Value
Model	223.41	14	15.96	80.66	<0.0001
A	1.61	1	1.61	8.16	0.0127
B	37.85	1	37.85	191.3	<0.0001
C	8.42	1	8.42	42.55	<0.0001
D	11.16	1	11.16	56.42	<0.0001
AB	0.023	1	0.023	0.12	0.7385
AC	0.029	1	0.029	0.15	0.708
AD	0.62	1	0.62	3.12	0.099
BC	0.17	1	0.17	0.85	0.3734
BD	2.04	1	2.04	10.34	0.0062
CD	0.99	1	0.99	5	0.0422
A^2	22.71	1	22.71	114.81	<0.0001
B^2	74.74	1	74.74	377.81	<0.0001
C^2	87.38	1	87.38	441.69	<0.0001
D^2	55.37	1	55.37	279.86	<0.0001
Residual	2.77	14	0.2		
Lack of fit	1.91	10	0.19	0.88	0.6044
Pure error	0.86	4	0.22		
Cor total	226.18	28			
R-squared	0.9878				
Pred R-squared	0.9455				
Adj R-squared	0.9755				

Note: differences were considered significant at the level of $p < 0.05$.

By response surface analysis, the EA extraction efficiency equation in relation to the main factors was determined to be y = 55.13 − 0.37A + 1.78B − 0.84C − 0.96D + 0.076AB − 0.085AC + 0.39AD − 0.20BC − 0.71BD + 0.50CD − 1.87A^2 − 3.39B^2 − 3.67C^2 − 2.92D^2. The partial regression coefficients of the primary terms in the order of B > D > C > A indicated that the most influential factor on the EA extraction efficiency was the extraction time, followed by the solid–liquid ratio, ethanol concentration, and extraction temperature. The ANOVA results showed that the experimental model was significant with a misfit of 0.604 and an R^2 of 0.988, which was similar to the predicted R^2 = 0.946, indicating that the experimental results were reliable.

Using Design-Expert 8.0.6.1 software, the contour lines and response surface maps of the corresponding quadratic regression equations were obtained (Figure 6). Discretization of the slope of the response surface and the contour of the response surface can directly reflect the interaction between the factors. It can be seen from the figure that the response surfaces of extraction time and liquid-solid ratio are very steep, indicating that extraction time and solid–liquid ratio have a significant effect on the extraction volume. In addition, the contours are elliptical in shape, indicating that the interaction between them is also very significant. The best process for extracting EA was determined to be a 1.20 solid–liquid ratio, 40% ethanol concentration, 80 °C extraction temperature, and 20 min extraction time.

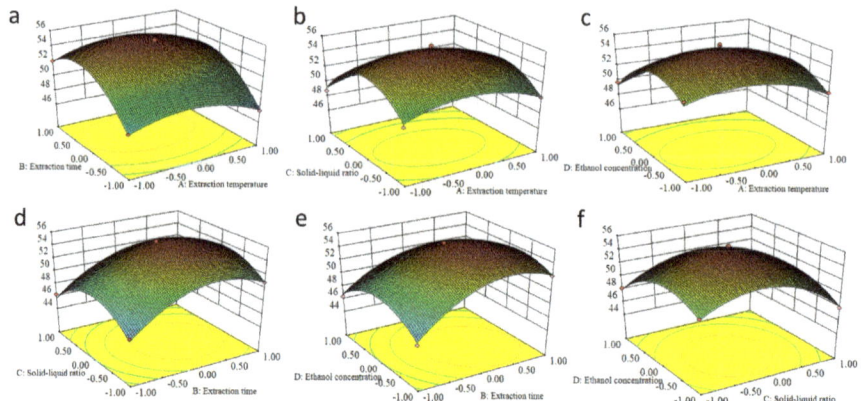

Figure 6. Response surface maps of the corresponding quadratic regression equations. (**a**) AB; (**b**) AC; (**c**) AD; (**d**) BC; (**e**) BD; (**f**) CD.

2.5. Purification of EA

The purification experiments were mainly performed by adsorption of macroporous resins, and the most suitable macroporous resin was selected by determining the static adsorption and resolution. HPD300 and HP20 had strong adsorption capacity for EA, and the adsorption capacity was stable after 5 h. The adsorption rates were about 65% and 63%, and the amounts of EA adsorbed on the resins were 13.77 mg/g and 13.43 mg/g, respectively. The results showed that the resolution of EA was completed after adding ethanol for 30 min, with the highest resolution of 93% and 88% for HP20 and HPD300, respectively (Figure 7). HP20 macroporous resin was selected for subsequent purification.

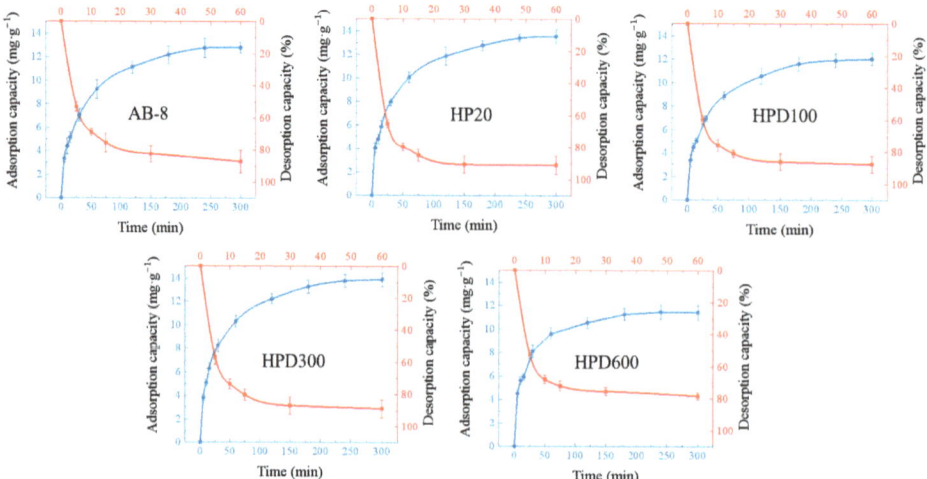

Figure 7. Adsorption and resolution curves with the five macroporous resins. The blue lines are the adsorption curves, and the red lines are the resolution curves.

In order to separate compounds, the adsorption force of macroporous resins depends on the physical adsorption between the macroporous resins and the adsorbed substances through van der Waals forces. Macroporous resins have the advantages of high extraction rate, non-toxicity, non-harmfulness, and non-pollution of the environment. Wang's group compared the adsorption capacity of different resins for EA, and finally chose HPD 600 for the first isolation and purification of the crude extract of EA [40]. In the experiment, the EA concentration measured at constant volume was 61%, and after the second purification by CG-161 resin, the final concentration of EA reached 80%.

The first purified powder collected after adsorption with HP20 macroporous resin contained 20% EA. The recovery of EA from the fruit was 85%. After that, the supernatant was extracted continuously (twice) by column adsorption, and the purified powder with 55% EA content was recovered. This powder was completely dissolved with NaOH and precipitated with HCl, and a precipitated powder with about 85% EA content was collected. Then, the powder was further dissolved in methanol, heated under reflux conditions and the precipitate was collected by centrifugation. The final high-purity powder with 90% EA content was obtained and used for the following evaluation of anticancer activity. Infrared spectra (pure) v_{max}/cm^{-1} 3474, 3155, 1721, 1618, 1582, 1510, 1446, 1398, 1374, 1326, 1260, 1194, 1111, 1038, 922, 875, 813, 757, 687, 634, 580, 535, and 460 (Figure S1). The retention time of EA in the UPLC was 12.38 min. EA retention time in UHPLC was 12.38 min, which was similar to the literature (Figure S2) [41].

2.6. Biological Evaluations

2.6.1. Anticancer Activity of EA In Vitro

We further evaluated the anticancer activity of the purified EA on the growth of the human cancer cell lines HeLa, HepG2, MCF-7, and A549 and normal cells (HUVECs) by MTT assay in vitro. The results are shown in Figure 8.

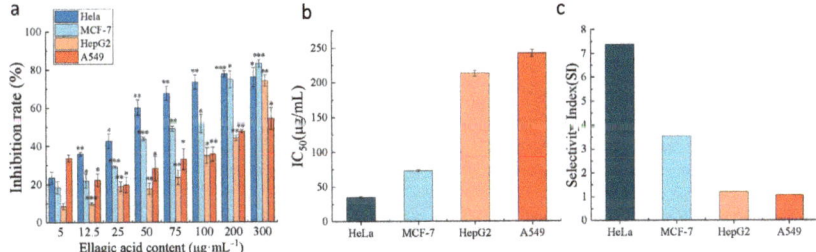

Figure 8. The anticancer activity of the purified EA extract. (**a**) The rates of inhibition of four types of cancer cells induced by EA; (**b**) IC$_{50}$ values of the purified EA extract against four types of cancer cells; (**c**) selectivity indices (SIs) of the purified EA extract. *** $p < 0.001$; ** $p < 0.01$; * $p < 0.05$.

According to Figure 8a, EA-mediated growth inhibition occurred in a dose-dependent manner. The highest inhibition rate was observed in HeLa cells with an IC$_{50}$ of 35 µg/mL, while in MCF-7 cells, the IC$_{50}$ was 73 µg/mL, in HepG2 cells, the IC$_{50}$ was 213 µg/mL, in A549 cells, the IC$_{50}$ was 242 µg/mL, and in HUVECs, the IC$_{50}$ was 258 µg/mL (Figure 8b). The toxicity of EA to the nonmalignant cell line (HUVECs) was also investigated to characterize the selectivity, which is expressed as the selectivity index (SI) (SI = (IC$_{50}$ for nonmalignant HUVECs)/(IC$_{50}$ for the human tumor cell lines)) [42], as illustrated in Figure 8c. An important consideration for future pharmacological applications is the SI. EA exhibits moderate to good cytotoxic activity against human cancer cells, with significantly enhanced selectivity for HeLa, MCF-7, HepG2, and A549 cells (SI value > 1). Li and colleagues further demonstrated the anticancer properties of EA in human cervical cancer cell lines by MTT assays. These authors confirmed that EA reduced the proliferation of human cervical cancer HeLa, SiHa, and C33A cells in a dose- and time-dependent manner, and the inhibitory effect was significantly more pronounced in HeLa cells than in SiHa and C33A cells [30]. In another study, it was previously reported that EA dose-dependently inhibited the growth of HeLa cells [43], which is consistent with our findings.

In order to investigate the apoptosis-inducing ability of EA in HeLa cells, we chose three EA concentrations (50, 25, and 12.5 µg/mL) that were close to the IC$_{50}$ of HeLa cells. Figure 9 is an image of normal HeLa cells in a logarithmic growth phase under a normal light microscope, with clear cell boundaries and moderately pike-shaped morphology. After incubation with different concentrations of EA for different times (24 and 48 h), the morphology and number of HeLa cells were observed under the light microscope. The results showed that the number of cells gradually decreased with the increase in culture concentration and time, and the cells became wrinkled, rounded, and lost their original morphology.

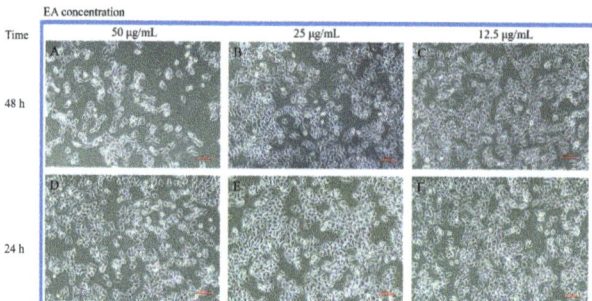

Figure 9. HeLa cells incubated with EA. (**A–C**) are images taken under a light microscope after incubation with 50, 25, and 12.5 µg/mL EA for 48 h, respectively; (**D–F**) for 24 h, respectively. Scale bar = 500 µm.

2.6.2. Induction of Apoptosis In Vitro

It is generally recognized that the mechanism of anticancer action of EA involves the regulation of apoptosis. Apoptosis is characterized by numerous morphological changes in the structure of the cell, together with many enzyme-dependent biochemical processes. The result of apoptosis is the removal of cells from the body with minimal damage to surrounding tissues. And the initiation of apoptosis depends on the activation of a series of cysteine-aspartate proteases called caspases [44].

To further investigate the exact mechanism by which EA inhibits the proliferation of HeLa cells, we used flow cytometry to assess the effect of EA on HeLa cell apoptosis. The results indicated that the apoptosis rate of HeLa cells was dose-dependent with EA concentration. The apoptosis rate was highest at about 67% when the EA concentration was 50 µg/mL, 45% when the EA concentration was 25 µg/mL, and 44% when the EA concentration was 12.5 µg/mL. The data showed (Figure 10) that EA significantly inhibited the proliferation of HeLa cells by inducing apoptosis.

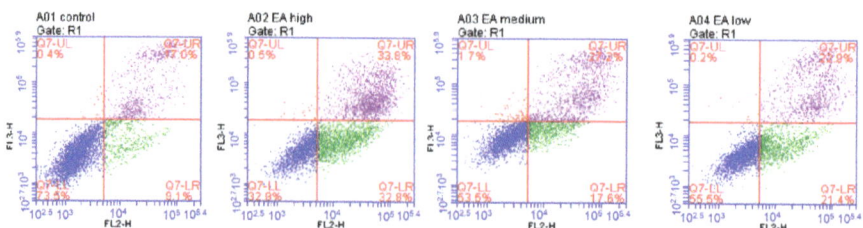

Figure 10. Apoptosis induced by EA analyzed by flow cytometry. HeLa cells incubated with DMSO were used as controls, while experimental cells were treated with 50, 25, and 12.5 µg/mL EA.

2.6.3. Confocal Fluorescence Imaging In Vitro

As mentioned above, EA can inhibit cell proliferation by inducing apoptosis. Therefore, we tried to visualize the induced apoptosis process by confocal fluorescence imaging (Figure 11).

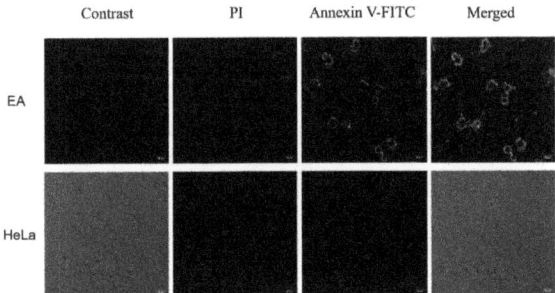

Figure 11. Confocal fluorescence microscopy images of HeLa cells incubated with 50 µg/mL EA for 48 h at 37 °C. Scale bar = 20 µm.

As D'Arcy reported, apoptosis can be distinguished from non-programmed forms of cellular necrosis by visual observation under a microscope and by a variety of molecular biology techniques including flow cytometry and DNA fragmentation assays using Annexin V-FITC staining [44]. After Annexin V-FITC staining, the cytoplasm displays green fluorescence and the PI after staining, the nucleus shows red fluorescence. Apoptotic cells stained only green fluorescence, necrotic cells stained green and red fluorescence, and normal cells did not fluoresce. Almost no green or red fluorescence signal was observed in the negative control, indicating that the cells were in a normal state. After treatment with EA (50 µg/mL) for 48 h at 37 °C, the green fluorescent signal was strong and the red fluorescent signal was weak in the cytoplasm, which indicated that EA had the ability to induce apoptosis.

2.6.4. Apoptosis Pathway Assay

In order to further determine the pathways by which EA inhibits the growth of HeLa cells, we studied the changes in the mRNA levels of genes associated with the apoptotic pathway. Changes in apoptosis-related pathway genes are shown in Figure 12. The results showed that *caspase*, *PTEN*, *TSC*, and *mToR* expression were up-regulated and *AKT*, *PDK1* expression were down-regulated, which showed a dose-dependent relationship with EA. *E6/E7* are two sequences encoded by HPV18 whose open reading frames are directly involved in cervical cancer cell growth and development. We further evaluated the *E6/E7* gene. The mRNA levels of *E6/E7* were determined to decrease gradually with the increase in EA incubation time and concentration. The phosphatase and tensin homolog (PTEN), which is deleted on chromosome 10, is a tumor suppressor that negatively regulates the AKT/PI3K with negative regulatory effects, and the AKT/PI3K signaling pathway is associated with tumorigenesis and apoptosis [45,46]. The mammalian target of rapamycin (mTOR) is involved with malignancy-associated genes, which can promote cancer cell proliferation and inhibit apoptosis [47]. TSC upstream of the mTOR signaling pathway, and the TSC1/TSC2 complex can inhibit mTOR activity [48]. The above results tentatively suggest that EA may inhibit cell growth through the above-related pathway.

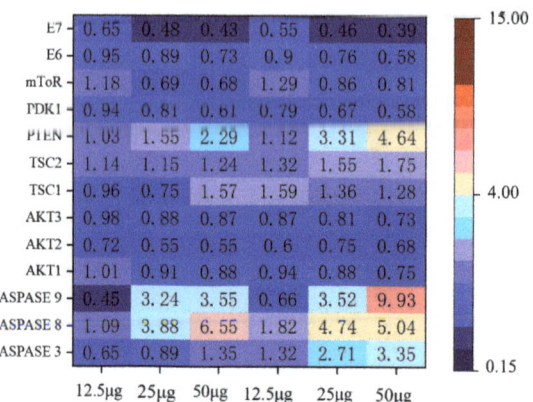

Figure 12. Heatmap of the inhibition of HeLa cell growth and apoptosis pathway-related genes after incubation with 12.5, 25, and 50 μg/mL EA for 24 h and 48 h.

3. Discussion

It has been shown that daily consumption of phenolic-rich foods has a preventive effect on some diseases [49,50], so it has a positive effect on the breeding of plants with high phenolic acid content. In this paper, we initially determined the trend of EA content during the growth and development process of Hull fruits; the results showed that Hull has high EA content. The highest EA content was 5.76 mg/g FW in the S1 period and the lowest EA content was in the S5 period. Because metabolites during fruit ripening depend on the expression of relevant genes and the action of biological enzymes [51], metabolomics and transcriptomics are of great significance for the study of metabolite accumulation. Therefore, elucidating the molecular mechanism of EA accumulation in blackberry fruits will have a positive effect on the targeted selection of superior varieties, and it will be beneficial to develop effective methods to improve fruit quality in response to market demand.

As verified by in vitro cell assay, the results indicated that EA could regulate the expression of E6/E7 genes through PTEN/AKT/mTOR/PI3K-related pathways and inhibit the growth and development of HeLa cells. In a few words, EA inhibits the growth of HeLa cells by inducing apoptosis. Apoptosis is a form of cell suicide in a physiological mode, resulting in controlled cell death. It plays a central role in cancer and can provide important information for studying behaviors related to development and homeostasis regulation. Consistent with Li's findings [30], E6/E7 is directly involved in the growth and development of cervical cancer cells, and EA has an inhibitory effect on its expression, so EA shows an inhibitory effect on HeLa. As per our previous report, polyphenol extract may interact with DNA in an intercalation mode to change or destroy DNA and cause apoptosis, and inhibit cell proliferation. When DNA damage is introduced into cells from exogenous or endogenous sources there is an increase in the amount of intracellular reactive oxygen species (ROS) that may be related to apoptosis [42]. EA is a kind of natural polyphenol, the further possible mechanism may be that EA can induce apoptosis by interacting with DNA in an intercalation mode, changing or destroying DNA. However, EA cannot be exploited for in vivo therapeutic applications in the current situation because of its poor water solubility and accordingly low bioavailability. Thus, further work to improve its water solubility and bioavailability will be needed in the future. Despite the fact that blackberry is one of the natural sources of EA, an edible berry rich in several phenolic acids, the digestive and absorptive transformation of EA after ingestion into the human body is necessary. As Lei [52] reported that EA in pomegranate leaf is rapidly absorbed and distributed as well as eliminated in rats. Zhou and co-workers determined the pharmacokinetics of oral EA in rats with rapid distribution and time to peak. The blood concentration peaked at 0.5 h with C_{max} = 7.29 μg/mL, and the drug concentration decreased to half of the original after 57 min of administration [53]. Therefore, increasing the drug concentration, prolonging the retention time of EA, and improving the bioavailability are of great significance in the research and development as well as utilization of botanical drugs.

4. Materials and Methods

4.1. Materials and Chemicals

Hull blackberry fruits were collected from the Baima Science Research Base of the Institute of Botany, Jiangsu Province, and Chinese Academy of Sciences (Nanjing, China), and the disease-free fruits were stored at −30 °C. EA standards (content > 96%, were used as control analysis; content > 98%, standard products). The total antioxidant capacity assay kit, DPPH free radical scavenging capacity assay kit, plant soluble sugar content test kit, Vitamin E assay kit, Vitamin C assay kit, and fructose assay kit (Nanjing Jiancheng Bioengineering Institute, Nanjing, China) were used. The macroporous resins HPD100, HPD300, HPD600, AB-8, and HP20 (Sobolai, Beijing, China) and acetonitrile, trichloroacetic acid, potassium bromide (KBr), Dulbecco's modified Eagle's medium (DMEM), fetal bovine serum (FBS), phosphate-buffered saline (PBS), 3-(4,5-dimethyl-2-thiazolyl)-2,5-diphenyl-2-H-tetrazolium bromide (MTT), dimethyl sulfoxide (DMSO), penicillin/streptomycin, trypsin, the RNA extraction kit (Keybionet, Nanjing, China), and Annexin V-FITC/PI (Beyotime, Shanghai, China) were purchased commercially. HeLa, HepG2, MCF-7, and A549 cells and HUVECs were kindly provided by Cell Bank, Chinese Academy of Sciences.

4.2. Measurement Method of EA

4.2.1. UV Spectrophotometric Method

The EA content was rapidly determined by UV spectrophotometry. EA is a phenolic acid that reacts with bases, and this complex has a maximum absorption peak of 357 nm [54]. According to this method the gradient concentration EA absorbance values were determined and the standard curve was plotted as in Figure 13. The standard curve gave the equation of y = 0.0531x + 0.0042 after fitting (R^2 = 0.9997).

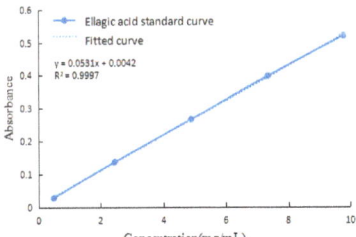

Figure 13. EA standard curve.

4.2.2. UHPLC Analysis

An Agilent 1260 Infinity II ultra-high performance liquid chromatography system was used for separation by Phenomenex Gemini 5u C18 column (250 mm × 4.60 mm, 5 μm). The mobile phase water(A)/acetonitrile(B) (A:B = 85:15) acidified to 0.05% (w/v) with trichloroacetic acid. The flow rate was 1 mL/min; the column temperature was 30 °C; the wavelength of 254 nm; and the injection volume of 10 μL [55].

4.3. Measurement of Fruit Quality Indexes

Ultrasound-assisted solvent extraction method was used to extract the anthocyanin in the fruits, and anthocyanin content was determined at 510 nm by UV spectrophotometry [56]. Determination of the total phenol content of the fruit was carried out by Floin–Ciocalteu method [57], absorbance value was measured at 750 nm, and the total phenol content in the sample was calculated by the standard curve y = 0.128x + 0.00045

($R^2 = 0.999$). The content of the remaining substances was determined according to the method of the kit instructions.

4.4. Single-Factor Experiments of EA Extraction from Blackberries

For each stage, 30 g of fruit was homogenized and prepared. Extraction conditions were as follows: the temperature of ultrasonic extraction was 50 °C, the time of ultrasonic extraction was 20 min, the solid–liquid ratio was 1:10, and the solvent was anhydrous ethanol. After the extraction, the extract was centrifuged at 7000 rpm for 5 min, and then 1 mL of the clarified supernatant was added with 4 mL of NaOH (0.1 mol/L), absorbance value was measured at 357 nm, so as to calculate the concentration of EA.

An analysis of four extraction process factors was performed to determine the effect of each factor on extraction efficiency in order to optimize the extraction process: solid–liquid ratio (1:5, 1:10, 1:15, 1:20, 1:25, 1:30, 1:35, and 1:40 (g:mL)), ethanol concentration (100%, 90%, 80%, 70%, 60%, 50%, 40%, 30%, 20%, and 10%), ultrasonic time (10 min, 20 min, 30 min, 40 min, and 50 min) and extraction temperature (50 °C, 60 °C, 65 °C, 70 °C, 75 °C, 80 °C, 85 °C).

4.5. Response Surface Factor Test

From the results of single-factor experiments, the Box–Behnken design in Design-Expert v8.0 software was used to optimize the extraction process with ethanol concentration (A), solid–liquid ratio (B), extraction time (C) and extraction temperature (D) as the independent variables, and amount of EA extracted as the dependent variable. Thus, −1, 0 and 1 denote the three levels of the independent variables. The experimental factors and levels were designed as shown in Table 3.

Table 3. Single-factor level experimental design.

Factors	Code	Coding Level		
		−1	0	1
Ethanol concentration	A	30%	40%	50%
Solid–liquid ratio	B	1:15	1:20	1:25
Extraction time	C	10 min	20 min	30 min
Extraction temperature	D	75 °C	80 °C	85 °C

4.6. EA Purification Experiment

After pretreatment, five macroporous resins of different polarities were selected, which include polar HPD600, weakly polar AB-8 and HPD300, and non-polar HP20 and HPD100. Next, 100 mL triangular flasks were filled with 3 g of the resins and 50 mL of the EA supernatant, and shaken for 5 min, 10 min, 15 min, 30 min, 60 min, 120 min, 180 min, 240 min, 300 min, and 360 min, at 150 rpm at room temperature. The EA content was determined from these data and the adsorption curves were plotted. We rinsed the EA-adsorbed resin with water to remove excess contaminants and liquid, and then added 50 mL of 60% ethanol and took samples at the same points to plot the resolution curves in the adsorption experiments. The most effective resin was selected for subsequent purification experiments.

The extracted supernatant was purified by column chromatography and eluted with 60% ethanol, and the primary purified EA powder was obtained after evaporation of ethanol and freeze-drying. The primary purified EA powder was mixed with 1 mol/L NaOH until it was completely dissolved, the pH was adjusted to 12~14, the pH was then adjusted to 2~4 by adding HCl, and EA was precipitated overnight at 4 °C. The EA precipitate was collected by centrifugation after secondary purification, and the secondary purified product was added to a methanol solution at a ratio of 1:100. After heating to reflux at 80 °C for 2 h, the solution was recrystallized overnight at 4 °C and collected. Finally, the relative content of EA was determined.

4.7. MTT Assay In Vitro

Human cervical cancer cells (HeLa), human non-small-cell lung cancer cells (A549), human breast cancer cells (MCF-7), and human liver cancer cells (HepG2) were cultured in vitro under 5% CO_2 at 37 °C. Cancer cells were added to 96-well plates at a density of 1×10^4 cells per well. After 12 h of incubation, the medium was removed and the cells were incubated with different EA concentrations (each concentration was repeated three times) for 48 h. Then, the medium was removed and a new medium containing MTT (1 mg/mL) was added and incubated for 4 h. The absorbance of each well was measured at 595 nm. Cell viability values were determined (at least three times) according to the following formula: cell viability (%) = absorbance of the experimental group/absorbance of the blank control group × 100% [54,57].

4.8. Induction of Apoptosis In Vitro

HeLa cells (1×10^6) were cultured in 35 mm dishes and incubated at 37 °C for 24 h. After adding EA at concentrations of 12.5, 25, and 50 μg/mL, the cells were incubated for 48 h (each concentration was repeated three times). DMSO (0.1%) was used as a control. The treated cells were washed, trypsinized (without EDTA (ethylene diamine tetraacetic acid), and centrifuged. Next, the cells were collected and resuspended in 500 μL of buffer solution loaded with 5 μL of Annexin V-FITC and 5 μL propidium iodide (PI), the cells were incubated for 5–15 min in the dark. Flow cytometry analysis was conducted with a single 488 nm argon laser and 80,000 events with a BD Accuri C6 flow cytometer and software (Becton, Dickinson and Company, Franklin Lakes, NJ, USA) [54].

4.9. qRT–PCR Detection

After treating the cells with the same procedure as in vitro apoptosis assessment, all the cells were collected to extract all the RNA according to the kit method and reverse transcribed to cDNA. cDNA was diluted to 400 ng/μL. The fluorescence quantification reaction (qPCR) system had a total volume of 15 μL (1 μL of cDNA, 0.6 μL of primers, 5.3 μL of ddH$_2$O, and 7.5 μL of mix). The primer sequences are detailed in Table 4.

Table 4. Primer sequences for quantitative fluorescence analysis.

Gene Name	Forward (5′-3′)	Reverse (5′-3′)	Amplification Length (bp)
Caspase 3	ACCAGTGGAGGCCGACTTCT	GCATGGCACAAAGCGACTGG	107
Caspase 8	ACCGAAACCCTGCAGAGGGA	CATCGCCTCGAGGACATCGC	78
Caspase 9	GATGCCCTGTGTCGGTCGAG	GTGGAGGCCACCTCAAACCC	139
AKT1	GCGGCACACCTGAGTACCTG	CAGGCGACCGCACATCATCT	113
AKT2	CAGAACACCAGGCACCCGTT	GCCCGCTCCTCTGTGAAGAC	143
AKT3	TGTCGAGAGAGCGGGTGTTC	TGGTGGCTGCATCTGTGATCC	198
PTEN	TCCCAGTCAGAGGCGCTATGT	CCGTCGTGTGGGTCCTGAAT	199
TSC1	AAGCTTGGGCCTGACACACC	CTGTCTCCCGCAGGGCTTTC	86
TSC2	ATCTGCAGCGTGGAGATGCC	GTGTACGGCAGGGAGATGGC	200
mTOR	GCCTTTCCTGCGCAAGATGC	GCGGGCACTCTGCTCTTTGA	85
PI3K	AGGAGATCGCTCTGGCCTCA	TGGCTCGGTCCAGGTCATCC	161
E7	GGACGGGCCAGATGGACAAG	GGGTTCGTACGTCGGTTGCT	122
E6	TGTGTCAGGCGTTGGAGACAT	ACCTCAGATCGCTGCAAAGT	82

4.10. Data Analysis

The analytical data were statistically analyzed using SPSS Statistics 16.0 ((IBM, Chicago, IL, USA) and one-way ANOVA at a level of reliability of 0.05%. Origin 2019b (OriginLab Crop., Northampton, MA, USA) was used to analyze the IC$_{50}$ values with linear fitting. All experiments were repeated three times.

5. Conclusions

As one of the earliest introduced blackberry varieties in China, the Hull variety is currently planted over a large area in Jiangsu Province [58]. Hull is an extremely productive variety, has a high resistance to stress, and is the parent of many bred blackberry varieties [59,60]. Research has shown that the aging process and the occurrence of some diseases are oxidative processes, and the daily consumption of phenolic acid-rich substances has a positive effect on the occurrence and alleviation of some diseases [61,62]. Blackberries are rich in a variety of antioxidant-active substances such as phenols, flavonoids, and vitamins [63]. Blackberry fresh fruits are not easy to store, so the trend of blackberry active substances as well as their extraction and purification have certain far-reaching significance for the development and utilization of blackberries. In this research, in order to further develop and utilize blackberry fruits in depth, the fruits were divided into different developmental periods according to their color. The results showed that the EA content decreased gradually with the growth of blackberry fruits. The total antioxidant capacity, DPPH radical scavenging capacity, and total phenols in the fruit showed similar trends to the EA content, which was the highest in the S1 stage. The anthocyanin and saccharides accumulated gradually with the growth and development of the fruits, and the highest content was found at the S5 stage. The extraction process of EA was optimized by single-factor and response surface test, and the high-purity blackberry EA powder was purified several times. The results showed that EA had an anticancer effect and inhibited the growth of HeLa cells by inducing apoptosis.

Supplementary Materials: The following supporting information can be downloaded at: https://www.mdpi.com/article/10.3390/ijms242015228/s1.

Author Contributions: Methodology, investigation, formal analysis, writing—original draft, J.W. and F.Z.; plant resources collection, statistical analysis—original draft, L.L. and W.W.; data curation, writing—review and editing, supervision, C.Z.; funding acquisition, supervision, W.L. All authors have read and agreed to the published version of the manuscript.

Funding: This work is supported by Jiangsu Province Key Project of R&D Plan (Modern Agriculture) (BE2020344), Chinese Central Financial Project for Extension and Demonstration of Forestry Technology (SU [2021]TG08), and Chinese Central Financial Project for Cooperative Extension of Major Agricultural Technology (2022-ZYXT-06).

Institutional Review Board Statement: Not applicable.

Informed Consent Statement: The authors declare that they have no known competing financial interests or personal relationships that could have appeared to influence the work reported in this paper.

Data Availability Statement: The datasets generated during and/or analyzed during the current study are available from the corresponding author upon reasonable request.

Conflicts of Interest: The authors declare no conflict of interest.

References

1. Morin, P.; Luke, R.H.; John, T.; Cindi, B.; Andy, M.; Renee, T.T.; John, R.C.; Margaret, W. Phenolics and volatiles in arkansas fresh-market blackberries (Rubus subgenus Rubus Watson). *ACS Food Sci. Technol.* **2022**, *2*, 1728–1737. [CrossRef]
2. Moraes, D.P.; Machado, M.L.; Farias, C.A.A.; Barin, J.S.; Zabot, G.L.; Lozano, S.J.; Ferreira, D.F.; Vizzotto, M.; Leyva Jimenez, F.J.; Da Silveira, T.L.; et al. Effect of microwave hydrodiffusion and gravity on the extraction of phenolic compounds and antioxidant properties of blackberries (*Rubus* spp.): Scale-up extraction. *Food Bioprocess. Technol.* **2020**, *13*, 2200–2216. [CrossRef]
3. Moghadam, D.; Zarei, R.; Tatar, M.; Khoshdel, Z.; Mashayekhi, F.J.; Naghibalhossaini, F. Antiproliferative and anti-telomerase effects of blackberry juice and berry-derived polyphenols on HepG2 liver cancer cells and normal human blood mononuclear cells. *Anticancer Agents Med. Chem.* **2022**, *22*, 395–403. [CrossRef] [PubMed]
4. Paczkowska-Walendowska, M.; Go'sciniak, A.; Szymanowska, D.; Szwajgier, D.; Baranowska-Wójcik, E.; Szulc, P.; Dreczka, D.; Simon, M.; Cielecka-Piontek, J. Blackberry leaves as new functional food screening antioxidant, anti-inflammatory and microbiological activities in correlation with phytochemical analysis. *Antioxid* **2021**, *10*, 1945. [CrossRef]

5. Wu, H.; Di, Q.R.; Zhong, L.; Zhou, J.Z.; Shan, C.J.; Liu, X.L.; Ma, A.M. Enhancement on antioxidant, anti-hyperglycemic and antibacterial activities of blackberry anthocyanins by processes optimization involving extraction and purification. *Front. Nutr.* **2022**, *9*, 1007691. [CrossRef]
6. Gil-Martínez, L.; Mut-Salud, N.; Ruiz-García, J.A.; Falcón-Piñeiro, A.; Maijó-Ferré, M.; Baños, A.; De la Torre-Ramírez, J.M.; Guillamón, E.; Verardo, V.; Gómez-Caravaca, A.M. Phytochemicals determination, and antioxidant, antimicrobial, anti-inflammatory and anticancer activities of blackberry fruits. *Foods* **2023**, *12*, 1505. [CrossRef]
7. Sharifi-Rad, J.; Quispe, C.; Castillo, C.M.S.; Caroca, R.; Lazo-Vélez, M.A.; Antonyak, H.; Polishchuk, A.; Lysiuk, R.; Oliinyk, P.; De Masi, L.; et al. Ellagic acid: A review on its natural sources, chemical stability, and therapeutic potential. *Oxid. Med. Cell Longev.* **2022**, *2*, 3848084. [CrossRef]
8. Wink, M. Modes of action of herbal medicines and plant secondary metabolites. *Medicines* **2015**, *2*, 251–286. [CrossRef]
9. Pedro, A.Z.; Pedro, A.Z.; Jorge, E.W.; Juan, J.B.; Juan, A.A.; Juan, C.C.; Cristóbal, N.A. Ellagitannins: Bioavailability, purification and biotechnological degradation. *Mini. Rev. Med. Chem.* **2018**, *18*, 1244–1252. [CrossRef]
10. Tošović, J.; Bren, U. Antioxidative action of ellagic acid-a kinetic DFT study. *Antioxid* **2020**, *9*, 587. [CrossRef]
11. Ivan, S.M.; Emilija, J.; Nikolic Vesna, N.D.; Mirjana, P.M.; Srdjan, R.J.; Ivana, S.M. The effect of complexation with cyclodextrins on the antioxidant and antimicrobial activity of ellagic acid. *Pharm. Dev. Technol.* **2018**, *24*, 410–418. [CrossRef]
12. Al-Mugdadi, S.F.H.; Al-Sudani, B.T.; Mohsin, R.A.; Mjali, A.J. Anticarcinogenic and antimicrobial activity effects of the ellagic acid extract. *Int. J. Res. Pharm. Sci.* **2019**, *10*, 1172–1180. [CrossRef]
13. Wang, Y.; Ren, F.; Li, B.; Song, Z.; Chen, P.; Ouyang, L. Ellagic acid exerts antitumor effects via the PI3K signaling pathway in endometrial cancer. *J. Cancer* **2019**, *10*, 3303–3314. [CrossRef] [PubMed]
14. Duan, J.; Li, Y.X.; Gao, H.H.; Yang, D.H.; He, X.; Fang, Y.L.; Zhou, G.B. Phenolic compound ellagic acid inhibits mitochondrial respiration and tumor growth in lung cancer. *Food Funct.* **2020**, *11*, 6332–6339. [CrossRef]
15. Gil, T.Y.; Hong, C.H.; An, H.J. Anti-Inflammatory effects of ellagic acid on keratinocytes via MAPK and STAT pathways. *Int. J. Mol. Sci.* **2021**, *22*, 1277. [CrossRef] [PubMed]
16. Ashutosh, G.; Ramesh, K.; Risha, G.; Singh, A.K.; Rana, H.K.; Pandey, A.K. Antioxidant, anti-inflammatory and hepatoprotective activities of Terminalia bellirica and its bioactive component ellagic acid against diclofenac induced oxidative stress and hepatotoxicity. *Toxicol. Rep.* **2021**, *8*, 44–52. [CrossRef]
17. Zahin, M.; Ahmad, I.; Gupta, R.C.; Aqil, F. Punicalagin and ellagic acid demonstrate antimutagenic activity and inhibition of benzo[a]pyrene induced DNA adducts. *BioMed Res. Int.* **2014**, *5*, 467465. [CrossRef]
18. Ramadan, D.T.; Ali, M.A.M.; Yahya, S.M.; El-Sayed, W.M. Correlation between Antioxidant/ antimutagenic and antiproliferative activity of some phytochemicals. *Anticancer Agents Med. Chem.* **2019**, *19*, 1481–1490. [CrossRef]
19. Lin, C.; Wei, D.Z.; Xin, D.W.; Pan, J.L.; Huang, M.Y. Ellagic acid inhibits proliferation and migration of cardiac fibroblasts by down-regulating expression of HDAC1. *J. Toxicol. Sci.* **2019**, *44*, 425–433. [CrossRef]
20. Javaid, N.; Shah, M.A.; Rasul, A.; Chauhdary, Z.; Saleem, U.; Khan, H.; Ahmed, N.; Uddin Md, S.; Mathew, B.; Behl, T.; et al. Neuroprotective effects of ellagic acid in alzheimer's disease: Focus on underlying molecular mechanisms of therapeutic potential. *Curr. Pharm. Des.* **2021**, *27*, 3591–3601. [CrossRef]
21. Antonio, J.A.; Carmen, G.G.; Emilio, O.; Aleix, S.V.; Iolanda, L. Ellagic acid as a tool to limit the diabetes burden: Updated evidence. *Antioxid* **2020**, *9*, 1226. [CrossRef]
22. Harikrishnan, H.; Jantan, I.; Alagan, A.; Haque, M.A. Modulation of cell signaling pathways by Phyllanthus amarus and its major constituents: Potential role in the prevention and treatment of inflammation and cancer. *Inflammopharmacology* **2020**, *28*, 1–18. [CrossRef] [PubMed]
23. Wang, L.; Shi, Y.; Wang, R.; Su, D.D.; Tang, M.F.; Liu, Y.D.; Li, Z.G. Antioxidant activity and healthy benefits of natural pigments in fruits: A review. *Int. J. Mol. Sci.* **2021**, *22*, 4945. [CrossRef]
24. Syed, U.; Ponnuraj, N.; Ganapasam, S. Ellagic acid inhibits proliferation and induced apoptosis via the Akt signaling pathway in HCT-15 colon adenocarcinoma cells. *Mol. Cell. Biochem.* **2015**, *399*, 303–313. [CrossRef]
25. Srigopalram, S.; Jayraaj, I.A.; Kaleeswaran, B.; Balamurugan, K.; Ranjithkumar, M.; Kumar, T.S.; Park, J.I.; Nou, I.S. Ellagic acid normalizes mitochondrial outer membrane permeabilization and attenuates inflammation-mediated cell proliferation in experimental liver cancer. *Appl. Biochem. Biotechnol.* **2014**, *173*, 2254–2266. [CrossRef]
26. Shi, L.; Gao, X.; Li, X.; Jiang, N.; Luo, F.; Gu, C.; Chen, M.; Cheng, H.; Liu, P. Ellagic acid enhances the efficacy of PI3K inhibitor GDC-0941 in breast cancer cells. *Curr. Mol. Med.* **2015**, *15*, 478–486. [CrossRef]
27. Mouad, E.; Irina, O.; Izumi, O.; Ilya, G.; Liang, W.G.V.; Stephen, P.; Anna, S.G. Ellagic acid induces apoptosis through inhibition of nuclear factor κB in pancreatic cancer cells. *World J. Gastroenterol.* **2019**, *14*, 3672–3680. [CrossRef]
28. Tan, Y.H.; Shudo, T.; Tomoki, Y.; Yuma, S.; Ying, S.J.; Chihiro, T.; Takemoto, Y.; Akira, K. Ellagic acid, extracted from Sanguisorba officinalis, induces G1 arrest by modulating PTEN activity in B16F10 melanoma cells. *Genes Cell Devot. Mol. Cell Mech.* **2019**, *24*, 688–704. [CrossRef]
29. Li, L.W.; Na, C.; Tian, S.Y.; Chen, J.; Ma, R.; Gao, Y.; Lou, G. Ellagic acid induces HeLa cell apoptosis via regulating signal transducer and activator of transcription 3 signaling. *Exp. Ther. Med.* **2018**, *16*, 29–36. [CrossRef]
30. Li, K.; Yin, R.; Wang, D.Q.; Li, Q.L. Human papillomavirus subtypes distribution among 2309 cervical cancer patients in West China. *Oncotarget* **2017**, *8*, 28502–28509. [CrossRef]

31. Zhang, J.J.; Cao, X.C.; Zheng, X.Y.; Wang, H.Y.; Li, Y.W. Feasibility study of a human papillomavirus E6 and E7 oncoprotein test for the diagnosis of cervical precancer and cancer. *J. Int. Med. Res.* **2018**, *46*, 1033–1042. [CrossRef] [PubMed]
32. Zhang, X.; Zhang, A.; Zhang, X.; Hu, S.Y.; Bao, Z.H.; Zhang, Y.H.; Jiang, X.A.; He, H.P.; Zhang, T.C. ERa-36 instead of ERa mediates the stimulatory effects of estrogen on the expression of viral oncogenes HPV E6/E7 and the malignant phenotypes in cervical cancer cells. *Virus Res.* **2021**, *306*, 198602. [CrossRef]
33. Negi, S.S.; Sharma, K.; Sharma, D.; Singh, P.; Agarwala, P.; Hussain, N.; Bhargava, A.; Das, P.; Agarwal, S. Genetic analysis of human papilloma virus 16 E6/E7 variants obtained from cervical cancer cases in Chhattisgarh, a central state of India. *Virusdisease* **2021**, *32*, 492–503. [CrossRef]
34. Wen, N.; Bian, L.H.; Gon, J.; Meng, Y.G. RPRD1B is a potentially molecular target for diagnosis and prevention of human papillomavirus E6/E7 infection-induced cervical cancer: A case-control study. *Asia-Pac. J. Clin. Oncol.* **2020**, *17*, 230–237. [CrossRef] [PubMed]
35. Butz, K.; Geisen, C.; Ullmann, A.; Spitkovsky, D.; Hoppe-Seyler, F. Cellular responses of HPV-positive cancer cells to genotoxic anti-cancer agents: Repression of E6/E7-oncogene expression and induction of apoptosis. *Int. J. Cancer* **1996**, *68*, 506–513. [CrossRef]
36. Zhao, F.Y.; Wang, J.L.; Wang, W.F.; Lyu, L.F.; Wu, W.L.; Li, W.L. The extraction and high antiproliferative effect of anthocyanin from gardenblue blueberry. *Molecules* **2023**, *28*, 2850. [CrossRef]
37. Hanis, N.A.A.; Aini, N.A.; Suzana, Y.; Mohd, Y.M.H. Ultrasonic extraction of 2-acetyl-1-pyrroline (2AP) from pandanus amaryllifolius roxb. Using ethanol as solvent. *Molecules* **2022**, *27*, 4906. [CrossRef]
38. Li, X.P. Study on Extraction, Refining and Oxidationresistant and Antimicrobiall Effects of Ellagic Acid from Red Raspberry. Ph.D. Thesis, Gansu Agriculture University, Lanzhou China, 2010.
39. Wang, J.H.; Yu, X.Y.; Liao, S.L.; Chen, S.K.; Zhao, Y.; Fu, Q. Optimization of extraction process of ellagic acid from raspberry. *For. By-Prod. Spéc. China* **2017**, *27*, 14–17. [CrossRef]
40. Wang, J.N. Separation and Purification of Ellagic Acid of and Its Effect on Lipid Peroxidation in *Lonicera caerulea* L. Ph.D Thesis, Harbin University Commerce, Harbin, China, 2018.
41. Paulo Isaac, D.A.; Edemilson, C.C.; Leonardo, L.B.; Joelma, A.M.P. Development and validation of a HPLC-UV method for the evaluation of ellagic acid in liquid extracts of *Eugenia uniflora* L. (Myrtaceae) leaves and its ultrasound-assisted extraction optimization. evidence-based complement. *Altern. Med.* **2017**, *2017*, 1501038. [CrossRef]
42. Zhao, F.Y.; Du, L.L.; Wang, J.L.; Liu, H.X.; Zhao, H.F.; Lyu, L.F.; Wang, W.F.; Wu, W.L.; Li, W.L. Polyphenols from Prunus mume: Extraction, purification and anticancer activity. *Food Funct.* **2023**, *14*, 4380–4391. [CrossRef]
43. Kumar, D.; Basu, S.; Parija, L.; Rout, D.; Manna, S.; Dandapat, J.; Debata, P.R. Curcumin and ellagic acid synergistically induce ROS generation, DNA damage, p53 accumulation and apoptosis in HeLa cervical carcinoma cells. *Biomed. Pharmacother.* **2016**, *6*, 31–37. [CrossRef] [PubMed]
44. Mark, S.D. Cell death: A review of the major forms of apoptosis, necrosis and autophagy. *Cell Biol. Int.* **2019**, *43*, 582–592. [CrossRef]
45. Feng, Y.Q.; Zou, W.; Hu, C.H.; Li, G.Y.; Zhou, S.H.; He, Y.; Ma, F.; Deng, C.; Sun, L.L. Modulation of CASC2/miR-21/PTEN pathway sensitizes cervical cancer to cisplatin. *Arch. Biochem. Biophys.* **2017**, *6*, 623–624. [CrossRef] [PubMed]
46. Du, G.H.; Cao, D.M.; Meng, L.Z. miR-21 inhibitor suppresses cell proliferation and colony formation through regulating the PTEN/AKT pathway and improves paclitaxel sensitivity in cervical cancer cells. *Mol. Med. Rep.* **2017**, *15*, 2713–2719. [CrossRef]
47. van Veelen, W.; Korsse, S.E.; van de Laar, L.; Peppelenbosch, M.P. The long and winding road to rational treatment of cancer associated with LKB1/AMPK/TSC/mTORC1 signaling. *Oncog* **2011**, *30*, 2289–2303. [CrossRef]
48. Ken, I.; Li, Y.; Xu, T.; Guan, K.L. Rheb GTPase is a direct target of TSC2 GAP activity and regulates mTOR signaling. *Genes Dev.* **2003**, *17*, 1829–1834. [CrossRef]
49. Wu, X.; Schauss, A.G. Mitigation of inflammation with foods. *J. Agric. Food Chem.* **2012**, *60*, 6703–6717. [CrossRef]
50. Jean-Gilles, D.; Li, L.; Ma, H.; Yuan, T.; Chichester, C.O.; Seeram, N.P. Anti-inflammatory effects of polyphenolic-enriched red raspberry extract in an antigen-induced arthritis rat model. *J. Agric. Food Chem.* **2012**, *60*, 5755–5762. [CrossRef]
51. Chen, Z.; Jiang, J.Y.; Shu, L.Z.; Li, X.B.; Huang, J.; Qian, B.Y.; Wang, X.D.; Li, X.; Chen, J.X.; Xu, H.D. Combined transcriptomic and metabolic analyses reveal potential mechanism for fruit development and quality control of Chinese raspberry (*Rubus chingii* Hu). *Plant Cell Rep.* **2021**, *40*, 1–24. [CrossRef]
52. Lei, F.; Xing, D.M.; Xiang, L.; Zhao, L.X.; Wang, W.; Zhang, L.J. Pharmacokinetic study of ellagic acid in rat after oral administration of pomegranate leaf extract. *Drug Evaluat.* **2005**, *2*, 38–41. [CrossRef]
53. Zhou, J.; Zhou, B.X.; Tu, J.; Zhang, C.; Luo, Y.; Liu, Y. Pharmacokinetic study of ellagic acid and gallic acid of *Punica granatum* L. husk extract in rats. *China Med. Herald.* **2015**, *12*, 19–23.
54. Zhao, H.F.; Lyu, L.F.; Zhang, C.H.; Wang, X.M.; Li, W.L.; Wu, W.L. Rubus'Ningzhi 3': A new blackberry cultivar. *J. Nanjing For. Univ.* **2020**, *44*, 231–232. [CrossRef]
55. Zhang, C.H.; Lyu, L.F.; Zhao, H.F.; Wang, X.M.; Li, W.L.; Wu, W.L. Rubus'Shuofeng': A new blackberry cultivar. *J. Nanjing For. Univ.* **2020**, *44*, 245–246. [CrossRef]
56. Chen, G.; Huang, L.S.; Xu, J.; Jian, S.P.; Wang, H.L. Ultrasonic-assisted extraction and antioxidant activity of antho cyanins from blackberry fruits. *Food Sci.* **2012**, *33*, 117–121.

57. Li, J.; Nie, J.Y.; Li, H.F.; Xu, G.F.; Wang, X.D.; Wu, Y.L.; Wang, Z.X. On determination conditions for total polyphenols in fruits and its derived products by Folin- phenol methods. *J. Fruit Sci.* **2008**, *25*, 126–131. [CrossRef]
58. Wu, W.L.; Sun, Z.J.; Cai, J.H. The five varieties of black poison are "Hull" and "Chester" and their cultivation techniques. *China Fruit* **1995**, *4*, 16–18. [CrossRef]
59. Zhang, Y.Z.; Wang, L.; Zhang, J.J.; Xiong, X.M.; Zhang, D.; Tang, X.M.; Luo, X.J.; Ma, Q.L. Vascular peroxide 1 promotes ox-LDL-induced programmed necrosis in endothelial cells through a mechanism involving β-catenin signaling. *Atheroscler* **2018**, *274*, 128–138. [CrossRef]
60. Zhao, F.Y.; Zhao, H.F.; Wu, W.L.; Wang, W.F.; Li, W.L. Research on anthocyanins from Rubus "Shuofeng" as potential antiproliferative and apoptosis-inducing agents. *Foods* **2023**, *12*, 1216. [CrossRef]
61. Croge, P.C.; Cuquel, L.F.; Pintro, T.M.P.; Biasi, L.A.; Claudine, M.B. Antioxidant capacity and polyphenolic compounds of blackberries produced in different climates. *HortScience* **2019**, *54*, 2209–2213. [CrossRef]
62. Neth, B.J.; Bauer, B.A.; Benarroch, E.E. The role of oxidative stress in Parkinson's disease. *Antioxyd* **2020**, *9*, 461–491. [CrossRef]
63. Mar, L.; Antonio, G.S.; Teresa, M.G.; Francisco, A.T.; Juan, C.E. Urolithins, ellagic acid-derived metabolites produced by human colonic microflora, exhibit estrogenic and antiestrogenic activities. *J. Agric. Food Chem.* **2006**, *54*, 1611–1620. [CrossRef]

Disclaimer/Publisher's Note: The statements, opinions and data contained in all publications are solely those of the individual author(s) and contributor(s) and not of MDPI and/or the editor(s). MDPI and/or the editor(s) disclaim responsibility for any injury to people or property resulting from any ideas, methods, instructions or products referred to in the content.

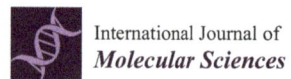

Article

Potentiation of Cisplatin Cytotoxicity in Resistant Ovarian Cancer SKOV3/Cisplatin Cells by Quercetin Pre-Treatment

Aseel Ali Hasan [1], Elena Kalinina [1,*], Julia Nuzhina [2,3], Yulia Volodina [4], Alexander Shtil [4] and Victor Tatarskiy [2,3]

[1] T.T. Berezov Department of Biochemistry, RUDN University, 6 Miklukho-Maklaya St., 117198 Moscow, Russia; ali.aseel.hasan@gmail.com
[2] Laboratory of Molecular Oncobiology, Institute of Gene Biology, Russian Academy of Sciences, 34/5 Vavilov Street, 119334 Moscow, Russia; julia.nuzhina@gmail.com (J.N.); tatarskii@gmail.com (V.T.)
[3] Center for Precision Genome Editing and Genetic Technologies for Biomedicine, Institute of Gene Biology, Russian Academy of Science, 34/5 Vavilov Street, 119334 Moscow, Russia
[4] Laboratory of Tumor Cell Death, Blokhin National Medical Research Center of Oncology, 24 Kashirskoye Shosse, 115478 Moscow, Russia; uvo2003@mail.ru (Y.V.); shtilaa@yahoo.com (A.S.)
* Correspondence: kalinina-ev@rudn.ru

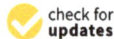

Citation: Hasan, A.A.; Kalinina, E.; Nuzhina, J.; Volodina, Y.; Shtil, A.; Tatarskiy, V. Potentiation of Cisplatin Cytotoxicity in Resistant Ovarian Cancer SKOV3/Cisplatin Cells by Quercetin Pre-Treatment. *Int. J. Mol. Sci.* **2023**, *24*, 10960. https://doi.org/10.3390/ijms241310960

Academic Editors: Marilena Gilca and Adelina Vlad

Received: 18 May 2023
Revised: 28 June 2023
Accepted: 29 June 2023
Published: 30 June 2023

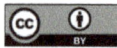

Copyright: © 2023 by the authors. Licensee MDPI, Basel, Switzerland. This article is an open access article distributed under the terms and conditions of the Creative Commons Attribution (CC BY) license (https://creativecommons.org/licenses/by/4.0/).

Abstract: Previously, we demonstrated that the overexpression of antioxidant enzymes (*SOD-1*, *SOD-2*, *Gpx-1*, *CAT*, and *HO-1*), transcription factor *NFE2L2*, and the signaling pathway (*PI3K/Akt/mTOR*) contribute to the cisplatin resistance of SKOV-3/CDDP ovarian cells, and treatment with quercetin (QU) alone has been shown to inhibit the expression of these genes. The aim of this study was to expand the previous data by examining the efficiency of reversing cisplatin resistance and investigating the underlying mechanism of pre-treatment with QU followed by cisplatin in the same ovarian cancer cells. The pre-incubation of SKOV-3/CDDP cells with quercetin at an optimum dose prior to treatment with cisplatin exhibited a significant cytotoxic effect. Furthermore, a long incubation with only QU for 48 h caused cell cycle arrest at the G1/S phase, while a QU pre-treatment induced sub-G1 phase cell accumulation (apoptosis) in a time-dependent manner. An in-depth study of the mechanism of the actions revealed that QU pre-treatment acted as a pro-oxidant that induced ROS production by inhibiting the thioredoxin antioxidant system Trx/TrxR. Moreover, QU pre-treatment showed activation of the mitochondrial apoptotic pathway (cleaved caspases 9, 7, and 3 and cleaved PARP) through downregulation of the signaling pathway (mTOR/STAT3) in SKOV-3/CDDP cells. This study provides further new data for the mechanism by which the QU pre-treatment re-sensitizes SKOV-3/CDDP cells to cisplatin.

Keywords: quercetin; cisplatin; antioxidant systems; antioxidant enzymes; signaling pathway; pro-oxidant effect

1. Introduction

Despite the significant strides that have been made towards the development of targeted anticancer therapies, chemotherapy remains the first-line treatment for most cancers [1,2]. Platinum-based antitumor drugs, such as cisplatin (CDDP) (Figure 1), are established chemotherapeutic agents in the treatment of a number of cancers and sarcomas; however, the development of cisplatin resistance is a major obstacle to curative cancer treatment [3]. Drug resistance phenomena can be developed through several mechanisms, such as the overexpression of drug efflux pumps, activation of DNA repair efficiency, escape of drug-induced apoptosis, active cell survival signals, and enhanced drug detoxifying systems [4,5].

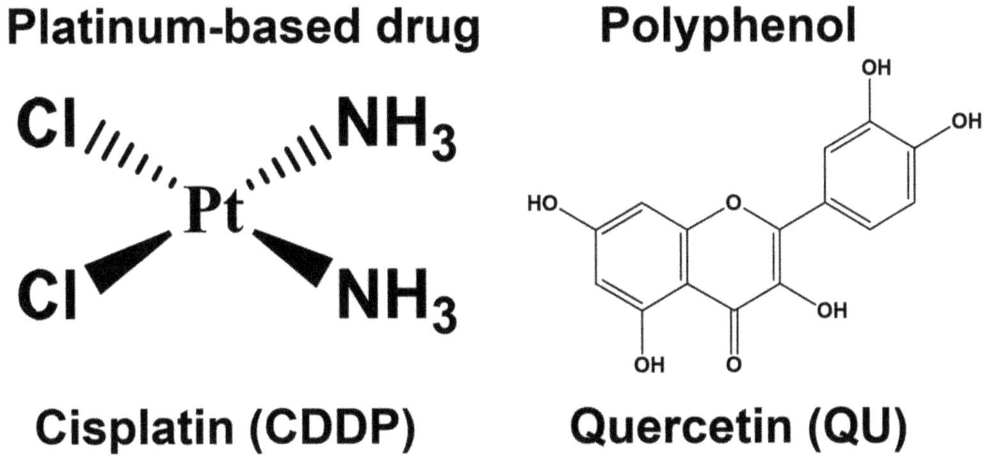

Figure 1. The chemical structures of the platinum-based drug (cisplatin; CDDP) and polyphenol (quercetin; QU).

Under normal physiological conditions, the cellular redox homeostasis ensures that the cells respond appropriately to endogenous and exogenous stimuli. The redox systems are perfectly suited to the regulation of the cell's life-or-death decisions [6]. Both antioxidant enzymes (superoxide dismutase (SOD), glutathione reductase (GR), catalase (CAT), etc.) and low molecular weight antioxidants are, effectively, inbuilt defense strategies to maintain cellular redox homeostasis during oxidative stress [7], which is defined as a disturbance in the balance between the generation of reactive oxygen and nitrogen species (RONS) and the antioxidant systems in the cell. The electron transport chain (ETC) in mitochondria and the NADPH oxidases (NOX) are the major endogenous sources of ROS, including the superoxide anion ($O_2^{\bullet-}$), hydrogen peroxide (H_2O_2), organic hydroperoxides (ROOH), the hydroxyl radical ($^{\bullet}OH$), and the peroxyl radical (ROO), inside the cell. Enzymatic antioxidant defense for ROS elimination occurs as a series of the following reactions: SODs catalyze the dismutation of the $O_2^{\bullet-}$ into H_2O_2. GPx catalyzes the detoxification of H_2O_2 by reduced glutathione (GSH). Further on, GR reduces oxidized glutathione (GSSG) to (GSH) using NADPH as the electron donor, while H_2O_2, which is found mainly in peroxisomes and cytosol, is neutralized by the CAT enzyme [8].

In addition to its role in defense against oxidative stress, the thioredoxin (Trx) system also regulates DNA synthesis, the cell cycle, and the apoptosis process in mammalian cells [9]. The over-activated Trx system, which contributes significantly to cancer progression and therapy resistance, has been recognized in several human tumors, including such highly aggressive types as lung, liver, pancreas, ovarian, and breast cancers. This antioxidant system is composed of cytosolic/nuclear and mitochondrial thioredoxin reductases (TrxR-1 and TrxR-2) and thioredoxins (Trx-1 and Trx-2), respectively. TrxR-1 and TrxR-2 are able to transfer electrons from NADPH to oxidized forms of Trx-1 and Trx-2, respectively, which reduce their substrates using a highly conserved dithiol form of the active site sequence [8]. Oxidized signal transducers and activators of transcription 3 (STAT3) dimers, being one of the Trx target proteins, receive electrons from a reduced Trx form to regenerate reduced STAT3 monomers. Upon Tyr705 phosphorylation, the transcriptionally active phosphorylated STAT3 (pSTAT3) homodimer is formed, which in turn translocates to the nucleus and interacts with specific DNA sequences to promote STAT3-dependent gene expression [10]. The accumulating evidence shows that the overexpression of STAT3, a transcription factor, has been observed in several cancer types and that it correlates with increased tumor cell proliferation, survival, self-renewal, tumor invasion, and angiogenesis, as well as higher cellular resistance to cisplatin [11,12]. Another important signaling pathway that correlates with pro-survival, the mechanistic target of rapamycin (mTOR) signaling, is also associated with CDDP resistance; it is necessary to phosphorylate STAT3 on serine^{727} to ensure its maximum activation [11].

A number of epidemiological studies have validated the fact that the consumption of dietary polyphenols, mainly quercetin (QU) (Figure 1), is inversely correlated with cancer incidence; this has been attributed to the antioxidant properties of QU, which prevent cancer through the increasing expression of antioxidant enzymes [13]. Moreover, QU exerts its anticancer activity by modulating cell cycle progression, reducing cell proliferation, and inhibiting angiogenesis and metastasis progression [14], as well as by promoting apoptosis and autophagy via the modification of various pathways, such as the PI3K/Akt/mTOR, Wnt/β-catenin, and MAPK/ERK1/2 pathways [15]. QU, a DNA intercalator, causes S-phase arrest during cell cycle progression and is consistent with the plausible induction of DNA damage following DNA intercalation within the cancer cells, which can eventually lead to the inducing of apoptosis [16]. In addition to these mechanisms, QU can also trigger apoptosis via various mechanisms that depend on the type of cancer cells. For instance, QU inhibited the growth of human A375SM melanoma cells through inducing apoptosis via activation of the JNK/P38 MAPK signaling pathway [17]. In vitro and in vivo mitochondrial-derived apoptosis following QU treatment in HL-60 AML cells was found to occur via reactive-oxygen-species-mediated ERK activation [18].

However, the clinical application of QU is limited due to its poor solubility, low bioavailability, poor permeability, and instability [19]. The bioavailability of quercetin can be significantly enhanced when it is consumed as an integral food component [20]. The bioavailability of QU can be improved by encapsulating it in polymer micelles. The intravenous administration of QU encapsulated in biodegradable monomethoxy poly (ethylene glycol)-poly (ε-caprolactone) (MPEG-PCL) micelles significantly inhibited the growth of established xenograft A2780S ovarian tumors through the activation of apoptosis and the inhibition of angiogenesis in vivo. This confirms the effectiveness of the clinical application of QU in the treatment of ovarian cancer [21].

QU also showed an anticancer effect on chemotherapy-resistant cells, such as CDDP, through the inhibition of the proliferation of ovarian carcinoma (SKOV3) and osteosarcoma (U2OS) human cell lines, as well as their cisplatin (CDDP)-resistant counterparts. Furthermore, the inhibition of the cyclin D1 level was associated with G1/S-phase alteration in QU-treated cells. CDK and cyclin inhibition by QU may be a viable therapeutic target in the ovarian CDDP-resistant cell line. Due to the ability of quercetin to overcome the resistance of cancers toward CDDP, a significant emphasis should be placed on using combinatory chemotherapy with cytotoxic drugs, particularly CDDP [22].

Despite the several studies which have investigated the anticancer effects of QU in in vitro and in vivo models, some of these effects have not been observed in ovarian cancer. However, to the best of our knowledge, the underlying mechanisms by which QU sensitizes ovarian cancer cells to CDDP, particularly those with acquired CDDP resistance, e.g., SKOV-3/CDDP, remain elusive and still need to be elucidated to a large extent. In the previous study, after treatment with QU alone, cisplatin-resistant SKOV-3/CDDP ovarian cancer cell lines exhibited inhibition in the gene expressions of antioxidant enzymes (*SOD-1, SOD-2, Gpx-1, CAT,* and *HO-1*), transcription factor *NFE2L2*, and the signaling pathway (*PI3K/Akt/mTOR*), which contribute to cisplatin-resistance in these cells [23].

In the present study, we attempted to explore the anticancer effects of QU pre-treatment on the CDDP-resistant ovarian adenocarcinoma human SKOV-3/CDDP cell line model. For the first time, we provide evidence that QU pre-treatment exerts pro-oxidant activity on the SKOV-3/CDDP cell line via alleviation of the protein expression of the cytosolic and mitochondrial thioredoxin antioxidant (Trx/TrxR) system that maintains STAT3 in a reduced/active state. We also identified the mechanism by which QU pre-treatment sensitizes SKOV-3/CDDP cells to cisplatin-induced apoptosis through a downregulation signaling (mTOR/STAT3) pathway. Thus, this research provides a better understanding of the mechanisms involved in QU-mediated CDDP sensitization in SKOV-3/CDDP ovarian cancer cells.

2. Results

2.1. QU Pre-Treatment Inhibits the Cell Survival of SKOV3 and SKVO3/CDDP Cell Lines

In our recently published research articles [23,24], IC$_{50}$ doses of the QU and CDDP under investigation in the SKOV3 human ovarian cancer cell line and the CDDP-resistant subline, SKVO3/CDDP, were screened as cell models. In order to determine whether QU pre-treatment impairs the CDDP resistance in the SKOV3/CDDP cell line, we designed an alternative QU pre-treatment strategy to compare it to the classical individual QU or CDDP treatment, assuming that the individual treatment with QU or CDDP does not exhibit an effect; the significant effect appears only when co-treatment is applied (Figure 2a).

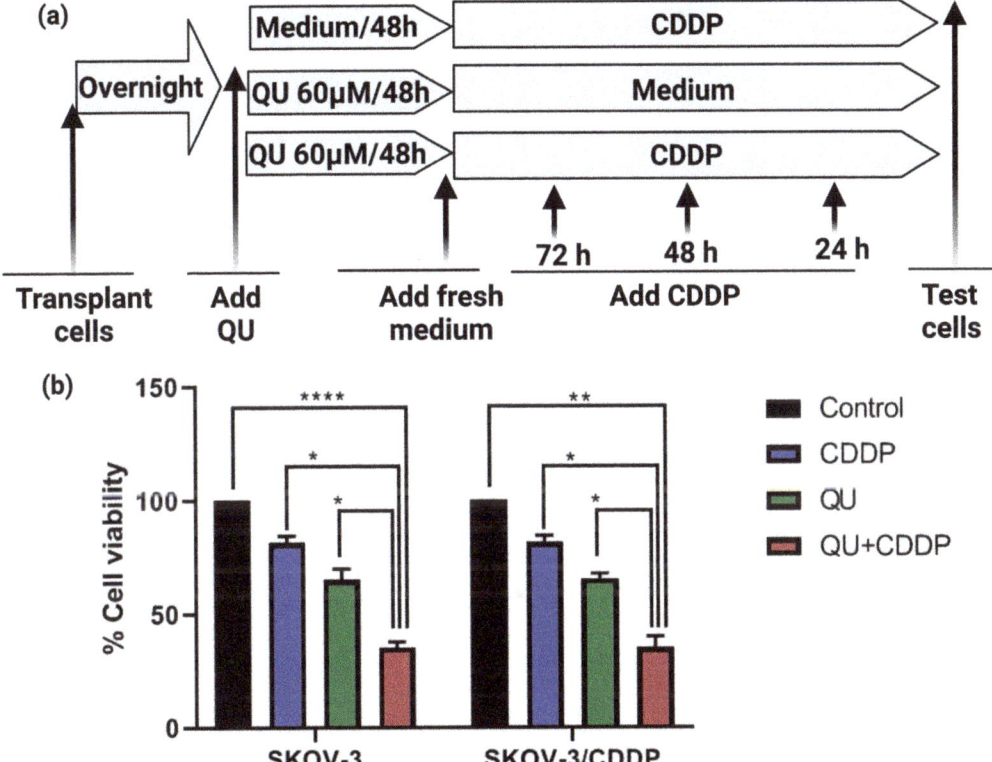

Figure 2. The QU effect on the viability of SKOV3 and SKOV3/CDDP cells. (a) Design of QU pre-treatment strategy. Both ovarian cancer cells were either treated individually with CDDP for 24, 48, and 72 h, or with QU for 48 h followed by replacement with fresh medium for an additional 24, 48, and 72 h, or pre-treated with QU for 48 h followed by CDDP for an additional 24, 48, and 72 h after changing medium. (b) QU pre-treatment effect on the CDDP efficacy. Both cells were treated with QU (60 µM) for 48 h followed by fresh medium for 72 h and/or CDDP (5 µM for SKOV-3 and 17 µM for SKOV-3/CDDP) for 72 h. Cell viability was assessed using an MTT assay. All data are presented as mean ± SEM and were evaluated using one-way ANOVA followed by Tukey's corrections for multiple comparisons between different treatments; * $p = 0.05/0.01$, ** $p = 0.005$, **** $p = 0.0001$.

Based on our data, we decided to use the optimum minimum and maximum effective doses of QU and CDDP as the reference values for QU (15 and 100 µM) for 24 h [23]

(Figure S1). However, we found that a long pre-incubation with a significantly non-toxic moderate dose (60 µM) of QU for 48 h was recognized as having an optimum effect on cell viability, enabling it to re-sensitize the SKOV-3/CDDP cisplatin-resistant human ovarian adenocarcinoma subline to CDDP, which was used in this experiment and further on in the rest of the experiments in this study. For instance, at 60 µM of QU for 48 h, followed by 5 µM (1/2 IC_{50}) for 72 h, CDDP significantly resulted in the inhibition (65% decrease; $p < 0.0001$) of the viability of the SKOV-3 cells, compared with CDDP (5 µM; 20% decrease) and QU (60 µM; 35% decrease) alone (Figure 2b).

However, in the SKOV-3/CDDP subline cells, CDDP at the doses of 5 µM and 10 µM did not result in any loss of viability, suggesting that these cells are endogenously resistant to CDDP compared to the SKOV-3 cells (Figure S2). The MTT assay revealed that the percentage of QU-treated cells decreased concomitantly when cisplatin was used at the dose of 34 µM (IC_{50}) and at 17 µM (1/2 IC_{50}) (Figure S2). Thus, for the SKOV-3/CDDP subline, the non-toxic dose of CDDP was optimized at 17 µM (1/2 IC_{50}). In a similar manner to the SKOV-3 cells, the pre-incubation of SKOV-3/CDDP subline cells with QU significantly resulted in the inhibition of cell survival (65% decrease at 17 µM concentration of CDDP for 72 h; $p < 0.005$), compared with the treatments with only CDDP (17 µM; 20% decrease) and QU (60 µM; 35% decrease) alone (Figure 2b). These data revealed that the pre-treatment with QU followed by CDDP effectively induced survival inhibition in both ovarian cancer cells.

2.2. QU Pre-Treatment Increases Sub-G1 Phase Cell Accumulation in SKOV3 and SKVO3/CDDP Cell Lines, with Increasing Apoptotic Cell Percentages

As cytotoxicity is frequently accompanied by cell cycle arrest, the impact of QU or CDDP alone and QU pre-treatment in SKOV-3 and SKOV-3/CDDP cells was evaluated by cell DNA content using PI staining for flow cytometry (Figure 3). The cell cycle analysis showed that at the lower dose of 5 µM (1/2 IC_{50} SKOV-3) of CDDP treatment, the SKOV-3 cells were arrested at the S phase (Figure 3a), while only at the higher dose of 17 µM (1/2 IC_{50} SKOV-3/CDDP) of CDDP were the SKOV-3/CDDP cells arrested at the S and G2/M phases and slightly accumulated at the sub-G1 phase in a time-dependent manner (Figure 3b). Compared to the control groups, the sub-G1 and G2/M phases of the SKOV-3 and SKOV-3/CDDP cells treated with only QU were time-dependently increased (Figure 3). Therefore, the effect of CDDP on cell cycle distribution in QU pre-treated cells was the induction of sub-G1 accumulation, which indicated apoptosis-associated chromatin degradation and the arrest of the cell cycle in the G2/M or S phases. For the SKOV-3 cells, the QU pre-treatment resulted in a significant increase in the sub-G1 phase, where it increased from 61 ± 1% at 24 h to 72.4 ± 2% at 48 h (Figure 3c). Meanwhile, in comparison, the percentage of cells in the sub-G1 phase at 72 h for the SKOV-3/CDDP cells was 53.5 ± 0.7% (Figure 3d). In our previous study [23], we revealed that the treatment of cells with only QU at a high dose (100 µM for 24 h) slightly increased the population of ovarian treated cells in the S and sub-G1 phases, while with a long incubation period, mainly of 48 h, QU significantly arrested the cell cycle at the G1/S phase and at the same time had no toxicity effect even after 72 h of incubation (Figure S3). Representative flow cytometry images for the cell cycle analysis are shown in (Figure 3).

Here, in addition to the pre-treatment strategy, we studied the synergistic approach by adding QU and CDDP at the same time for 24 h, 48 h, and 72 h and analyzed the effect of this combination on the cell cycle. Unexpectedly, the results of the cell cycle showed that the synergistic approach in SKOV-3/CDDP leads to an arrested cell cycle in the G2/M or S phases without a significant increase in the sub-G1 phase, even after the long incubation (Figure S4). On the other hand, QU pre-treatment significantly increased the percentage of cells in the sub-G1 phase and the sensitivity of the cisplatin-resistant ovarian cancer cells SKOV-3/CDDP to CDDP even after replacing QU with a fresh medium for a period of 24, 48, and 72 h.

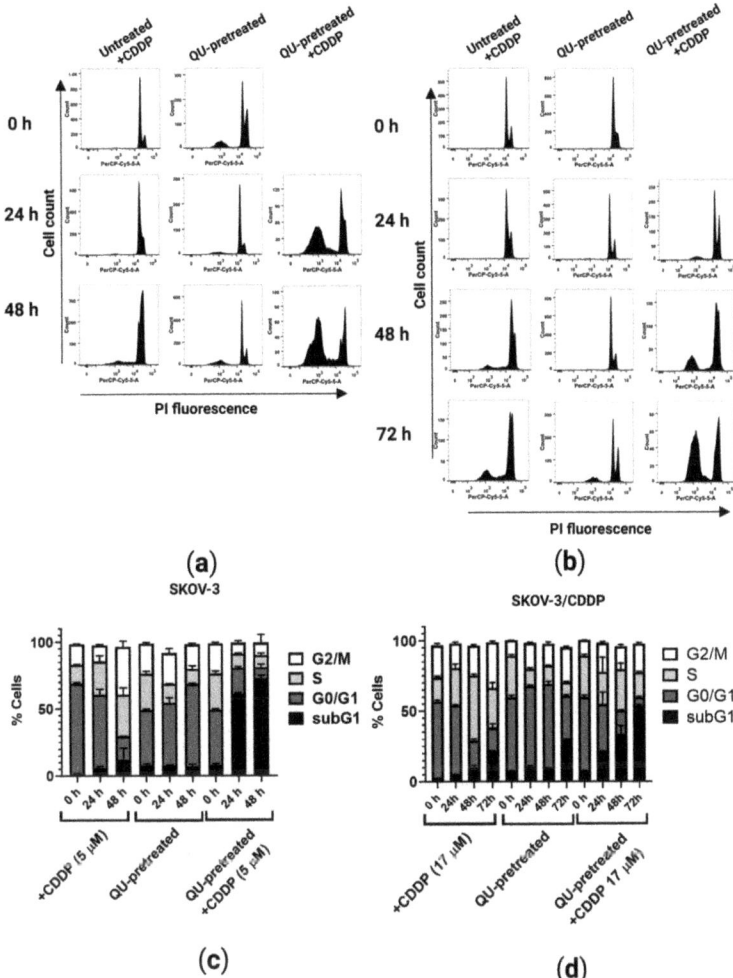

Figure 3. Cell cycle progression of ovarian cancer cells treated with QU and/or CDDP. Cells were incubated with QU (60 μM) for 48 h and then fresh medium and/or CDDP (5 μM for SKOV-3 and 17 μM for SKOV-3/CDDP) were added for further 24, 48, and 72 h incubation. After this exposure period, cell DNA content analysis with PI staining was performed by flow cytometry. (**a**) Representative flow cytometry dot plots; SKOV-3 and (**b**) SKOV-3/CDDP. (**c**) Representative flow cytometry histograms; SKOV-3 and (**d**) SKOV-3/CDDP.

2.3. QU Pre-Treatment Induces Cellular Reactive Oxygen Species (ROS) Production by CDDP in SKVO3/CDDP Cell Line

To investigate whether the accumulation of both ovarian cancer cells in sub-G1 by QU pre-treatment was due to the induction of oxidative stress, intracellular ROS production was evaluated by using the CellROX Deep Red assay (Figure 4). Our study suggested that QU pre-treatment could induce earlier ROS production; therefore, we investigated the change in the ROS level in pre-treated ovarian cancer cells. The treatment with QU alone for 24 h and 48 h was found to reduce the ROS levels in comparison to those of the control group in both types of cells (Figure 4). Following CDDP exposure for 4 h, no increase in ROS levels was observed in either the SKOV-3 or the SKOV-3/CDDP cells (Figure 4). In SKOV-3, after 24 h, CDDP triggered the ROS generation up to four-fold

(17 ± 2.9% cells against 4 ± 0.3% in the control), whereas in the SKOV3/CDDP cells it was only up to three-fold; this can be explained by the high level of antioxidant system in the resistant cells [23] (Figure 4b). The QU pre-treatment reduced the effect of CDDP through decreasing the intracellular ROS to the control level in SKOV-3 (Figure 4b). Conversely, in SKOV-3/CDDP, the proportion of the fluorescent cells was 5 ± 1% and 9 ± 1% in the untreated cells and the CDDP group, respectively, whereas the QU pre-treated cells had 23 ± 1% fluorescent cells (Figure 4b).

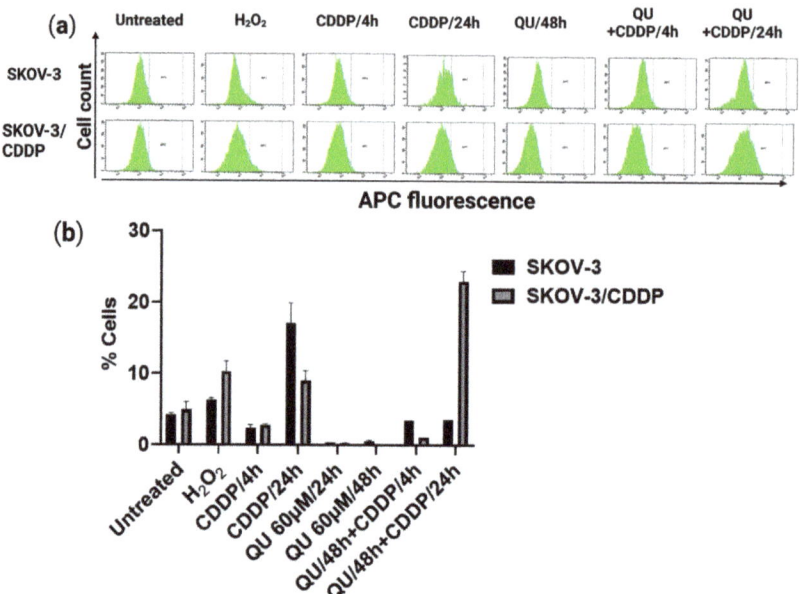

Figure 4. ROS flow cytometry detection in ovarian SKOV-3 and SKOV-3/CDDP cells under QU and CDDP treatment. (**a**) Intracellular ROS level upon either QU or CDDP treatment alone and QU pre-treatment. Both cultured cells were treated with either 60 μM QU (48 h) or 5 μM and 17 μM CDDP (24 h) and QU pre-treatment (48 h), followed by 5μM or 17 μM CDDP (24 h) for SKOV-3 and SKOV-3/CDDP, respectively, and subjected to ROS detection with CellROX Deep Red staining using flow cytometry. (**b**) Quantitative analysis of CellROX Deep Red probe-positive cells.

According to these results, we evaluated the increase in the pro-oxidant effect of QU pre-treatment concomitant with ROS production in the SKOV-3/CDDP cells. Interestingly, this polyphenol compound had an antioxidant effect at 24 and 48 h and a pro-oxidant effect only in the pre-treatment group. These results provide support for the proposal that QU pre-treatment increased the sensitivity of CDDP-resistant ovarian cancer SKOV-3/CDDP cells to CDDP and induced the accumulation of SKOV-3/CDDP cells in sub-G1 by promoting ROS formation.

2.4. QU Pre-Treatment Alleviates Protein Expression of Thioredoxin Antioxidant System Trx/TrxR, as Well as the mTOR/STAT3 Signaling Pathway in SKVO3/CDDP Cell Line

To further elucidate whether the inducing of the accumulation of SKOV-3/CDDP cells in sub-G1 and ROS production by QU pre-treatment is mediated through modulation of the antioxidant system and signaling pathway, the protein expression level associated with sensitivity to CDDP was assessed in ovarian cells using Western blot analysis. Our study identified that the expressions of the important thioredoxin antioxidant system Trx/TrxR, as well as the mTOR/STAT3 signaling pathway, were dramatically higher in the SKOV-3/CDDP subline cells compared with those in the SKOV-3 cells (Figure 5a–c). This suggests that the overexpression of these proteins makes a significant contribution to the development of SKOV-3/CDDP cells in their acquiring of resistance to CDDP. Previously, we used SKOV-3 and SKOV-3/CDDP subline cells to analyze the effect of two different doses (15 μM and 100 μM) of QU in modulating antioxidant enzymes (*SOD-1*, *SOD-2*, *Gpx-1*, *CAT*, and *HO-1*), transcription factor *NFE2L2*, and the protein kinase pathway (*PI3K/Akt/mTOR*) gene expression levels [23].

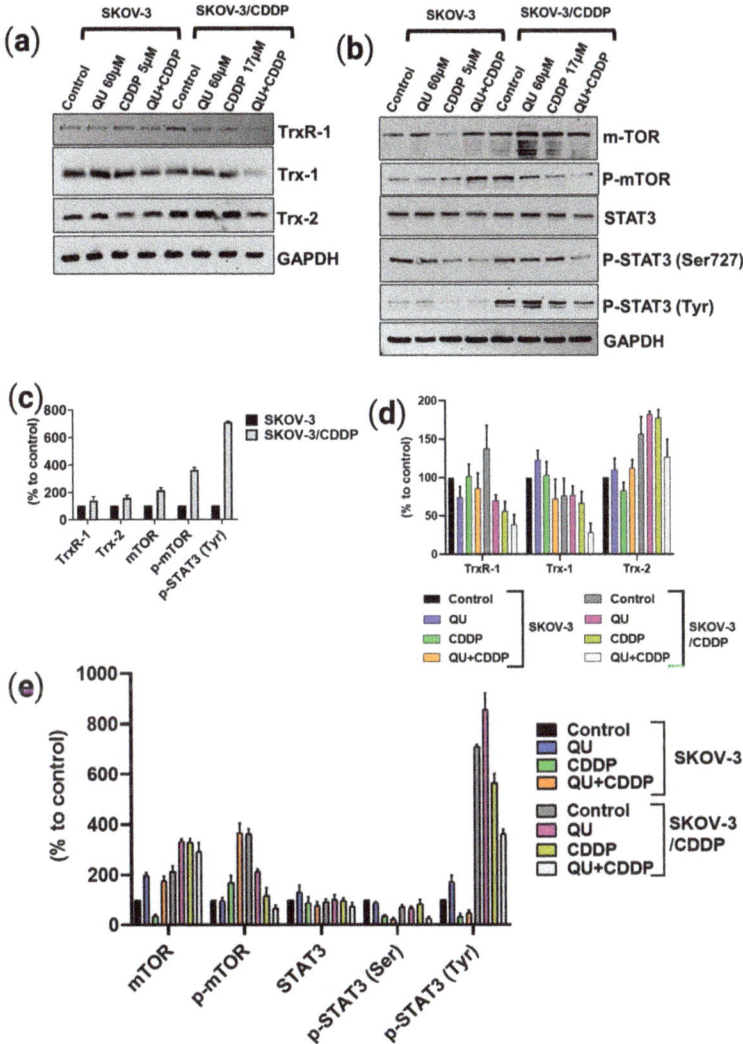

Figure 5. The effect of QU pre-treatment on Trx/TrxR system and mTOR/STAT3 signaling pathway protein expression in ovarian cancer cells using Western blot analysis. Expression of (**a**) Trx/TrxR and (**b**) mTOR/STAT3 protein level in ovarian SKOV-3/CDDP cancer cells compared to SKOV-3 cells. (**c**–**e**) Densitometry results. (**c**) SKOV-3 and SKOV-3/CDDP controls. (**d**) Trx/TrxR system. (**e**) mTOR/STAT3 signaling pathway. The ovarian cancer cells were treated with 60 μM QU (48 h), 5 μM (24 h), or 17μM (48 h) CDDP, or pre-treated with 60 μM QU followed by 5 μM or 17 μM CDDP (24 h and 48 h) for SKOV-3 and (**d**) SKOV-3/CDDP cells, respectively. GAPDH was used as loading control. Values represent mean ± SD (*n* = 3).

In the present experiment, we analyzed the most effective dose of QU followed by CDDP in modulating the antioxidant system and protein kinase signaling pathway proteins. Compared with individual action, the highest inhibition effect in SKOV-3/CDDP subline cells that led to their increased sensitivity to CDDP was observed in the protein expression levels after incubation with 60 µM QU for 48 h, followed by 5 µM CDDP for 24 h in SKOV-3 and 17 µM CDDP for 48 h in SKOV-3/CDDP (Figure 5a,b,d,e). The expression levels of the cytosolic and mitochondrial Trx/TrxR system and the active phosphorylated forms of the mTOR/STAT3 proteins in the SKOV-3/CDDP subline cells were effectively decreased by the QU pre-treatment.

2.5. QU Pre-Treatment Triggers Apoptotic Mitochondrial Pathway in SKOV3 and SKVO3/CDDP Cell Lines

To determine whether the growth inhibition and accumulation of both ovarian cancer cells in sub-G1 by pre-treatment with QU were due to the induction of apoptosis, cell apoptosis was assessed by flow cytometry based on Annexin-V/PI double staining analysis. In contrast to the control group, a single treatment of CDDP mildly induced apoptosis at an average of 0.9 ± 0.1 and 4 ± 0.6% in the SKOV-3 cells and at an average of 2.5 ± 0.4 and 2 ± 0.1% in the SKOV-3/CDDP cells for 24 h and 48 h, respectively. QU monotherapy slightly reduced the live cells and slightly increased apoptosis to an average of ~3 ± 0.4% and ~1.5 ± 0.4% in SKOV-3 and SKOV-3/CDDP, respectively, compared to the untreated cells (Figure 6a,b).

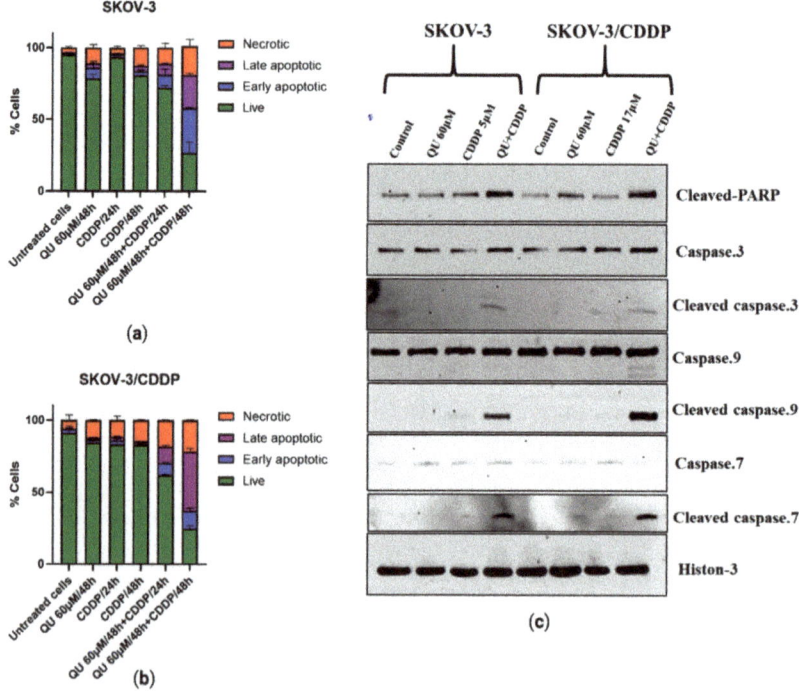

Figure 6. QU-pre-treatment-induced apoptosis in ovarian cancer cells. (**a**) Percent of apoptotic SKOV-3 and (**b**) SKOV-3/CDDP cell lines after treatment with either QU or CDDP and QU pre-treatment for different time periods, 24 and 48 h. (**c**) Representative Western blotting analysis of cleaved caspase-9,7,3 and C-PARP proteins in ovarian cancer cells treated with QU and/or CDDP. Histone was used as loading control. Values represent mean ± SD (n = 3).

Apoptosis was induced by QU pre-treatment, which induced necrotic cells in a time-dependent manner (Figure 6a,b). As the incubation time increased, the proportions of Annexin V+/PI− (early stage of apoptosis) and Annexin V+/PI+ (late stage of apoptosis) QU pre-treated ovarian cells were significantly higher than the CDDP and QU groups (Figure 6a,b); in particular, apoptosis was induced by approximately $20.3 \pm 3\%$ in the SKOV-3 QU pre-treated cells after 48 h, compared with the single-drug treatment group (Figure 6a). The results also indicated that QU sensitization prior to treatment with CDDP in the SKOV-3/CDDP cells substantially increased the percentage of apoptosis by $\sim 41.5 \pm 2\%$ as compared to the treatment with CDDP, with only $2 \pm 0.1\%$ apoptosis after 48 h (Figure 6b).

To further detect the mechanisms behind the apoptotic process induced by treatments using either QU or CDDP and QU pre-treatment, we investigated the expression of specific apoptosis marker proteins (cleaved caspase-9,7,3 and cleaved PARP) with Western blot in both cancer cells. Compared with the loading control histone protein, the levels of cleaved caspase-9, -7, and -3 proteins in both cells were observed only in the QU-pre-treated cells, while the QU pre-treatment induced a high expression of cleaved PARP in both cell lines compared with the mono-treatments (Figure 6c). In other words, these results demonstrated that QU pre-treatment effectively inhibited cell growth by increasing apoptosis in ovarian cancer cells. Taken together, the cell death effect of the studied QU compound was mediated by inhibition of the mTOR/STAT3 pathway, as well as stimulation of the ROS-mediated caspase-3, -7, and -9 activations.

3. Discussion

Ovarian cancer is a continuing health problem that accounts for a significant portion of mortality among women around the world [25,26]. In current clinical practice, surgery combined with chemotherapy based on platinum compounds is considered the standard therapeutic strategy for ovarian cancer [27]. CDDP is one of the most effective chemotherapeutic agents for ovarian cancer; however, resistance to this chemotherapeutic drug is a major obstacle to curative cancer therapy. Ovarian cancer cells develop resistance to anticancer drugs through various mechanisms, including DNA damage repair, cell metabolism, oxidative stress, cell cycle regulation, apoptotic pathways, and abnormal signaling pathways [28]. Due to their various beneficial properties, polyphenols are potential therapeutic candidates in cancer when combined with classical antitumor agents such as cisplatin [29]. For instance, QU could prevent ovarian cancer with its anti-inflammatory, pro-oxidative, and antiproliferation effects, and cell cycle arrest [26]. Discovering the main quercetin mechanisms that reduce cisplatin resistance is important for improving cancer treatment. However, the role of quercetin in SKOV-3/CDDP has not yet been completely investigated.

We initially focused on the effect of QU alone on the ovarian adenocarcinoma SKOV-3/CDDP cell lines to establish a baseline for comparison with our later study [23]. Hence, we hypothesized that the pre-exposure to QU might impair cisplatin resistance in ovarian adenocarcinoma cell lines. In the present study, we utilized two adenocarcinoma cell lines, i.e., the SKOV-3 (wild type) and SKOV-3/CDDP cisplatin-resistant sublines. Optimum doses for treatment were decided for QU and CDDP after examining the IC_{50} values from our previously published data [23,24]. Pre-treatment with QU at low (15 µM) and high doses (100 µM) for 24 h followed by CDDP showed an antiproliferative effect in the SKOV-3/CDDP cisplatin-resistant subline, as well as in the SKOV-3 wild cells, and it showed a sensitization of the resistant subline to the cytotoxicity of CDDP (Figure S1), while a long incubation for 48 h showed a maximum antiproliferative effect (Figure 2b).

The pre-treatment of leiomyosarcoma cells with epigallocatechin-3-gallate, a polyphenol compound, for 24 h failed to alter the S-phase cell cycle arrest induced by CDDP and to modulate the CDDP effects on mitochondrial function [30]. Furthermore, a recent study revealed that the higher efficacy of the prolonged pemetrexed pre-treatment of malignant pleural mesothelioma (MPM) for 48 h induced a cell cycle arrest, mainly in the G2/M phase, the accumulation of persistent DNA damage, and the induction of a senescence phenotype, thereby sensitizing cancer cells to subsequent CDDP treatment [31]. In our study, the treatment of ovarian cancer cells with only QU for 24 h was shown to lead to a slightly increasing cell cycle in the S phase, whereas a long treatment for 48 h significantly induced a cell cycle arrest in the G1/S phase (Figure S3). The conditions of a long treatment for 48 h significantly induced the cells to accumulate in sub-G1 after treatment with CDDP and increased the sensitization of the SKOV-3/CDDP subline to the subsequent CDDP treatment (Figure 3b,d). The sensitization of the ovarian cells to CDDP was observed when the polyphenols, curcumin or QU, were added synergistically with CDDP, as well as when they were added 24 h before [32]. In this study, two strategies (synergistic and pre-treatment) were designed. The result revealed that the SKOV-3/CDDP cells failed to enter into the sub-G1 phase even after a long incubation using the synergistic approach, while the cells effectively accumulated in sub-G1 using the QU pre-treatment strategy (Figure S4). Our strategy allowed the progression of the QU-treated cells into the S phase, whereby re-exposure of the QU-exhausted cells to CDDP after washing out the QU from the culture medium was sufficient to increase the duration of the S phase, which in turn led to further cell damage. The evaluation of this pre-treatment therapy in cisplatin-resistant ovarian cancer cells may lead to more efficient CDDP treatment.

The antioxidant or pro-oxidant properties of polyphenol compounds depend predominantly on the number and positions of the substituent hydroxyl groups, along with their redox metal (Cu, Fe) chelating capacity. For example, the higher number of hydroxyl groups, including the 3-OH group of the C ring of polyphenols in the presence of Cu(II) ions, act as potential anticancer agents with moderate pro-oxidant activity, causing DNA damage via interaction with DNA and ROS formation via the Fenton reaction. Otherwise, the slight pro-oxidant activity of polyphenols acts as a preventive anticancer therapeutic agent via the inducing of cellular antioxidant systems, including antioxidant enzymes, and the synthesis of low-molecular-weight antioxidants, such as glutathione [33]. In this study, QU could not effectively induce ROS generation, while CDDP slightly induced the ROS level in the SKOV/CDDP cells. However, QU pre-treatment effectively triggered the generation of ROS in the SKOV-3/CDDP cells. These data indicate that the increased oxidative stress induced by QU pre-treatment may have activated an apoptotic cascade in the SKOV-3/CDDP cells (Figure 4) and inhibited expression of antioxidant proteins and the signaling pathway (Figure 5a,b,d,e). Alternatively, QU pre-treatment in SKOV-3 acts as an antioxidant by decreasing ROS formation and inducing the expression of antioxidant proteins (Figure 5a,d) and the signaling of the mTOR/STAT3 pathway (Figure 5b,e). In the SKOV-3/CDDP cells, the oxidative stress was also monitored by the measuring of the antioxidant system and the signaling pathway at the protein levels.

In addition to altered proliferation, the cell cycle, oxidative stress, cell metabolism, increased ability to repair DNA damage, and reduced susceptibility to apoptosis, ovarian cancer cells develop resistance to anticancer drugs through various other mechanisms, defined as enhancement expression and alteration of signaling pathways [28]. In addition to the generation of ROS species, we also monitored the changes in the oxidative stress response proteins. Therefore, the marker proteins that were highly correlated with cellular sensitivity to CDDP were screened. Notably, we previously [23] provided the molecular evidence that antioxidant enzymes (*SOD-1, SOD-2, Gpx-1, CAT,* and *HO-1*), transcription factor *NFE2L2*, and the PI3K/Akt/mTOR signaling pathway are upregulated in SKOV-3/CDDP subline cells compared to normal line SKOV-3 cells and found that these gene expressions were associated with CDDP tolerance. The individual treatment with QU revealed marked downregulation in the expression of these genes. Our results suggest that QU pre-treatment has the potential to increase sensitivity to CDDP in SKOV-3/CDDP subline cells by regulating oxidative stress (ROS generation) and cell apoptosis via the antioxidant system and the signaling pathway.

Hence, we assessed the pro-oxidative therapeutic potential effect of QU pre-treatment on the antioxidative system. The thioredoxin system (Trx/TrxR) is essential to maintaining cellular redox homeostasis in living organisms through detoxification of harmful metabolites, i.e., ROS; however, the overexpression of the Trx-dependent system can also contribute to the intensifying of the process of oncogenesis, such as by the enhancement of tumor growth, angiogenesis, and resistance to therapy via the modulation of both the gene expression and the cell signaling pathways that lead to the regulation of apoptotic pathways in cancer cells [34]. Compared to SKOV-3, which exhibits normal Trx/TrxR protein expressions, SKOV-3/CDDP subline cells display unique overexpression in both the cytosolic (TrxR-1) and mitochondrial (Trx-2) protein levels, which are directly associated with resistance to cisplatin (Figure 5c). Accumulating evidence suggests that the tumoral activity of the Trx-dependent system can be modulated by natural polyphenolic compounds, which act as Trx/TrxR system inhibitors [34]. The inhibitory effect of QU depends on many factors, including concentration, NADPH, and the time of exposition and involvement in an attack on the reduced COOH-terminal active site sequence -Gly-Cys-Sec-Gly of TrxR. The inhibition of TrxR activity is associated with the oxidization of Trx in the cells [35]. As expected, QU pre-treatment effectively reduced the levels of thioredoxin system (Trx-1, TrxR-1, and Trx-2) proteins in the SKOV-3/CDDP cells (Figure 5a,d).

Furthermore, STAT3 and its two phosphorylated forms (on Ser^{727} and Tyr^{705}) were also found to be inhibited at the protein (Figure 5b,e) level by the QU pre-treatment in the SKOV-3/CDDP subline cells. Several TrxR-1 inhibitors also block the signal transducers and activators of transcription 3 (STAT3) activity via accumulation of oxidized STAT3, which blocks STAT3-dependent transcription [10,36] and induces cancer cell death [10]. Due to the thiol groups in the Cys residues in the active sites, reduced Trx catalyzes the reduction in disulfide bonds within oxidized target proteins [36,37], such as STAT3 [36].

Previously, SKOV-3/CDDP subline cells were shown to overexpress the *mTOR* gene, which was downregulated after treatment with QU [23]. A recent study demonstrated a significant correlation between STAT3 and mTOR overexpression, which underlies cancer-mediated drug resistance and cancer progression. Furthermore, the phosphorylation of STAT3 on Ser^{727} is regulated by mTOR [11]. Our data support the findings of the study; in particular, both STAT3 and mTOR were overexpressed in SKOV-3/CDDP compared with SKOV-3, and after QU pre-treatment, SKOV-3/CDDP showed inhibition of two phosphorylated STAT3 isoforms at Ser^{727} and Tyr^{705}, as well as the inhibition of phospho-mTOR Ser^{2448}. This was followed by mTOR/STAT3 pathway inactivation, which ultimately inhibits proliferation and induces caspase-dependent apoptosis in ovarian SKOV-3/CDDP cancer cells.

Apoptotic cell death can be triggered by inhibition of the mTOR/STAT3 signaling pathways that are closely linked with tumor progression. Moreover, inducing cell cycle arrest by enhancing the p53 phosphorylation and apoptosis pathway after treatment with QU in HPV-positive human cervical-cancer-derived cells may be one of the key mechanisms underlying the inhibition of cell proliferation in cancer cells [38]. Annexin V/PI staining showing early and late apoptotic cells suggests the activation of apoptosis following pre-exposure to QU (Figure 6a,b). The results of this study also indicated that QU pre-treatment induces SKOV-3 and SKOV-3/CDDP cell death through the mitochondria-dependent apoptosis pathway, where mitochondrial dysfunction, increased PARP cleavage, and activation of caspase-9,-7,-3 are critical events for apoptosis (Figure 6c). QU showed induction in both necrosis and apoptosis cell death in various cancer cells, including SCC-9 oral cancer cells [39] and prostate cancer over a period of time [40]. Apoptosis was induced by QU pre-treatment, and necrotic cells were induced in a time-dependent manner (Figure 6a,b). The proposed anti-cancer and sensitizing mechanisms of QU pre-treatment are summarized in Figure 7.

Taken together, the anticancer and chemosensitizing effects of QU pre-treatment are associated with the inducing of ROS-mediated apoptosis and the alleviation of the protein expressions that are highly correlated with cellular sensitivity to cisplatin, including antioxidant enzymes and the signaling pathway.

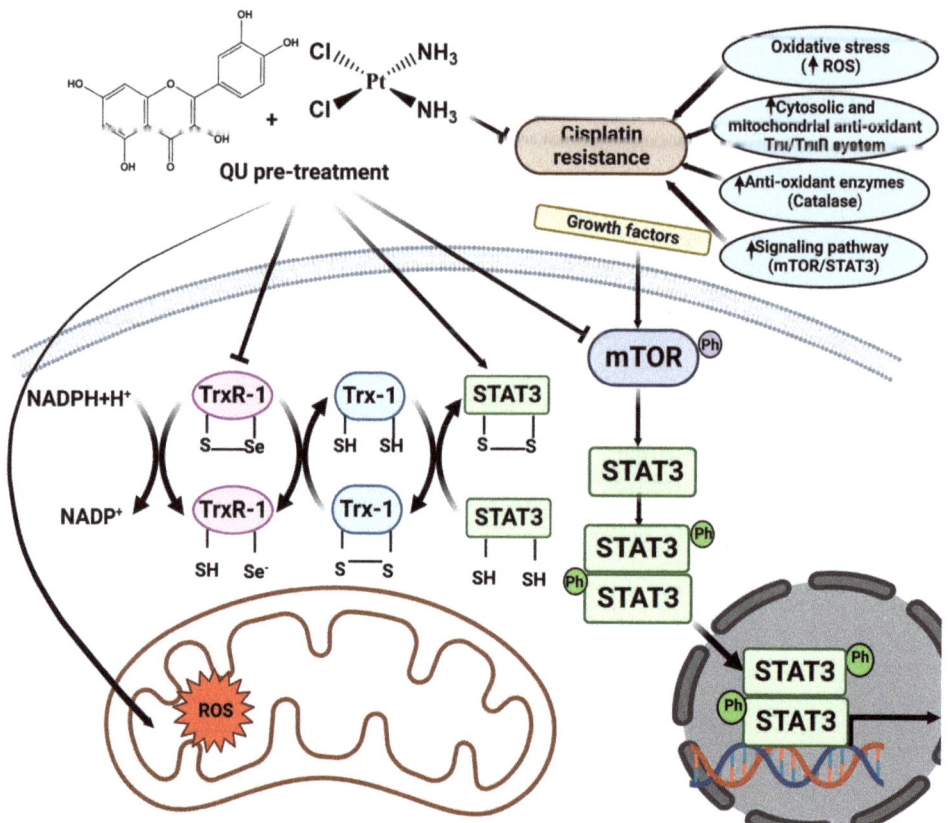

Figure 7. Ovarian SKOV-3/CDDP cells develop resistance to cisplatin through various mechanisms, including oxidative stress, enhanced antioxidant thioredoxin (Trx/TrxR) system, and abnormal signaling pathways. QU pre-treatment has been shown to influence various targets, including Trx/TrxR anti-oxidant system and signaling pathways involved in tumor development and progression. This antioxidant system is composed of thioredoxin reductases (TrxR), thioredoxins (Trx-1), and nicotinamide adenine dinucleotide phosphate (NADPH). Reduced Trx is maintained by TrxR, which accept reducing equivalents from NADPH to the oxidized forms of Trx, that in turn catalyze the reduction of disulfides (s-s) within oxidized cellular proteins, such as (STAT3). Inhibition of TrxR by QU pre-treatment results in the accumulation of oxidized STAT3, which prevents STAT3-dependent transcription. QU pre-treatment also targets mTOR. Inhibition of mTOR is associated with inhibition of phosphorylation of STAT-3 at both Ser^{727} and Tyr^{705} that collectively inhibit SKOV-3/CDDP cell survival and proliferation.

4. Materials and Methods

4.1. Reagents

The chemicals used in the experiments were purchased from the following suppliers: cisplatin (cis-platinum (ii)-diamine dichloride (CDDP; Teva, Tel Aviv-Yafo, Israel)); 3-(4,5-dimethylthiazol-2-yl)-2,5-diphenyl tetrazolium bromide (MTT) (PanEco); and quercetin (QU) (3,3′,4′,5,7-pentahydroxyflavone) from (Acros Organics, Geel, Belgium). The chemical structures of CDDP and QU are illustrated in (Figure 1). The purity of QU was [97% (HPLC)]. The stock quercetin solution was immediately prepared before use by dissolving these test agents in dimethyl sulfoxide (DMSO) at 100 mM concentration.

4.2. Cell Culture

The SKOV-3 non-resistant human ovarian adenocarcinoma and SKOV-3/CDDP cisplatin-resistant subline cells were obtained from the All-Russian Scientific Center for Molecular Diagnostics and Treatment. The SKOV-3 and SKOV-3/CDDP cells were cultured in DMEM cell culture media supplemented with 10% heat-inactivated fetal bovine serum (HealthCare, Chicago, IL, USA), 2 mM L-glutamine, 100 U/mL penicillin, and 50 µg/mL streptomycin. All the cells were incubated at 37 °C under 5% CO^2 in a humidified incubator.

4.3. Cell Viability (MTT Assay)

The inhibitory effect of the pre-treatment of QU followed by CDDP on ovarian cancer cells was assessed using the MTT assay. The SKOV-3 and SKOV-3/CDDP cells were seeded into 96-well plates (Nunc, ThermoFisher Scientific, Waltham, MA, USA) at a density of 5×10^3 cells per well overnight in triplicates. After the incubation period with QU, the culture medium was replaced with a fresh medium, and the cells were then treated with (5 µM, 1/2 IC_{50}, for SKOV-3) or (17 µM, 1/2 IC_{50}, for SKOV-3/CDDP) of CDDP for 72 h. The culture medium was again replaced with a fresh medium and 20 µL; 5 mg/mL MTT was added to each well; and the plates were further incubated at 37 °C for 4 h, allowing the viable cells to reduce the yellow MTT to dark blue formazan crystals. The supernatant was removed, and the formazan crystals were dissolved in 100 µL DMSO and mixed thoroughly prior to determination of the absorbance at a wavelength of 570 nm using a Multiscan FC plate reader (Thermo Scientific, Waltham, MA, USA). Cell viability was calculated according to the following equation: cell viability (%) = (absorbance of experiment group/absorbance of control group) × 100. The IC_{50} was developed by an inhibition curve and recorded as the mean ± standard deviation of three independent experiments.

4.4. Cell Cycle Assay

The distribution of the cell cycle was analyzed by flow cytometry using the FACS Canto II (BD Biosciences, Franklin Lakes, NJ, USA). The SKOV-3 and SKOV-3/CDDP cells in the logarithmic growth phase were seeded at a density of 1.5×10^5 cells/well in a 6-well plate, incubated at 37 °C, 5% CO_2 until adherent, and treated with CDDP alone and QU alone or followed by CDDP, as described above. After incubation, the cells were harvested and washed once with phosphate-buffered saline (PBS). The pellets were then lysed in the solution containing 0.1% sodium citrate, 0.3% NP-40, 50 µg/mL RNAse A, and 10 µg/mL PI. The cells were analyzed using a BD FACS Canto II flow cytometer in a PE channel. Ten thousand 'events' were acquired per each sample. The data were analyzed using the FACSDiva program (BD Biosci., Franklin Lakes, NJ, USA).

4.5. Intracellular Reactive Oxygen Species (ROS) Assay

The intracellular ROS level was measured to detect the anti- or pro-oxidant effect of QU pre-treatment on the SKOV-3/CDDP subline cells. ROS Deep Red dye (RDR; Cellular Reactive Oxygen Species Detection Assay Kit; Abcam, Cambridge, UK) was used to assess the production of ROS. CellROX Deep Red dye freely penetrates into cells, which in turn are oxidized by ROS into a highly fluorescent color. Briefly, the SKOV-3 and SKOV-3/CDDP cells were seeded at a density of 1.5×10^5 cells/well in a 6-well plate, treated with CDDP alone for 4 h or 24 h, QU alone for 24 h or 48 h or followed by CDDP for 4 h or 24 h, and 5 mM H_2O_2, as a positive control, (Ecotex, Moscow, Russia; a reference ROS inducer) for 30 min separately. After incubation, the cells were finally stained with 5 µg/mL CellROX Deep Red dye for 40 min at 37 °C in the dark and analyzed on a BD FACSCanto II (BD Biosciences, Franklin Lakes, NJ, USA) flow cytometer in the APC channel (filter 660/20). The data were analyzed using the FACSDiva program (BD Biosciences). The ROS production for each compound was represented as the percentage based on the shift of the RDR fluorescence in the drug-treated vs. untreated control cells. Ten thousand fluorescent 'events' were acquired per each sample.

4.6. Western Blotting Analysis

Proteins from the treated cells were extracted using RIPA lysis buffer (50 mM Tris-HCl pH 7.4, 1% NP-40, 0.1% sodium dodecylsulfate, 150 mM NaCl, 1 mM EDTA) containing a protein inhibitor cocktail and 2 mM phenylmethylsulfonyl fluoride, then kept on ice for 30 min and centrifuged at 10,000× g for 15 min. The total protein in the lysates was quantitated by the Bradford method [41]. The proteins were resolved by 10–15% SDS-PAGE (40 mg total protein/lane) and transferred onto a 0.2 mm nitrocellulose membrane (GE Healthcare Bio-Sci., Chicago, IL, USA). The membranes were blocked with 5% skimmed milk in 1× TBST (Tris-buffered saline with 0.1% Tween-20), incubated for 2 h, and then probed overnight at 4 °C with the indicated primary rabbit antibodies against catalase; mTOR; phospho-mTOR (S^{2448}); Trx1; TrxR-1(Abcam (Cambridge, MA, USA)); Trx-2; STAT3; phospho-STAT3 (Tyr^{705} and ser^{727}) (Sigma-Aldrich (St. Louis, MO, USA)); caspase 3; caspase 7; caspase 9, PARP; the cleaved caspase 3 (Asp^{175}); cleaved caspase 7; cleaved caspase 9 (Asp^{330}); cleaved PARP (Asp^{214}); and Histon-3/GAPDH (as reference proteins) (Cell Signaling Technology, Danvers, MA, USA)). Next, the membranes were washed twice with 1× TBST and incubated with secondary antirabbit antibodies conjugated with horseradish peroxidase (HRP) (Cell Signaling Tech., Danvers, MA, USA) for 1 h at room temperature. The immunoreactive bands were visualized by enhanced chemiluminescence using the Image Quant LAS 4000 system (GE Healthcare, Chicago, IL, USA).

4.7. Apoptotic Programmed Cell Death Analysis

Apoptosis was measured using the Annexin V-FITC apoptosis detection kits (Thermo Fisher Scientific Inc., Waltham, MA, USA). The SKOV-3 and SKOV-3/CDDP cells in the logarithmic growth phase were seeded at a density of 1.5×10^5 cells/well in a 6-well plate, incubated overnight at 37 °C, 5% CO_2, and treated with CDDP alone or QU alone and followed by cisplatin. The cells were harvested and washed once with PBS and once with 1× binding buffer. The pellets were then resuspended in 100 µL 1× binding buffer, stained with 5 µL of fluorochrome-conjugated Annexin V-APC or FITC, and incubated for 10–15 min at room temperature in the dark. After adding 2 mL of 1× binding buffer, the samples were centrifuged at 400–600 g for 5 min at room temperature. The supernatants were removed; the cells were re-suspended in 200 µL of 1× binding buffer; 5 µL of propidium iodide (PI) staining solution was added and incubated for 5–15 min on ice and analyzed by flow cytometry on a BD FACSCanto II (BD Biosciences, Franklin Lakes, NJ, USA) in the APC channel (filter 660/20 for detection of Annexin V-positive cells) and in the PerCP-Cy™5.5 channel (filter 695/40 for PI-positive cells). The data were analyzed using the FACSDiva program (BD Biosci.).

4.8. Statistical Analysis

All the in vitro data presented herein are presented as the mean ± standard deviation (SD). Each of the experiments was repeated at least three times ($n = 3$). Statistical analysis and graphs were generated using GraphPad Prism 8.0 software (San Diego, CA, USA).

5. Conclusions

The in vitro data show that polyphenol QU increases the sensitivity of SKOV-3/CDDP cisplatin-resistant human ovarian adenocarcinoma subline cells to cisplatin due to their biological effects, including alteration of the cell cycle, classical pro-oxidation, upregulation of ROS and downregulation of the thioredoxin antioxidant system (Trx/TrxR), and cell signaling (mTOR/STAT3) suppression, which collectively lead to the enhancement of the mitochondrial apoptotic pathway (Cas9, 7, and 3 and PARP). To confirm these results, further studies should be conducted using other cell lines that are resistant not only to cisplatin but also to other chemical drugs; future experiments are needed to validate the effect of QU pre-treatment in vivo to assess their potential to reverse cisplatin resistance in cell lines.

Supplementary Materials: The following supporting information can be downloaded at: https://www.mdpi.com/article/10.3390/ijms241310960/s1.

Author Contributions: Conceptualization, visualization, data curation, resources, software, statistical analysis, A.A.H. and V.T.; writing—original draft preparation, A.A.H.; methodology, A.A.H., J.N., Y.V., and V.T.; writing—review and editing, A.A.H., E.K., and V.T.; supervision, A.A.H., E.K., A.S., and V.T.; funding acquisition, V.T. All authors have read and agreed to the published version of the manuscript.

Funding: This work was supported by grant 075-15-2019-1661 from the Ministry of Science and Higher Education of the Russian Federation.

Institutional Review Board Statement: Not applicable.

Informed Consent Statement: Not applicable.

Data Availability Statement: Not applicable.

Acknowledgments: This paper has been supported by the RUDN University Strategic Academic Leadership Program. The figures were created with BioRender.com software.

Conflicts of Interest: The authors declare no conflict of interest.

References

1. Peng, L.; Zhu, H.; Wang, J.; Sui, H.; Zhang, H.; Jin, C.; Leping, L.; Xu, T.; Miao, R. MiR-492 Is Functionally Involved in Oxaliplatin Resistance in Colon Cancer Cells LS174T via Its Regulating the Expression of CD147. *Mol. Cell. Biochem.* **2015**, *405*, 73–79. [CrossRef]
2. Bukowski, K.; Kciuk, M.; Kontek, R. Mechanisms of Multidrug Resistance in Cancer Chemotherapy. *Int. J. Mol. Sci.* **2020**, *21*, 3233. [CrossRef]
3. Makovec, T. Cisplatin and beyond: Molecular Mechanisms of Action and Drug Resistance Development in Cancer Chemotherapy. *Radiol. Oncol.* **2019**, *53*, 148–158. [CrossRef] [PubMed]
4. Zhang, T.; Yuan, Q.; Gu, Z.; Xue, C. Advances of Proteomics Technologies for Multidrug-Resistant Mechanisms. *Future Med. Chem.* **2019**, *11*, 2573–2593. [CrossRef] [PubMed]
5. Saha, S.; Adhikary, A.; Bhattacharyya, P.; Das, T.; Sa, G. Death by Design: Where Curcumin Sensitizes Drug-Resistant Tumours. *Anticancer Res.* **2012**, *32*, 2567–2584. [PubMed]
6. Trachootham, D.; Lu, W.; Ogasawara, M.A.; Rivera-dell Valle, N.; Huang, P. Redox Regulation of Cell Survival. *Antioxid. Redox Signal.* **2008**, *10*, 1343–1374. [CrossRef]
7. Zandi, P.; Schnug, E. Reactive Oxygen Species, Antioxidant Responses and Implications from a Microbial Modulation Perspective. *Biology* **2022**, *11*, 155. [CrossRef]
8. Jovanović, M.; Podolski-Renić, A.; Krasavin, M.; Pešić, M. The Role of the Thioredoxin Detoxification System in Cancer Progression and Resistance. *Front. Mol. Biosci.* **2022**, *9*, 883297. [CrossRef]
9. Ouyang, Y.; Peng, Y.; Li, J.; Holmgren, A.; Lu, J. Modulation of Thiol-Dependent Redox System by Metal Ions via Thioredoxin and Glutaredoxin Systems. *Metallomics* **2018**, *10*, 218–228. [CrossRef] [PubMed]
10. Busker, S.; Qian, W.; Haraldsson, M.; Espinosa, B.; Johansson, L.; Attarha, S.; Kolosenko, I.; Liu, J.; Dagnell, M.; Grandér, D.; et al. Irreversible TrxR1 Inhibitors Block STAT3 Activity and Induce Cancer Cell Death. *Sci. Adv.* **2020**, *6*, eaax7945. [CrossRef]
11. Morelli, A.P.; Tortelli, T.C.; Mancini, M.C.S.; Pavan, I.C.B.; Silva, L.G.S.; Severino, M.B.; Granato, D.C.; Pestana, N.F.; Ponte, L.G.S.; Peruca, G.F.; et al. STAT3 Contributes to Cisplatin Resistance, Modulating EMT Markers, and the MTOR Signaling in Lung Adenocarcinoma. *Neoplasia* **2021**, *23*, 1048–1058. [CrossRef]
12. Sun, C.-Y.; Nie, J.; Huang, J.-P.; Zheng, G.-J.; Feng, B. Targeting STAT3 Inhibition to Reverse Cisplatin Resistance. *Biomed. Pharmacother.* **2019**, *117*, 109135. [CrossRef] [PubMed]
13. Maiuolo, J.; Gliozzi, M.; Carresi, C.; Musolino, V.; Oppedisano, F.; Scarano, F.; Nucera, S.; Scicchitano, M.; Bosco, F.; Macri, R.; et al. Nutraceuticals and Cancer: Potential for Natural Polyphenols. *Nutrients* **2021**, *13*, 3834. [CrossRef] [PubMed]
14. Tang, S.-M.; Deng, X.-T.; Zhou, J.; Li, Q.-P.; Ge, X.-X.; Miao, L. Pharmacological Basis and New Insights of Quercetin Action in Respect to Its Anti-Cancer Effects. *Biomed. Pharmacother.* **2020**, *121*, 109604. [CrossRef] [PubMed]
15. Reyes-Farias, M.; Carrasco-Pozo, C. The Anti-Cancer Effect of Quercetin: Molecular Implications in Cancer Metabolism. *Int. J. Mol. Sci.* **2019**, *20*, 3177. [CrossRef] [PubMed]
16. Srivastava, S.; Somasagara, R.R.; Hegde, M.; Nishana, M.; Tadi, S.K.; Srivastava, M.; Choudhary, B.; Raghavan, S.C. Quercetin, a Natural Flavonoid Interacts with DNA, Arrests Cell Cycle and Causes Tumor Regression by Activating Mitochondrial Pathway of Apoptosis. *Sci. Rep.* **2016**, *6*, 24049. [CrossRef]
17. Kim, S.-H.; Yoo, E.-S.; Woo, J.-S.; Han, S.-H.; Lee, J.-H.; Jung, S.-H.; Kim, H.-J.; Jung, J.-Y. Antitumor and Apoptotic Effects of Quercetin on Human Melanoma Cells Involving JNK/P38 MAPK Signaling Activation. *Eur. J. Pharmacol.* **2019**, *860*, 172568. [CrossRef]

18. Lee, W.-J.; Hsiao, M.; Chang, J.-L.; Yang, S.-F.; Tseng, T.-H.; Cheng, C.-W.; Chow, J.-M.; Lin, K.-H.; Lin, Y.-W.; Liu, C.-C.; et al. Quercetin Induces Mitochondrial-Derived Apoptosis via Reactive Oxygen Species-Mediated ERK Activation in HL-60 Leukemia Cells and Xenograft. *Arch. Toxicol.* **2015**, *89*, 1103–1117. [CrossRef]
19. Cai, X.; Fang, Z.; Dou, J.; Yu, A.; Zhai, G. Bioavailability of Quercetin: Problems and Promises. *Curr. Med. Chem.* **2013**, *20*, 2572–2582. [CrossRef]
20. Kaşıkcı, M.B.; Bağdatlıoğlu, N. Bioavailability of Quercetin. *Curr. Res. Nutr. Food Sci.* **2016**, *4*, 146–151. [CrossRef]
21. Gao, X.; Wang, B.; Wei, X.; Men, K.; Zheng, F.; Zhou, Y.; Zheng, Y.; Gou, M.; Huang, M.; Guo, G.; et al. Anticancer Effect and Mechanism of Polymer Micelle-Encapsulated Quercetin on Ovarian Cancer. *Nanoscale* **2012**, *4*, 7021–7030. [CrossRef] [PubMed]
22. Catanzaro, D.; Ragazzi, E.; Vianello, C.; Caparrotta, L.; Montopoli, M. Effect of Quercetin on Cell Cycle and Cyclin Expression in Ovarian Carcinoma and Osteosarcoma Cell Lines. *Nat. Prod. Commun.* **2015**, *10*, 1365–1368. [CrossRef] [PubMed]
23. Hasan, A.A.S.; Kalinina, E.V.; Tatarskiy, V.V.; Volodina, Y.L.; Petrova, A.S.; Novichkova, M.D.; Zhdanov, D.D.; Shtil, A.A. Suppression of the Antioxidant System and PI3K/Akt/MTOR Signaling Pathway in Cisplatin-Resistant Cancer Cells by Quercetin. *Bull. Exp. Biol. Med.* **2022**, *173*, 760–764. [CrossRef] [PubMed]
24. Kalinina, E.V.; Hasan, A.A.S.; Tatarskiy, V.V.; Volodina, Y.L.; Petrova, A.S.; Novichkova, M.D.; Zhdanov, D.D.; Nurmuradov, N.K.; Chernov, N.N.; Shtil, A.A. Suppression of PI3K/Akt/MTOR Signaling Pathway and Antioxidant System and Reversal of Cancer Cells Resistance to Cisplatin under the Effect of Curcumin. *Bull. Exp. Biol. Med.* **2022**, *173*, 371–375. [CrossRef]
25. Momenimovahed, Z.; Tiznobaik, A.; Taheri, S.; Salehiniya, H. Ovarian Cancer in the World: Epidemiology and Risk Factors. *Int. J. Women's Health* **2019**, *11*, 287–299. [CrossRef] [PubMed]
26. Vafadar, A.; Shabaninejad, Z.; Movahedpour, A.; Fallahi, F.; Taghavipour, M.; Ghasemi, Y.; Akbari, M.; Shafiee, A.; Hajighadimi, S.; Moradizarmehri, S.; et al. Quercetin and Cancer: New Insights into Its Therapeutic Effects on Ovarian Cancer Cells. *Cell Biosci.* **2020**, *10*, 32. [CrossRef]
27. Cortez, A.J.; Tudrej, P.; Kujawa, K.A.; Lisowska, K.M. Advances in Ovarian Cancer Therapy. *Cancer Chemother. Pharmacol.* **2018**, *81*, 17–38. [CrossRef]
28. Yang, L.; Xie, H.-J.; Li, Y.-Y.; Wang, X.; Liu, X.-X.; Mai, J. Molecular Mechanisms of Platinum-based Chemotherapy Resistance in Ovarian Cancer (Review). *Oncol. Rep.* **2022**, *47*, 82. [CrossRef]
29. Vladu, A.F.; Ficai, D.; Ene, A.G.; Ficai, A. Combination Therapy Using Polyphenols: An Efficient Way to Improve Antitumoral Activity and Reduce Resistance. *Int. J. Mol. Sci.* **2022**, *23*, 10244. [CrossRef] [PubMed]
30. Dhima, I.T.; Peschos, D.; Simos, Y.V.; Gkiouli, M.I.; Palatianou, M.E.; Ragos, V.N.; Kalfakakou, V.; Evangelou, A.M.; Karkabounas, S.C. Modulation of Cisplatin Cytotoxic Activity against Leiomyosarcoma Cells by Epigallocatechin-3-Gallate. *Nat. Prod. Res.* **2018**, *32*, 1337–1342. [CrossRef]
31. Karatkevich, D.; Deng, H.; Gao, Y.; Flint, E.; Peng, R.-W.; Schmid, R.A.; Dorn, P.; Marti, T.M. Schedule-Dependent Treatment Increases Chemotherapy Efficacy in Malignant Pleural Mesothelioma. *Int. J. Mol. Sci.* **2022**, *23*, 11949. [CrossRef]
32. Chan, M.M.; Fong, D.; Soprano, K.J.; Holmes, W.F.; Heverling, H. Inhibition of Growth and Sensitization to Cisplatin-Mediated Killing of Ovarian Cancer Cells by Polyphenolic Chemopreventive Agents. *J. Cell. Physiol.* **2003**, *194*, 63–70. [CrossRef] [PubMed]
33. Jomová, K.; Hudecova, L.; Lauro, P.; Simunkova, M.; Alwasel, S.H.; Alhazza, I.M.; Valko, M. A Switch between Antioxidant and Prooxidant Properties of the Phenolic Compounds Myricetin, Morin, 3′,4′-Dihydroxyflavone, Taxifolin and 4-Hydroxy-Coumarin in the Presence of Copper(II) Ions: A Spectroscopic, Absorption Titration and DNA Damage Study. *Molecules* **2019**, *24*, 4335. [CrossRef] [PubMed]
34. Jastrząb, A.; Skrzydlewska, E. Thioredoxin-Dependent System. Application of Inhibitors. *J. Enzym. Inhib. Med. Chem.* **2021**, *36*, 362–371. [CrossRef]
35. Lu, J.; Papp, L.V.; Fang, J.; Rodriguez-Nieto, S.; Zhivotovsky, B.; Holmgren, A. Inhibition of Mammalian Thioredoxin Reductase by Some Flavonoids: Implications for Myricetin and Quercetin Anticancer Activity. *Cancer Res.* **2006**, *66*, 4410–4418. [CrossRef]
36. Chun, K.-S.; Jang, J.-H.; Kim, D.-H. Perspectives Regarding the Intersections between STAT3 and Oxidative Metabolism in Cancer. *Cells* **2020**, *9*, 2202. [CrossRef] [PubMed]
37. Yu, Y.; Di Trapani, G.; Tonissen, K.F. Thioredoxin and Glutathione Systems: Cancer Cells' Defensive Weapons Against Oxidative Stress. In *Handbook of Oxidative Stress in Cancer: Mechanistic Aspects*; Chakraborti, S., Ray, B.K., Roychoudhury, S., Eds.; Springer Nature Singapore: Singapore, 2022; pp. 2407–2420. ISBN 9789811594106.
38. Clemente-Soto, A.; Salas-Vidal, E.; Milan-Pacheco, C.; Sánchez-Carranza, J.; Peralta-Zaragoza, O.; González-Maya, L. Quercetin Induces G2 Phase Arrest and Apoptosis with the Activation of P53 in an E6 Expression-independent Manner in HPV-positive Human Cervical Cancer-derived Cells. *Mol. Med. Rep.* **2019**, *19*, 2097–2106. [CrossRef]
39. Haghiac, M.; Walle, T. Quercetin Induces Necrosis and Apoptosis in SCC-9 Oral Cancer Cells. *Nutr. Cancer* **2005**, *53*, 220–231. [CrossRef]
40. Ward, A.B.; Mir, H.; Kapur, N.; Gales, D.N.; Carriere, P.P.; Singh, S. Quercetin Inhibits Prostate Cancer by Attenuating Cell Survival and Inhibiting Anti-Apoptotic Pathways. *World J. Surg. Oncol.* **2018**, *16*, 108. [CrossRef] [PubMed]
41. Bradford, M.M. A Rapid and Sensitive Method for the Quantitation of Microgram Quantities of Protein Utilizing the Principle of Protein-Dye Binding. *Anal. Biochem.* **1976**, *72*, 248–254. [CrossRef]

Disclaimer/Publisher's Note: The statements, opinions and data contained in all publications are solely those of the individual author(s) and contributor(s) and not of MDPI and/or the editor(s). MDPI and/or the editor(s) disclaim responsibility for any injury to people or property resulting from any ideas, methods, instructions or products referred to in the content.

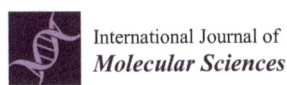

Article

The Synergistic Effect of Proanthocyanidin and HDAC Inhibitor Inhibit Breast Cancer Cell Growth and Promote Apoptosis

Tsz Ki Wang [1,2], Shaoting Xu [1,2], Yuanjian Fan [1,2], Jing Wu [1,2], Zilin Wang [1,2], Yue Chen [2,3] and Yunjian Zhang [1,*]

1. Department of Breast Surgery, The First Affiliated Hospital of Sun-Yat Sen University, Guangzhou 510080, China; wangtszki@mail2.sysu.edu.cn (T.K.W.)
2. Laboratory of Surgery, The First Affiliated Hospital of Sun-Yat Sen University, Guangzhou 510080, China
3. Department of Thyroid Surgery, The First Affiliated Hospital of Sun-Yat Sen University, Guangzhou 510080, China
* Correspondence: zhyunj2@mail.sysu.edu.cn; Tel.: +86-20-8760-8212

Abstract: Histone deacetylase inhibitor (HDACi) is a drug mainly used to treat hematological tumors and breast cancer, but its inhibitory effect on breast cancer falls short of expectations. Grape seed proanthocyanidin extract (GSPE) with abundant proanthocyanidins (PAs) has been explored for its inhibition of HDAC activity in vitro and in vivo. To enhance HDACi's effectiveness, we investigated the potential of PA to synergistically enhance HDACi chidamide (Chi), and determined the underlying mechanism. We evaluated the half-inhibitory concentration (IC50) of PA and Chi using the cell counting kit 8 (CCK8), and analyzed drugs' synergistic effect with fixed-ratio combination using the software Compusyn. Breast cancer cell's phenotypes, including short-term and long-term proliferation, migration, invasion, apoptosis, and reactive oxygen species (ROS) levels, were assessed via CCK8, clone-formation assay, wound-healing test, Transwell Matrigel invasion assay, and flow-cytometry. Protein–protein interaction analysis (PPI) and KEGG pathway analysis were used to determine the underlying mechanism of synergy. PA + Chi synergistically inhibited cell growth in T47D and MDA-MB-231 breast cancer cell lines. Short-term and long-term proliferation were significantly inhibited, while cell apoptosis was promoted. Ten signaling pathways were identified to account for the synergistic effect after RNA sequencing. Their synergism may be closely related to the steroid biosynthesis and extracellular matrix (ECM) receptor interaction pathways. PA + Chi can synergistically inhibit breast cancer cell growth and proliferation, and promote apoptosis. These effects may be related to steroid biosynthesis or the ECM receptor pathway.

Keywords: histone deacetylase inhibitor; breast cancer; proanthocyanidins; synergistic effect; cell proliferation; apoptosis; steroid biosynthesis; extracellular matrix receptor pathway

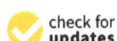

Citation: Wang, T.K.; Xu, S.; Fan, Y.; Wu, J.; Wang, Z.; Chen, Y.; Zhang, Y. The Synergistic Effect of Proanthocyanidin and HDAC Inhibitor Inhibit Breast Cancer Cell Growth and Promote Apoptosis. *Int. J. Mol. Sci.* **2023**, *24*, 10476. https://doi.org/10.3390/ijms241310476

Academic Editors: Marilena Gilca and Adelina Vlad

Received: 6 May 2023
Revised: 13 June 2023
Accepted: 17 June 2023
Published: 22 June 2023

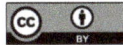

Copyright: © 2023 by the authors. Licensee MDPI, Basel, Switzerland. This article is an open access article distributed under the terms and conditions of the Creative Commons Attribution (CC BY) license (https://creativecommons.org/licenses/by/4.0/).

1. Introduction

Breast cancer is the most common cancer among women worldwide, with over 2.26 million reported cases out of a total of 9.23 million female cancer cases. Chinese women account for about 18.5% of these cases [1]. Approximately 70% of breast cancer cases are estrogen-receptor-positive (ER+), but many patients develop primary or secondary resistance to hormone therapy [2,3].

Histone deacetylase (HDAC) inhibitors are adjunctive drugs that can help cancer cells regain sensitivity to hormone therapy [4]. HDAC is an enzyme that regulates histone lysine residue acetylation, thereby altering gene expressions by modifying the spatial structure of DNA [5–7]. In malignancies, tumor-suppressor genes were transcription inhibited and resulted in tumor progression [8]. HDAC inhibitors (HDACi) have been used to treat late-stage breast cancer, but their effectiveness varies among patients, highlighting the importance of identifying the responders to this treatment [9–13]. Therefore, investigating the mechanism by which HDACi affect breast cancer cells is of significant importance. Chidamide (or named tucidinostat, CS055; Chi) is a novel synthetic benzamide-type selective HDACi developed in China that targets type I and IIa HDACs (HDAC1, HDAC2, HDAC3 and HDAC10). Although it is included in the second-line treatment regimen in the Chinese Society of Clinical Oncology (CSCO) guidelines based on successful results from the ACE study, the clinical effectiveness of HDACi in solid tumors has been limited [14,15]. Therefore, exploring methods to enhance the efficacy of HDACi is warranted.

Proanthocyanidins (PAs) are flavonoids that are widely found in fruits, plant peels, seeds, and processed beverages, such as green tea, black tea, and grape seed extract (GSE/GSPE) [16–22]. PAs have been shown to have multiple therapeutic effects in both malignant and normal tissues, including anti-angiogenesis, pro-apoptosis, and epigenetic changes. Combining PAs with other drugs can also enhance the effects of the other drugs [23,24]. Previous studies have reported that GSPE regulates histone acetylation and decreases HDAC activity in both in vivo and in vitro settings, whether used individually or in combination [23,25]. Therefore, the use of a safe and easily accessible PA as an HDACi sensitizer to promote the effect of the HDACi could hold significant promise for patients with advanced breast cancer.

This study aimed to investigate the synergistic inhibitory effect of the combined administration of PA and Chi in the treatment of breast cancer. In addition, we aimed to identify potential targets or pathways associated with the synergistic anti-tumor growth and development effects of this combination therapy through transcriptome sequencing and bioinformatic analysis. The findings could provide a new therapeutic direction for HDACi as an adjuvant drug in treating advanced breast cancer.

2. Results

2.1. Proanthocyanidin in Combination with an HDACi Exerts Synergistic Anti-Tumor Effects on Breast Cancer Cell Lines

(a) Breast cancer cell line selection based on HDAC expression screening from a single-cell RNA expression profile

Chidamide (Chi) is an HDACi primarily used in patients with ER+ breast cancer. To select a suitable cell line for our experiments, we screened a single-cell RNA sequencing profile of four commonly used ER+ breast cancer cell lines (BT474, MCF7, T47D, and ZR751) in the Gene Expression Omnibus (GEO) database. We observed variations in the expression levels of *HDAC1*, *HDAC2*, *HDAC3* and *HDAC10* mRNAs targeted by chidamide among the ER+ breast cancer cell lines. Notably, the T47D cell line exhibited significant expression of *HDAC1* and *HDAC3* genes compared to the other cell lines, as shown in the violin plot (Figure 1a). Therefore, we selected the T47D cell line and the widely accessible triple-negative breast cancer (TNBC) cell line MDA-MB-231 as the primary cell lines for subsequent experiments.

(b) Proanthocyanidins and chidamide synergistically inhibit breast cancer cell growth

To evaluate the inhibitory effects of applied drugs, we first determined the half-inhibitory concentrations (IC50) of grape seed extract powder (the main component is PA) and Chi, separately. The IC50 of PA for the T47D cell line was 90.74 µg/mL, and the IC50 of Chi was 9.778 µM (Figure S1a,b). In MDA-MB-231 cells, the IC50 of PA was 87.9 µg/mL, and that of Chi was 3.096 µM (Figure S1c,d). These findings indicated that both drugs exhibit growth-inhibiting effects on breast cancer cell lines of different molecular types. Based on the IC50 values, we tested various combinations of PA and Chi and analyzed them using a synergistic model. We observed a synergistic inhibitory effect when treating T47D cells with a PA and Chi ratio of 18.5 to 1 (18.5:1) (Figure 1b, Table 1). Similarly, MDA-MB-231 cells showed a synergistic effect at a ratio of 50 to 1 (50:1) (Figure 1c, Table 2).

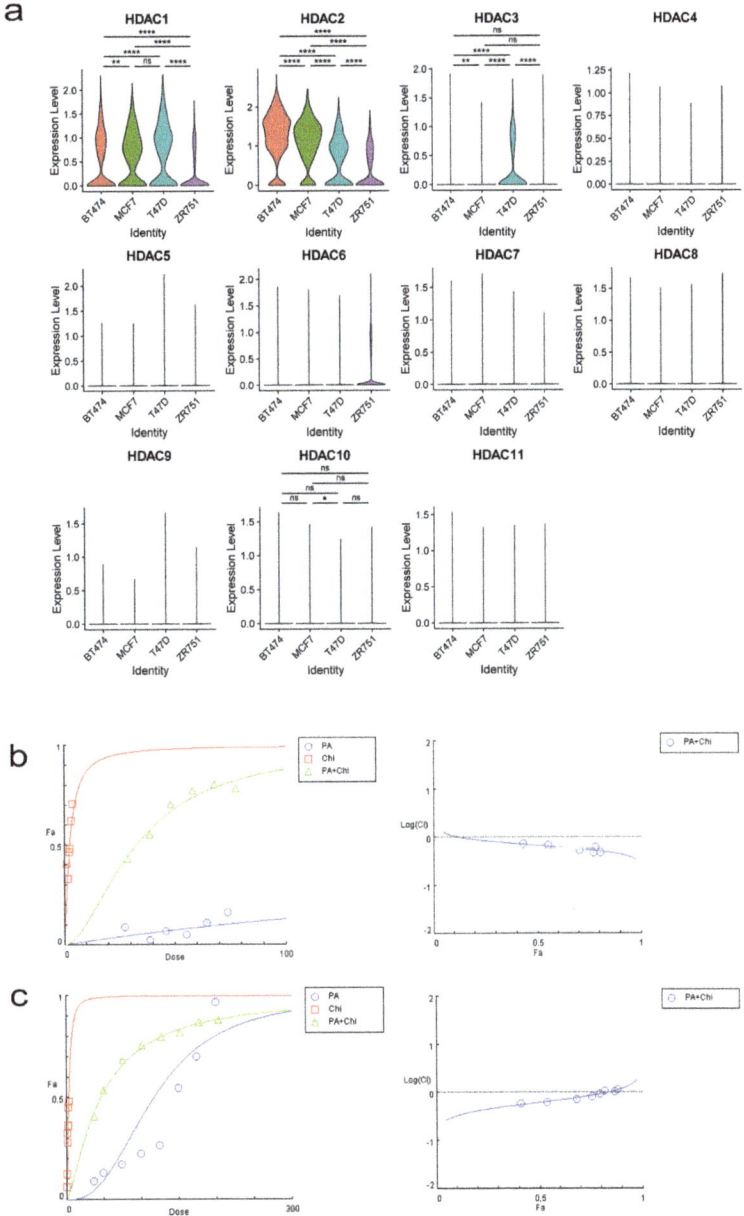

Figure 1. (**a**) Violin plot depicting the expression levels of HDACs in commonly used estrogen-positive breast cancer cell lines (BT474, MCF7, T47D, and ZR751). (For gene expression level, n = 2158 (BT474), n = 839 (MCF7), n = 825 (T47D), and n = 943 (ZR751). ^{ns} $p > 0.05$, * $p < 0.05$, ** $p < 0.01$, or **** $p < 0.0001$, statistical significances were assessed by one-way ANOVA after the D'Agostino-Pearson normality test). (**b**) Cell inhibition curve and logarithmic combination index (LogCI) value after treating T47D cells with a proanthocyanidin and chidamide (PA + Chi) ratio of 18.5 to 1. LogCI value < 0 indicates synergistic effect between drugs. (**c**) Cell inhibition curve and LogCI value after treating MDA-MB-231 cells with a PA + Chi ratio of 50 to 1.

Table 1. The fractional effect and CI value of T47D cell after treatment with 18.5:1 ratio of proanthocyanidins and chidamide.

Combination (Drug A + Drug B)	PA Dose (μg/mL)	Chi Dose (μM)	Total Dose (PA + Chi)	Fractional Effect (Fa)	CI Value
Grape seed proanthocyanidin extract (GSPE/PA) + Chidamide (Chi)	27.75	1.5	29.25	0.433	0.75492
	37	2	39.00	0.552	0.70197
	46.25	2.5	48.75	0.705	0.53421
	55.5	3	58.50	0.773	0.49223
	64.75	3.5	68.25	0.806	0.49523
	74	4	78.00	0.783	0.62861

Combination index (CI) values were calculated using Compusyn (version 1.0). CI value < 1 indicates synergistic effect between drugs, and CI value > 1 indicates antagonistic effect between drugs.

Table 2. The fractional effect and CI value of MDA-MB-231 cells after treatment with 50:1 ratio of proanthocyanidins and chidamide.

Combination (Drug A + Drug B)	PA Dose (μg/mL)	Chi Dose (μM)	Total Dose (PA + Chi)	Fractional Effect (Fa)	CI Value
Grape seed proanthocyanidin extract (GSPE/PA) + Chidamide (Chi)	37.5	0.75	38.25	0.410	0.60335
	50	1	51.00	0.536	0.64555
	75	1.5	76.50	0.685	0.73750
	100	2	102.00	0.758	0.84109
	125	2.5	127.50	0.797	0.95470
	150	3	153.00	0.819	1.07840
	175	3.5	178.50	0.870	1.06536
	200	4	204.00	0.881	1.16653

Combination index (CI) values were calculated using Compusyn (version 1.0). CI value < 1 indicates synergistic effect between drugs, and CI value > 1 indicates antagonistic effect between drugs.

2.2. Analysis of the Cell Function of Proanthocyanidin in the Synergistic HDACi Inhibition of Breast Cancer Cell Growth

(a) Cell proliferation was significantly inhibited by treatment with PA + Chi

To investigate the impact of the combination of PA and Chi on breast cancer development, we conducted several tests to assess cancer cells' phenotypic changes. Initially, we used the CCK8 assay to evaluate the short-term proliferation capacity of T47D cells after monotherapy (PA or Chi) or combination therapy (PA + Chi) at 0, 3, 4, 5, and 7 days. The results showed that cell proliferation rate in the PA + Chi group was lower than in the PA or Chi treatment groups. Furthermore, the differences in cell proliferation among the groups increased in significance with an increase in culture time ($p < 0.05$) (Figures 2a and S2a,b).

(b) Clone-formation was dramatically inhibited by treatment with PA + Chi

The number of cell colonies formed in the PA + Chi group (133 ± 40) was significantly lower than in the control, PA, or Chi group (467 ± 92, 386 ± 100, 806 ± 131, respectively) (all, $p < 0.05$). Moreover, there were statistically significant differences between the control group and PA group, the PA group and Chi group, and the Chi group and PA + Chi group (Figure 2b). These findings suggested that the combination of PA + Chi can effectively reduce the long-term proliferation ability of T47D breast cancer cells.

(c) Wound healing was not different in cells treated with PA, Chi, or PA + Chi

To evaluate cell migration ability, a wound-healing experiment was conducted 72 h after treatment with PA, Chi, and PA + Chi. In the T47D cell line, the results showed no significant difference in cell scratch healing ability within all groups (Figure 2c, $p > 0.05$). This finding suggested that the synergistic effect of PA + Chi does not manifest by altering migration ability.

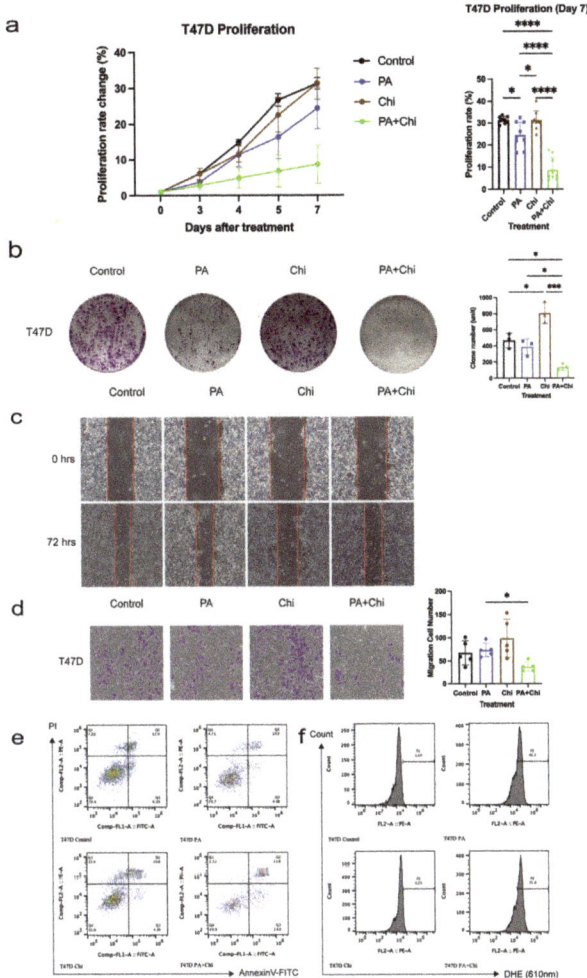

Figure 2. (**a**) Proliferation curves of T47D cells treated with proanthocyanidins (PA), chidamide (Chi), and their combination (PA + Chi), and the difference at day 7 after treatment. (For proliferation rate (%), $n = 9$ (Control), $n = 9$ (PA), $n = 9$ (Chi), and $n = 9$ (PA + Chi). * $p < 0.05$, or **** $p < 0.0001$). (**b**) Clone formation assay showing the number of cell colonies formed by T47D cells treated with PA, Chi, PA + Chi, and the control group. (For clone number present in histogram, $n = 3$ (Control), $n = 3$ (PA), $n = 3$ (Chi), and $n = 3$ (PA + Chi). * $p < 0.05$, or *** $p < 0.001$). (**c**) Wound-healing assay results comparing T47D cell migration from 0 h to 72 h after treatment with PA, Chi, and PA + Chi. (×40) (**d**) Transwell assay evaluating the invasive ability of T47D cells treated with PA, Chi, PA + Chi, and the control group. Representative photographs and quantification of migrated cells through the upper chamber are shown. The number of cells adhering to the outside membrane after 48 h was counted in five randomly selected views (×200; For migration cell number, $n = 5$ (Control), $n = 5$ (PA), $n = 5$ (Chi), and $n = 5$ (PA + Chi). * $p < 0.05$). (**e**) Apoptosis levels of T47D cells treated with PA, Chi, or PA + Chi compared to the control group. Upper left: control; upper right: PA; bottom left: Chi; bottom right: PA + Chi. (**f**) Percentage increase in reactive oxygen species (ROS) in T47D cells treated with PA, Chi, and PA + Chi. No synergistic effect on ROS percentage change was observed. Statistical analysis for all quantitative multi-group comparisons in the histograms was performed using one-way ANOVA (Brown-Forsythe and Welch ANOVA tests for data with non-equal standard deviations).

(d) No significant differences in cancer cell invasion inhibition via PA + Chi

To investigate the impact of PA + Chi on cell invasion ability, we conducted the Transwell Matrigel invasion assay using each drug individually and in combination (PA + Chi). The results demonstrated that compared to treatment with individual drugs, the number of cells invading through the Transwell permeable membrane (containing Matrigel gel) was lower in the PA + Chi group. However, only the difference between the PA group and the PA + Chi group reached statistical significance ($p < 0.05$), while no statistical differences were observed among other groups ($p > 0.05$) (Figure 2d). This finding suggested that the synergistic effect of PA + Chi does not directly inhibit tumor invasion, but may be mediated through the associated suppression of tumor growth.

(e) PA + Chi effectively promotes apoptosis

Flow cytometry was used to access apoptotic changes in T47D cells following treatment with PA, Chi, and PA + Chi. The results revealed no significant difference in the proportion of apoptotic cells between the control group (6.39% early apoptosis; 12.0% late apoptosis) and the PA group (4.68% early apoptosis; 10.9% late apoptosis). Notably, the Chi group exhibited a significant increase in late apoptosis (4.3% early apoptosis; 20.8% late apoptosis), with levels approximately two times that of the control group. The PA + Chi group demonstrated a significant elevation in both early and late stage apoptotic cells (14.9% early apoptosis; 31.8% late apoptosis), collectively accounting for half of all cells analyzed (Figure 2e). These findings conferred that the combination of PA + Chi may enhance cell apoptotic ability.

(f) The level of reactive oxygen species (ROS) Was similar between cells treated with PA and PA + Chi

The ROS detection kit and flow cytometry were employed to analyze the alterations in ROS level in T47D cells following treatment with PA, Chi, and PA + Chi. The results showed that the ROS levels in the control and Chi-treated groups were relatively low (1.44% and 6.23%, respectively), with no significant difference between the two groups. Remarkably, the cell treated with PA and PA + Chi exhibited a significant increase in ROS level (66.7% and 71.9%, respectively) compared to the control group. However, there was no significant difference in ROS levels between the two groups (Figure 2f), indicating that the elevation in ROS was primarily caused by PA, and PA + Chi did not have a synergistic effect on ROS levels.

2.3. Differential Gene Expression (DEG) Analysis and Gene Enrichment Analysis of RNA-Sequencing

To identify the pathways associated with the synergistic action of PA + Chi in breast cancer cells, transcriptome sequencing of twelve samples of T47D cell lines in four groups (control, PA, Chi, and PA + Chi) was performed. Genes showing a differential expression greater than 2-fold were identified using OmicShare tools. Genes that exhibited differential expression only in the PA or Chi treatment groups were excluded. A Wayne diagram was then constructed to illustrate the distribution of DEGs across the different groups, after excluding genes that were differentially expressed in the control group. As shown in the Wayne diagram, there were 38 DEGs in the PA group, 203 DEGs in the Chi group, and 436 DEGs in the PA + Chi group. After deducting the 187 genes found in the PA group and the Chi group, 247 genes remained in the PA + Chi group, potentially exerting a synergistic effect (Figure 3a).

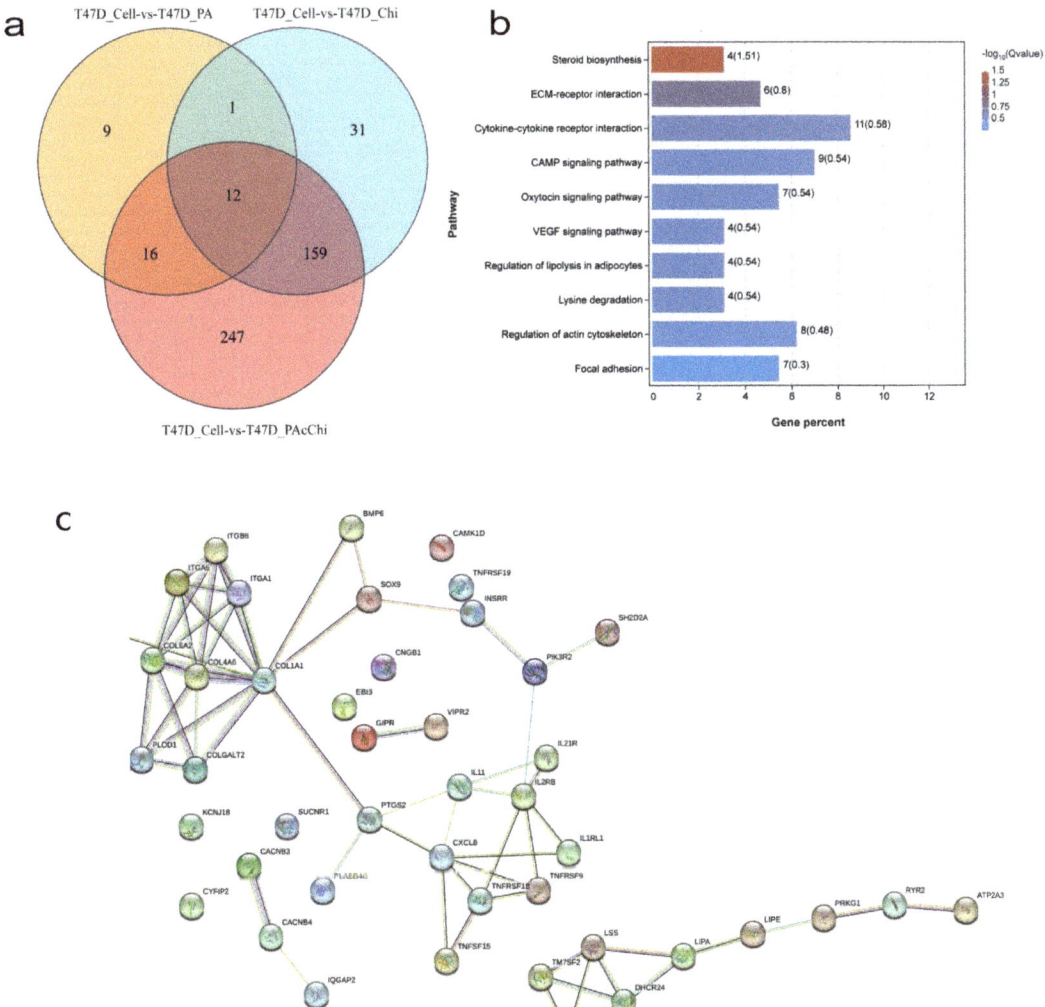

Figure 3. (**a**) Venn diagram illustrating the overlap of differentially expressed gene (DEG) in T47D cells treated with drugs. (**b**) Significantly associated pathways, up-regulated or down-regulated, possibly involved in the synergistic effect of proanthocyanidin (PA) and chidamide (Chi) on breast cancer cell characteristics or functions. (**c**) Protein–protein interaction (PPI) analysis of 48 DEGs related to T47D cells' characteristics or functions using the STRING online tool.

To elucidate the pathways associated with the synergistic effect of PA + Chi in breast cancer, we performed a bioinformatic gene enrichment analysis of the 247 genes identified as potential candidates for synergy based on the transcriptome sequencing data. We also performed comprehensive pathway annotations, the widely used KEGG database. By analyzing pathways at the B-level classification, we identified 21 candidate pathways with a nominal $p < 0.05$ (Table 3). Further comparative analysis allowed us to identify the top 10 pathways, which encompassed 48 genes related to tumor function, growth, and development. These pathways included steroid biosynthesis pathway, extracellular matrix (ECM) receptor interaction pathway, cytokine–cytokine receptor interaction pathway, cAMP signaling pathway, oxytocin signaling pathway, VEGF signaling pathway, regulation of lipolysis in adipocytes pathway, lysine degradation pathway, regulation of actin cytoskeletal pathway, and adhesion plaque pathway (Figure 3b). To gain deeper insights into these pathways, protein–protein interaction (PPI) analysis was performed to examine the interplay between genes involved. The results indicated that the steroid biosynthesis pathway and ECM receptor interaction pathway were the most promising pathways associated with the synergistic effect of PA + Chi (Figure 3c).

Table 3. Significant up-regulated or down-regulated pathways associated with synergistic PA + Chi synergistic effect in drug-treated breast cancer cell T47D.

Pathway(s)	Syn-DEGs (128)	* p-Value(s)
Arrhythmogenic right ventricular cardiomyopathy	7	0.00018945
Steroid biosynthesis	4	0.00025239
Hypertrophic cardiomyopathy	7	0.00051916
ECM-receptor interaction	6	0.00258582
Human papillomavirus infection	12	0.00626547
Cytokine–cytokine receptor interaction	11	0.00643997
cAMP signaling pathway	9	0.00842445
Oxytocin signaling pathway	7	0.01070732
Platelet activation	6	0.01383732
Dilated cardiomyopathy	7	0.014181
Small cell lung cancer	5	0.01420596
VEGF signaling pathway	4	0.01536765
Regulation of lipolysis in adipocytes	4	0.01536765
Mucin type O-glycan biosynthesis	3	0.01713699
Glycosaminoglycan biosynthesis—keratan sulfate	2	0.01862032
Lysine degradation	4	0.01888023
Protein digestion and absorption	5	0.02191461
Regulation of actin cytoskeleton	8	0.02415313
Bladder cancer	3	0.02580077
Focal adhesion	7	0.04042669
Cardiac muscle contraction	4	0.04997453

* All pathways mentioned are significantly different (* $p < 0.05$) in KEGG analysis; p-values are aligned in ascending order.

3. Discussion

Breast cancer is a complex disease characterized by abnormal cell proliferation involving genetic and epigenetic changes. However, the clinical application of HDACi as a therapy for breast cancer is limited due to frequent toxicity and adverse effects, including those involving the blood, lymphatic, and gastrointestinal systems [26]. To overcome this challenge, the combination of a polyphenoic compound, PA, and HDACi, such as Chi, has been proposed as a strategy to enhance the therapeutic effect and reduce toxicity.

The findings of this study provide evidence, for the first time, that the combination of PA and Chi effectively inhibits breast cancer cells' short-term and long-term proliferation, promotes apoptosis, and thus hold promise as a potential treatment for advanced breast cancer. Moreover, the synergistic effect observed in breast cancer cells was associated with the modulation of steroid biosynthesis and ECM receptor interaction pathways.

The metabolic alterations observed in malignancies involve changes in lipid metabolism, and steroid biosynthesis plays a critical role in lipid production, with genetic alterations associated with hormone-related tumors, such as breast and prostate cancer [27–29]. In our study, we observed significant changes in the expression of genes that participated in steroid biosynthesis, including *LSS*, *DHCR24*, *TM7SF2*, and *LIPA*, after treatment with PA + Chi. Previous research has demonstrated the inhibitory effect of PAs on lipid metabolism and the expression of steroid metabolism-related enzymes, which can suppress breast cancer carcinogenesis [30–32]. Based on these findings, we hypothesize that the synergistic effect of PA + Chi on the steroid biosynthesis pathway contributes to their anti-tumor activity.

Furthermore, we identified significant changes in genes related to ECM receptor interaction pathway, including *COL1A1*, *COL4A6*, *COL6A2*, *ITGA1*, *ITGA5*, and *ITGB6*, which are essential for cell support, signaling, invasion, and metastasis [33], suggesting that the modulation of the ECM receptor pathway may also contribute to the synergistic effect of PA + Chi on breast cancer cells.

Our study has certain limitations that need to be acknowledged. First, we did not confirm the entire pathway and specific genes involved in the observed synergistic effect. Additionally, it is important to consider the post-transcriptional regulation effect of HDACi, as it functions as an acetylation regulator. Further investigation employing techniques, such as short-hairpin RNA to interfere with specific gene expression and conducting in vivo experiments are warranted to validate the underlying mechanism of action of PA + Chi on steroid biosynthesis and ECM receptor pathways in breast cancer cells.

In conclusion, our results suggest that the combination of PA and the HDACi Chi may be a promising therapeutic approach for breast cancer. The mechanistic insights gained from our study provide valuable information for the development of novel strategies to treat advanced breast cancer, including drug-resistant forms of diseases.

4. Materials and Methods

4.1. Data Download, Processing, and Downstream Analysis

The raw data of single-cell RNA sequencing profile (GSE173634) were downloaded from the Gene Expression Omnibus (GEO) database. The count matrix data were processed using the Seurat package (version 4.1.1) of R software (version 4.1.3). A Seurat object was created and selected luminal cell types, including BT474, MCF7, T47D, and ZR751 for downstream analysis. The VlnPlot() function was used to investigate the expression levels of HDAC genes in each cell type.

4.2. Half Inhibitory Concentration Analysis (IC50) of Drugs Using the Cell Counting Kit 8 (CCK8)

The T47D cell line was obtained from our laboratory. The MDA-MB-231 cell line was obtained from Peking Union Medical College Cell Resource Center (Beijing, China). T47D and MDA-MB-231 cells were cultured in T25 flasks. Cells were then seeded into 96-well plates at a density of 5000–7000 cells/well, and cultured in logarithmic growth phase for 2 days. Once the cells adhered, 200 μL of 10% serum DMEM/1640 medium containing gradient concentrations of PA, Chi, or PA + Chi was added to each well, and the plates were incubated at 37 °C in a 5% CO_2 incubator. After 72 h, 10% of CCK8 solution was added to each well, and the plates were incubated at 37 °C and 5% CO_2 for approximately 2 h. The absorbance of each well at 450 nm was then measured using a microplate reader. Cell viability and IC50 values were calculated based on the absorbance readings.

4.3. Synergistic Effect Model Calculation and Short-Term Proliferation Analysis

The initial steps were similar to the cell IC50 analysis, wherein absorbance was measured and calculated as the cell inhibition rate. The obtained inhibition rates were then entered into the Compusyn1.0 software to determine the synergistic model.

For proliferation detection, cells in the logarithmic growth phase were seeded into 96-well plates at a density of 500–1000 cells/well and allowed to attach for 2 days. Subsequently, 10% serum DMEM medium containing a specific proportion of PA, Chi, or PA + Chi was added to each well, and the plates were cultured in an incubator at 37 °C and 5% CO_2. The cell proliferation rate was calculated.

4.4. Long-Term Proliferation Analysis via Clone Formation

Cells in the logarithmic growth phase (500–1000) were seeded onto 6-well plates and incubated for 2 days until they attached to the surface. Then, the cells were treated with varying proportions of PA, Chi, or PA + Chi for approximately 2 weeks. After the formation of monoclonal colonies, the cells were fixed with 4% paraformaldehyde for 20 min and stained with 0.5% crystal violet for 15 min. At least 50 individual cells per monoclonal colony were counted in each well using ImageJ software (Version 1.8.0.172).

4.5. Cell Migration Analysis via Wound Healing Assay

Approximately 100 µL of cells was seeded from a T25 flask onto a 6-well plate. After 2 days of incubation, three horizontal and vertical lines were drawn to divide the wells. Then, 5% serum DMEM medium containing a specific proportion of PA, Chi, or PA + Chi was added and the plates were incubated. Samples were collected at 0 and 72 h for photography and analysis.

4.6. Cell Invasion Analysis Using Transwell Matrigel Invasion Assay

For cell invasion assays, approximately 10,000 T47D cells were seeded in 200 µL of no-serum medium onto the upper chamber of Transwell inserts coated with Matrigel. Then, 400 µL of 10% DMEM was added to the lower chamber of the Transwell. The chambers were incubated at 37 °C in a 5% CO2 incubator. After 48 h, the Transwell chambers were removed, and the cells were fixed and stained with 4% paraformaldehyde and 0.5% crystal violet, respectively. The number of invaded cells in five randomly selected fields of view for each chamber was counted and compared.

4.7. Cell Apoptosis and Intracellular Reactive Oxygen Species (ROS) Analysis via Flow Cytometry

The Annexin V-FITC/PI staining kit was used to detect cell apoptosis. For flow cytometry, the excitation light wavelength was set to 488 nm, FITC fluorescence was detected by a passband filter with a wavelength of 515 nm, and PI was detected by a filter with a wavelength greater than 560 nm. Cells in the right quadrant were compared.

To detect ROS levels, treated cells were incubated with a diluted 10 µM DHE fluorescent probe, allowing the samples to come into full contact with the probe. Flow cytometry was used to detect the fluorescence intensity at an excitation wavelength of 535 nm and emission wavelength of 610 nm. The P2 channel was used to delineate the ROS levels within the cells.

4.8. Gene Enrichment Analysis and KEGG Analysis of RNA Sequencing

Following the administration of treatments, transcriptome sequencing data were obtained from 12 samples with 3 replicates in 4 groups of T47D cells. The OmicShare tools (www.omicshare.com/tools) from Gene Denovo were used to identify differentially expressed genes (DEGs) in the treated groups compared to the control group, using a DEG threshold of FDR < 0.05 and FC $\pm$ 2. The DEGs were then grouped, and a Wayne diagram was drawn to select the synergistic-related DEGs. Common pathway annotation data were also used to identify significantly enriched signaling pathways.

4.9. Protein–Protein Interaction Analysis

The protein–protein interaction analysis was performed using the STRING online tool (version 11.5, https://cn.string-db.org/, accessed on 24 March 2023).

4.10. Statistical Analysis

Synergistic models with fractional effect (Fa) and CI values were analyzed using Compusyn (version 1.0), which is a simple computerized analytical simulation based on the median-effect principle of the mass-action law and its combination index theorem [34]. Statistical analyses in tumor growth and functions analysis part were conducted using GraphPad Prism9 software. Multi-comparisons between data were performed using one-way ANOVA (Brown–Forsythe and Welch ANOVA tests for data, which have non-equal standard deviations), and statistical significance was set at $p < 0.05$. Statistical analyses in KEGG pathways were previously mentioned. All statistical analyses in figures including p-value(s) were marked in figure legends.

5. Conclusions

In conclusion, our study demonstrates that the combination of PA and Chi exhibits a synergistic anti-tumor effect on hormone receptor-positive and triple-negative breast cancer cell lines. This combination effectively inhibited short-term and long-term tumor cell proliferation, while promoting apoptosis. These findings suggested that the mechanism underlying the synergistic effect of PA + Chi may be associated with these tumor phenotypes. Furthermore, our results indicate a potential involvement of the steroid biosynthesis pathway and ECM receptor interaction pathway in mediating the synergism observed with PA + Chi treatment.

Supplementary Materials: The following supporting information can be downloaded at https://www.mdpi.com/article/10.3390/ijms241310476/s1.

Author Contributions: Conceptualization, T.K.W. and Y.Z.; methodology, T.K.W.; software, T.K.W. and S.X.; validation, T.K.W., S.X., J.W. and Y.Z.; formal analysis, T.K.W.; investigation, T.K.W., S.X., Y.F., Z.W. and Y.C.; resources, T.K.W. and S.X.; data curation, T.K.W.; writing—original draft preparation, T.K.W.; writing—review and editing, T.K.W., S.X., Y.F., J.W. and Y.Z.; visualization, T.K.W.; supervision, Y.Z.; project administration, T.K.W. and Y.Z.; funding acquisition, Y.Z. All authors have read and agreed to the published version of the manuscript.

Funding: This research was financially supported by the National Natural Science Foundation of China (81872344).

Institutional Review Board Statement: Not applicable.

Informed Consent Statement: Not applicable.

Data Availability Statement: The data presented in this study are available on request from the corresponding author. The data are not publicly available due to privacy issues.

Acknowledgments: We express our sincere gratitude to technicians, colleagues, and classmates in the Laboratory of Surgery and the Precise Medicine Research Institute of The First Affiliated Hospital of Sun-Yat Sen University for their invaluable technical support. Thanks to the Guangzhou Baoxing Biological Technology Company Limited and Shenzhen Chipscreen Biosciences Company Limited for providing us with experimental materials and drugs.

Conflicts of Interest: The authors declare no conflict of interest. The funders had no role in the design of the study; in the collection, analyses, or interpretation of data; in the writing of the manuscript; or in the decision to publish the results.

References

1. World Health Organization International Agency for Research of Cancer—2020 of Incidence and Mortality of Cancer. Available online: https://www.iarc.who.int/faq/latest-global-cancer-data-2020-qa/ (accessed on 24 June 2022).
2. Légaré, S.; Basik, M. Minireview: The Link between ERα Corepressors and Histone Deacetylases in Tamoxifen Resistance in Breast Cancer. *Mol. Endocrinol.* **2016**, *30*, 965–976. [CrossRef]
3. Ring, A.; Dowsett, M. Mechanisms of tamoxifen resistance. *Endocr. Relat. Cancer* **2004**, *11*, 643–658. [CrossRef]
4. Johnston, S.R. Enhancing Endocrine Therapy for Hormone Receptor-Positive Advanced Breast Cancer: Cotargeting Signaling Pathways. *J. Natl. Cancer Inst.* **2015**, *107*, djv212. [CrossRef]
5. Nagy, L.; Kao, H.Y.; Chakravarti, D.; Lin, R.J.; Hassig, C.A.; Ayer, D.; Schreiber, S.L.; Evans, R.M. Nuclear receptor repression mediated by a complex containing SMRT, mSin3A, and histone deacetylase. *Cell* **1997**, *89*, 373–380. [CrossRef] [PubMed]
6. Hong, L.; Schroth, G.P.; Matthews, H.R.; Yau, P.; Bradbury, E.M. Studies of the DNA binding properties of histone H4 amino terminus. Thermal denaturation studies reveal that acetylation markedly reduces the binding constant of the H4 "tail" to DNA. *J. Biol. Chem.* **1993**, *268*, 305–314. [CrossRef]
7. Spartalis, E.; Athanasiadis, D.I.; Chrysikos, D.; Spartalis, M.; Boutzios, G.; Schizas, D.; Garmpis, N.; Damaskos, C.; Paschou, S.A.; Ioannidis, A.; et al. Histone Deacetylase Inhibitors and Anaplastic Thyroid Carcinoma. *Anticancer. Res.* **2019**, *39*, 1119–1127. [CrossRef]
8. Milano, A.; Chiofalo, M.G.; Basile, M.; Salzano de Luna, A.; Pezzullo, L.; Caponigro, F. New molecular targeted therapies in thyroid cancer. *Anticancer Drugs* **2006**, *17*, 869–879. [CrossRef] [PubMed]

9. Seo, J.; Min, S.K.; Park, H.R.; Kim, D.H.; Kwon, M.J.; Kim, L.S.; Ju, Y.-S. Expression of Histone Deacetylases HDAC1, HDAC2, HDAC3, and HDAC6 in Invasive Ductal Carcinomas of the Breast. *J. Breast Cancer* **2014**, *17*, 323–331. [CrossRef]
10. Duong, V.; Licznar, A.; Margueron, R.; Boulle, N.; Busson, M.; Lacroix, M.; Katzenellenbogen, B.S.; Cavaillès, V.; Lazennec, G. ERalpha and ERbeta expression and transcriptional activity are differentially regulated by HDAC inhibitors. *Oncogene* **2006**, *25*, 1799–1806. [CrossRef]
11. Munster, P.N.; Thurn, K.T.; Thomas, S.; Raha, P.; Lacevic, M.; Miller, A.; Melisko, M.; Ismail-Khan, R.; Rugo, H.; Moasser, M.; et al. A phase II study of the histone deacetylase inhibitor vorinostat combined with tamoxifen for the treatment of patients with hormone therapy-resistant breast cancer. *Br. J. Cancer* **2011**, *104*, 1828–1835. [CrossRef] [PubMed]
12. Yardley, D.A.; Ismail-Khan, R.R.; Melichar, B.; Lichinitser, M.; Munster, P.N.; Klein, P.M.; Cruickshank, S.; Miller, K.D.; Lee, M.J.; Trepel, J.B. Randomized phase II, double-blind, placebo-controlled study of exemestane with or without entinostat in postmenopausal women with locally recurrent or metastatic estrogen receptor-positive breast cancer progressing on treatment with a nonsteroidal aromatase inhibitor. *J. Clin. Oncol.* **2013**, *31*, 2128–2135. [CrossRef]
13. Connolly, R.M.; Zhao, F.; Miller, K.D.; Lee, M.-J.; Piekarz, R.L.; Smith, K.L.; Brown-Glaberman, U.A.; Winn, J.S.; Faller, B.A.; Onitilo, A.A.; et al. E2112: Randomized Phase III Trial of Endocrine Therapy Plus Entinostat or Placebo in Hormone Receptor-Positive Advanced Breast Cancer. A Trial of the ECOG-ACRIN Cancer Research Group. *J. Clin. Oncol.* **2021**, *39*, 3171–3181. [CrossRef]
14. Zhou, Y.; Wang, Y.N.; Zhang, K.; Zhu, J.; Ning, Z. Chidamide reverses epidermal growth factor induced endocrine resistance in estrogen receptor-positive breast cancer. *J. Shenzhen Univ. Sci. Eng.* **2018**, *35*, 339–344. [CrossRef]
15. Jiang, Z.; Li, W.; Hu, X.; Zhang, Q.; Sun, T.; Cui, S.; Wang, S.; Ouyang, Q.; Yin, Y.; Geng, C.; et al. Tucidinostat plus exemestane for postmenopausal patients with advanced, hormone receptor-positive breast cancer (ACE): A randomised, double-blind, placebo-controlled, phase 3 trial. *Lancet Oncol.* **2019**, *20*, 806–815. [CrossRef]
16. Gu, L.; Kelm, M.A.; Hammerstone, J.F.; Beecher, G.; Holden, J.; Haytowitz, D.; Prior, R.L. Screening of foods containing proanthocyanidins and their structural characterization using LC-MS/MS and thiolytic degradation. *J. Agric. Food Chem.* **2003**, *51*, 7513–7521. [CrossRef] [PubMed]
17. Pastrana-Bonilla, E.; Akoh, C.C.; Sellappan, S.; Krewer, G. Phenolic Content and Antioxidant Capacity of Muscadine Grapes. *J. Agric. Food Chem.* **2003**, *51*, 5497–5503. [CrossRef]
18. Graham, H.N. Green tea composition, consumption, and polyphenol chemistry. *Prev. Med.* **1992**, *21*, 334–350. [CrossRef] [PubMed]
19. Bell, J.R.C.; Donovan, J.L.; Wong, R.; Waterhouse, A.L.; German, J.B.; Walzem, R.L. (+)-Catechin in human plasma after ingestion of a single serving of reconstituted red wine. *Am. J. Clin. Nutr.* **2000**, *71*, 103–108. [CrossRef] [PubMed]
20. Ferraz da Costa, D.C.; Pereira Rangel, L.; Quarti, J.; Santos, R.A.; Silva, J.L.; Fialho, E. Bioactive Compounds and Metabolites from Grapes and Red Wine in Breast Cancer Chemoprevention and Therapy. *Molecules* **2020**, *25*, 3531. [CrossRef] [PubMed]
21. Wang, T.K.; Xu, S.; Li, S.; Zhang, Y. Proanthocyanidins Should Be a Candidate in the Treatment of Cancer, Cardiovascular Diseases and Lipid Metabolic Disorder. *Molecules* **2020**, *25*, 5971. [CrossRef]
22. Rosato, R.R.; Almenara, J.A.; Grant, S. The histone deacetylase inhibitor MS-275 promotes differentiation or apoptosis in human leukemia cells through a process regulated by generation of reactive oxygen species and induction of p21CIP1/WAF1 1. *Cancer Res.* **2003**, *63*, 3637–3645. [PubMed]
23. Gao, Y.; Tollefsbol, T.O. Combinational Proanthocyanidins and Resveratrol Synergistically Inhibit Human Breast Cancer Cells and Impact Epigenetic-Mediating Machinery. *Int. J. Mol. Sci.* **2018**, *19*, 2204. [CrossRef] [PubMed]
24. Carriere, P.P.; Kapur, N.; Mir, H.; Ward, A.B.; Singh, S. Cinnamtannin B-1 inhibits cell survival molecules and induces apoptosis in colon cancer. *Int. J. Oncol.* **2018**, *53*, 1442–1454. [CrossRef]
25. Downing, L.E.; Ferguson, B.S.; Rodriguez, K.; Ricketts, M.L. A grape seed procyanidin extract inhibits HDAC activity leading to increased Pparα phosphorylation and target-gene expression. *Mol. Nutr. Food Res.* **2017**, *61*, 1600347. [CrossRef]
26. Kim, Y.H.; Bagot, M.; Pinter-Brown, L.; Rook, A.H.; Porcu, P.; Horwitz, S.M.; Whittaker, S.; Tokura, Y.; Vermeer, M.; Zinzani, P.L.; et al. Mogamulizumab versus vorinostat in previously treated cutaneous T-cell lymphoma (MAVORIC): An international, open-label, randomised, controlled phase 3 trial. *Lancet Oncol.* **2018**, *19*, 1192–1204. [CrossRef]
27. Snaebjornsson, M.T.; Janaki-Raman, S.; Schulze, A. Greasing the Wheels of the Cancer Machine: The Role of Lipid Metabolism in Cancer. *Cell Metab.* **2020**, *31*, 62–76. [CrossRef] [PubMed]
28. Miller, W.L. Steroidogenesis: Unanswered Questions. *Trends Endocrinol. Metab.* **2017**, *28*, 771–793. [CrossRef]
29. Ferraldeschi, R.; Sharifi, N.; Auchus, R.J.; Attard, G. Molecular pathways: Inhibiting steroid biosynthesis in prostate cancer. *Clin. Cancer Res.* **2013**, *19*, 3353–3359. [CrossRef]
30. Zhou, Q.; Han, X.; Li, R.; Zhao, W.; Bai, B.; Yan, C.; Dong, X. Anti-atherosclerosis of oligomeric proanthocyanidins from Rhodiola rosea on rat model via hypolipemic, antioxidant, anti-inflammatory activities together with regulation of endothelial function. *Phytomedicine* **2018**, *51*, 171–180. [CrossRef]
31. Shi, Y.; Jia, M.; Xu, L.; Fang, Z.; Wu, W.; Zhang, Q.; Chung, P.; Lin, Y.; Wang, S.; Zhang, Y. miR-96 and autophagy are involved in the beneficial effect of grape seed proanthocyanidins against high-fat-diet-induced dyslipidemia in mice. *Phytother. Res.* **2019**, *33*, 1222–1232. [CrossRef]
32. Song, X.; Siriwardhana, N.; Rathore, K.; Lin, D.; Wang, H.C. Grape seed proanthocyanidin suppression of breast cell carcinogenesis induced by chronic exposure to combined 4-(methylnitrosamino)-1-(3-pyridyl)-1-butanone and benzo[a]pyrene. *Mol. Carcinog.* **2010**, *49*, 450–463. [CrossRef] [PubMed]

33. Dzobo, K.; Senthebane, D.A.; Dandara, C. The Tumor Microenvironment in Tumorigenesis and Therapy Resistance Revisited. *Cancers* **2023**, *15*, 376. [CrossRef] [PubMed]
34. Chou, T.C. Theoretical basis, experimental design, and computerized simulation of synergism and antagonism in drug combination studies. *Pharmacol. Rev.* **2006**, *58*, 621–681. [CrossRef] [PubMed]

Disclaimer/Publisher's Note: The statements, opinions and data contained in all publications are solely those of the individual author(s) and contributor(s) and not of MDPI and/or the editor(s). MDPI and/or the editor(s) disclaim responsibility for any injury to people or property resulting from any ideas, methods, instructions or products referred to in the content.

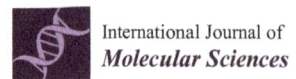 International Journal of
Molecular Sciences

Article

Relevance of Phytochemical Taste for Anti-Cancer Activity: A Statistical Inquiry

Teodora-Cristiana Grădinaru [1], Marilena Gîlcă [1,*], Adelina Vlad [2] and Dorin Dragoș [3,4]

1. Department of Functional Sciences I/Biochemistry, Faculty of Medicine, Carol Davila University of Medicine and Pharmacy, 050474 Bucharest, Romania; teodora.gradinaru@drd.umfcd.ro
2. Department of Functional Sciences I/Physiology, Faculty of Medicine, Carol Davila University of Medicine and Pharmacy, 050474 Bucharest, Romania; adelina.vlad@umfcd.ro
3. Department of Medical Semiology, Faculty of Medicine, Carol Davila University of Medicine and Pharmacy, 020021 Bucharest, Romania; dorin.dragos@umfcd.ro
4. 1st Internal Medicine Clinic, University Emergency Hospital Bucharest, Carol Davila University of Medicine and Pharmacy, 050098 Bucharest, Romania
* Correspondence: marilena.gilca@umfcd.ro

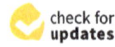

Citation: Grădinaru, T.-C.; Gîlcă, M.; Vlad, A.; Dragoș, D. Relevance of Phytochemical Taste for Anti-Cancer Activity: A Statistical Inquiry. *Int. J. Mol. Sci.* **2023**, *24*, 16227. https://doi.org/10.3390/ijms242216227

Academic Editor: Raffaele Capasso

Received: 23 September 2023
Revised: 6 November 2023
Accepted: 10 November 2023
Published: 12 November 2023

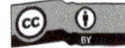

Copyright: © 2023 by the authors. Licensee MDPI, Basel, Switzerland. This article is an open access article distributed under the terms and conditions of the Creative Commons Attribution (CC BY) license (https://creativecommons.org/licenses/by/4.0/).

Abstract: Targeting inflammation and the pathways linking inflammation with cancer is an innovative therapeutic strategy. Tastants are potential candidates for this approach, since taste receptors display various biological functions, including anti-inflammatory activity (AIA). The present study aims to explore the power different tastes have to predict a phytochemical's anti-cancer properties. It also investigates whether anti-inflammatory phytocompounds also have anti-cancer effects, and whether there are tastes that can better predict a phytochemical's bivalent biological activity. Data from the PlantMolecularTasteDB, containing a total of 1527 phytochemicals, were used. Out of these, only 624 phytocompounds met the inclusion criterion of having 40 hits in a PubMed search, using the name of the phytochemical as the keyword. Among them, 461 phytochemicals were found to possess anti-cancer activity (ACA). The AIA and ACA of phytochemicals were strongly correlated, irrespective of taste/orosensation or chemical class. Bitter taste was positively correlated with ACA, while sweet taste was negatively correlated. Among chemical classes, only flavonoids (which are most frequently bitter) had a positive association with both AIA and ACA, a finding confirming that taste has predictive primacy over chemical class. Therefore, bitter taste receptor agonists and sweet taste receptor antagonists may have a beneficial effect in slowing down the progression of inflammation to cancer.

Keywords: taste; taste receptors; bitter; sweet; cancer; anti-inflammatory; phytochemical

1. Introduction

Taste receptors (TASRs) are sensory molecular structures specialized for detecting the five basic tastes: sweet, sour, salty, bitter, and umami. Receptors for sweet, umami, and bitter tastes belong to the G protein-coupled receptor superfamily, while salty and sour taste receptors are ion channels [1,2]. Although certain traditional medical systems (e.g., Ayurveda, Traditional Chinese Medicine) consider pungency and astringency to be fundamental tastes, modern science does not recognize them as basic taste sensations. Instead, they are classified as trigeminal orosensations that belong to chemesthesis, which is defined as a general sensitivity of the mucosal surfaces or skin [3]. Certain members of the transient receptor potential (TRP) channels family are the main transducers of chemestetic sensations [4]. A growing body of evidence shows that TASRs, as well as other orosensation transducers (e.g., TRPs), have widespread extraoral expressions (e.g., liver, pancreas, stomach, heart, brain, respiratory system, kidney, urinary bladder, adipose tissue, thyroid, gonads, spermatozoa, lymphocytes) and play important non-gustative, tissue-specific biological roles, such as the regulation of gastrointestinal functions, immunity, endocrine secretions, muscle relaxation, etc. [3,5–7]. Tastants binding to TASRs activate downstream signaling pathways in the target cells, leading eventually to either a gustatory chemosensation or to various extra-gustatory effects. They may be exogenous (e.g., nutrients, phytochemicals, xenobiotics) or endogenous (e.g., bile acids) compounds [8], and are characterized by an extreme structural and functional heterogeneity [9]. The functional diversity of TASR agonists led to the hypothesis that tastants have pharmacological significance and may even, in the future, become drug-like effectors in the treatment of various diseases [10–12].

Several studies have shown a direct involvement of bitter taste receptors in inflammatory processes. For instance, TAS2R16 expression is elevated in inflammatory conditions, and salicin, a TAS2R16 agonist, antagonizes NF-kB signaling [13]. Tiroch et al. demonstrated that resveratrol exhibits its anti-inflammatory activities (IL-6 targeting pathway) through the activation of TAS2R50 [14].

There is also increasing evidence about the multifaceted involvement of bitter taste receptors in cancer [15,16]. Recent studies have shown that bitter taste receptors are expressed differently in cancerous tissues compared to normal, cancer-free tissues [17–20]. In most cases, the expression of these receptors is downregulated. Additionally, overexpression of TAS2R has been shown to have anti-cancer effects [19].

Cancer represents a massive healthcare burden worldwide [21]. Intense research efforts have been focused on finding new methods of intervention in cancer prevention and treatment, in the quest for new therapeutic molecular targets that can modulate mechanisms involved in carcinogenesis. Targeting various pathways linking inflammation with cancer represents such an innovative therapeutic strategy.

In relation to cancer, inflammation can be either beneficial or detrimental to the body. Acute inflammation has been shown to inhibit tumor growth and is effective in treating various types of cancers, including bladder and colorectal cancers [22,23]. However, chronic inflammation can predispose the body towards cancer development. Chronic inflammation sustains and stimulates every step of carcinogenesis by promoting mutagenesis, tumor immune escape, inactivation of tumor suppressors, cell proliferation, etc., whereas cancer initiates, facilitates, and maintains local inflammatory processes through the chemoattraction of inflammatory cells, damage-associated molecular patterns, and hypoxia, which favors tumor growth and dissemination [24–26]. For instance, chronic gastritis increases the risk of stomach cancer [26–28]. Scientists estimate that at least 20–25% of cancers are produced or influenced by chronic inflammation [29,30], which may be linked to chronic infections with various viruses [31–34], Helicobacter pylori [35], autoimmune diseases [36], metabolic disorders [37], or exposure to various chemicals [38,39]. Tumor-promoting inflammation and genomic instability were considered to be the first two main "enabling characteristics" or oncogenic drivers which allow evolving preneoplastic cells to develop and acquire the aberrant phenotypic traits in the course of tumor growth and progression. Since then, other "enabling characteristics" have emerged (e.g., non-mutational epigenetic reprogramming, polymorphic microbiomes), adding more complexity to the cancer pathogenesis [40,41].

Several molecular targets, including transcription factors (e.g., NF-kB, STAT-3, AP-1), enzymes (e.g., COX-2, MAPK), and receptors (e.g., E series of prostaglandin receptors—EP receptors) were found to be simultaneously involved in inflammation and carcinogenesis, as well as in the progression of chronic inflammation towards cancer [25,42–46].

Plants are a huge reservoir of health-promoting compounds. At least 60% of approved anti-cancer drugs are derived from medicinal plants [47]. Bitter phytochemicals have displayed anti-cancer activity (ACA) in many in vitro and in vivo studies, with some of them showing the direct contribution of TAS2Rs activation to this effect [18–20]. In several cases (e.g., resveratrol, curcumin, kaempferol, epigallocatechin gallate) this ACA of bitter phytocompounds was proven to be achieved by also acting on inflammatory signaling pathways [48–52]. Regarding the anti-inflammatory potential of phytochemicals, our group has previously shown that bitter phytocompounds have a higher probability of displaying anti-inflammatory activity (AIA), when compared to non-bitter phytocompounds, while a sweet taste is negatively correlated with this activity [53]. In another study, we reported that the taste of phytocompounds is a better predictor of the ethnopharmacological activities of the medicinal plants than the phytochemical class [54].

By using data mining and statistical tools, the current research aims to determine whether there is any concordance between the taste or chemical class of phytocompounds and their evidence-based ACA, as well as between evidence-based ACA and AIA of phytocompounds. If there is a positive AIA-ACA agreement, the study will investigate whether taste or chemical class can predict this. Finally, the study aims to determine which attribute of phytocompounds (either chemical class or taste) better predicts a potential AIA-ACA agreement.

2. Results

Our analysis relies on the information gathered and made public in the PlantMolecularTasteDB (PMTDB) (http://plantmoleculartastedb.org, accessed on 1 February 2023), a previously published work, a database which contains a total of 1527 phytocompounds [9]. PMTDB is the largest database dedicated to individual plant-derived tastants (referred to as "phytotastants" in this paper) and orosensation-active phytochemicals among all the databases focused on flavor chemistry. In contrast, most databases are mixed collections of tastants (natural and synthetic, phytocompounds and synthetic drugs) or odorants [55], despite being sometimes larger (e.g., ChemTastesDB) [56].

The total number of phytocompounds included in the statistical analysis was 624: 429 with proven AIA and ACA, 82 with proven AIA but no ACA, 32 with proven ACA but not AIA, and 81 without either AIA or ACA. The total number of phytocompounds that fulfilled the inclusion criterion (a minimum of 40 hits in a PubMed search using the name of the phytotastant as the keyword, for details see Section 4, Materials and Methods) was obviously higher than that found in our previous study, mentioned in the Introduction section [53]. Hydroxy-α-sanshool, caffeic acid ethyl ester, kaempferol-3-O-β-galactopyranoside, guaiaverin, and clovamide are a few examples of such newly introduced phytotastants in our statistical analysis.

Regarding the update of data on AIA recorded in the PMTDB, we took notice of new studies about the AIA of various compounds that were available after the PMTDB was publicly open (e.g., isoschaftoside [57], cis-aconitic acid [58]).

2.1. The Correlation between Anti-Inflammatory/Anti-Cancer Activity and Taste/Chemical Class

Among the six tastes/orosensations included in our study (bitter, sweet, sour, salty, pungent, astringent), only bitter taste had a statistically significant positive association with both AIA and ACA. This was reflected by the greater-than-one odds ratio (OR) with a 95% confidence interval (CI) not including one. Conversely, sweet taste had a statistically significant negative association with ACA, as reflected by the less-than-one OR with a 95% confidence interval not including one. Sweet taste might have a negative association with AIA, but the p-value for this latter association was higher than the threshold calculated according to Bonferroni correction (Table 1).

Among the chemical classes, only flavonoids have a statistically significant positive association with both AIA and ACA (OR > 1.95% CI 3.03–324.24). By contrast, the saccharides and alkaloids have a negative association with AIA, and saccharides and amino acids have a negative association with ACA, as reflected by the less-than-one OR with a 95% CI not including one (Table 2).

Table 1. The correlation between anti-inflammatory/anti-cancer activity and taste. Legend: PDA = pharmacodynamic activity, AIA—anti-inflammatory activity, ACA—anti-cancer activity. Note: The third column contains the number of phytocompounds in each of the 4 cells of the 2 × 2 tables used for performing Fisher's exact test: a = taste-yes, AIA/ACA-yes; b = taste-yes, AIA/ACA-no; c = taste-no, AIA/ACA-yes; d = taste-no, AIA/ACA-no. As multiple comparisons were performed, the significance level (commonly set at 0.05) was lowered according to Bonferroni correction: the corrected significance level was 0.0035 (i.e., 0.05 divided by 14, the number of comparisons). Statistically significant results are in bold type.

Taste/Orosensation	PDA	(a, b, c, d)	Odds Ratio (OR)	95% Confidence Interval for OR	p-Value
Astringent	ACA	(75, 17, 386, 146)	1.67	0.97–2.99	0.073
Bitter (flavonoids only)	ACA	(57, 0, 5, 2)	Infinity	—	0.01
Bitter	**ACA**	**(324, 90, 137, 73)**	**1.92**	**1.32–2.77**	$\mathbf{7 \times 10^{-4}}$
Pungent	ACA	(64, 18, 397, 145)	1.3	0.75–2.32	0.42
Salty	ACA	(2, 2, 459, 161)	0.35	0.04–3.4	0.28
Sour	ACA	(29, 19, 432, 144)	0.51	0.28–0.95	0.039
Sweet	**ACA**	**(55, 45, 406, 118)**	**0.36**	**0.23–0.56**	$\mathbf{1 \times 10^{-5}}$
Umami	ACA	(4, 5, 457, 158)	0.28	0.07–1.11	0.057
Astringent	AIA	(82, 10, 429, 103)	1.97	1.01–4.13	0.056
Bitter	**AIA**	**(353, 61, 158, 52)**	**1.9**	**1.25–2.88**	**0.003**
Pungent	AIA	(70, 12, 441, 101)	1.34	0.71–2.66	0.44
Salty	AIA	(3, 1, 508, 112)	0.66	0.07–17.56	0.55
Sour	AIA	(37, 11, 474, 102)	0.72	0.36–1.53	0.43
Sweet	AIA	(73, 27, 438, 86)	0.53	0.32–0.88	0.016
Umami	AIA	(6, 3, 505, 110)	0.44	0.11–2.16	0.21

Table 2. The correlation between anti-cancer/anti-inflammatory activity and chemical classes. Legend: ACA—anti-cancer activity, AIA—anti-inflammatory activity, chemClass—chemical class. Note: The third column contains the number of phytocompounds in each of the 4 cells of the 2 × 2 tables built on the model mentioned in Section 4 (used for performing Fisher's exact test): a = chemClass-yes, AIA/ACA-yes; b = chemClass-yes, AIA/ACA-no; c = chemClass-no, AIA/ACA-yes; d = chemClass-no, AIA/ACA-no. As multiple comparisons were performed, the significance level (commonly set at 0.05) was lowered according to Bonferroni correction: the corrected significance level was 0.001 (i.e., 0.05 divided by 42, the number of comparisons). Statistically significant results are in bold type.

Chemical Class	PDA	(a, b, c, d)	Odds Ratio (OR)	95% Confidence Interval for OR	p-Value
alkaloids	ACA	(71, 37, 390, 126)	0.62	0.4–0.98	0.04
flavonoids	**ACA**	**(62, 2, 399, 161)**	**12.48**	**3.58–76.76**	$\mathbf{7 \times 10^{-7}}$
flavonoid glycosides	ACA	(33, 4, 428, 159)	3.06	1.15–10.28	0.032
saccharides	**ACA**	**(14, 18, 447, 145)**	**0.25**	**0.12–0.52**	**0.0002**
amino acids	**ACA**	**(9, 21, 452, 142)**	**0.14**	**0.06–0.3**	$\mathbf{3 \times 10^{-7}}$
monoterpenoids	ACA	(21, 6, 440, 157)	1.25	0.51–3.44	0.82
triterpenoids	ACA	(20, 2, 441, 161)	3.65	0.97–23.34	0.082
coumarins	ACA	(20, 1, 441, 162)	7.33	1.33–155.28	0.022
sesquiterpenoids	ACA	(18, 3, 443, 160)	2.16	0.68–9.33	0.31

Table 2. Cont.

Chemical Class	PDA	(a, b, c, d)	Odds Ratio (OR)	95% Confidence Interval for OR	p-Value
phenolic others	ACA	(16, 3, 445, 160)	1.92	0.6–8.33	0.43
phenolic acids	ACA	(14, 4, 447, 159)	1.24	0.42–4.45	1
short aliphatic acids	ACA	(9, 9, 452, 154)	0.34	0.13–0.9	0.028
tannins	ACA	(14, 1, 447, 162)	5.07	0.89–109.2	0.13
diterpenoids	ACA	(12, 2, 449, 161)	2.15	0.54–14.29	0.54
sulfur compounds	ACA	(8, 6, 453, 157)	0.46	0.15–1.45	0.21
monoterpenoid glycosides	ACA	(12, 1, 449, 162)	4.32	0.74–94.12	0.2
steroid glycosides	ACA	(10, 1, 451, 162)	3.59	0.59–79.2	0.3
fatty acids	ACA	(8, 2, 453, 161)	1.42	0.32–9.89	1
phenolic acid esters	ACA	(7, 3, 454, 160)	0.82	0.21–3.96	0.73
phenylpropanoids (others) *	ACA	(7, 3, 454, 160)	0.82	0.21–3.96	0.73
triterpenoid glycosides	ACA	(9, 1, 452, 162)	3.22	0.52–71.78	0.47
alkaloids	**AIA**	**(74, 34, 437, 79)**	**0.39**	**0.25–0.64**	**0.0002**
flavonoids	**AIA**	**(63, 1, 448, 112)**	**15.72**	**3.03–324.24**	**5×10^{-5}**
flavonoid glycosides	AIA	(34, 3, 477, 110)	2.61	0.87–10.89	0.12
saccharides	**AIA**	**(16, 16, 495, 97)**	**0.2**	**0.09–0.41**	**2×10^{-5}**
amino acids	AIA	(25, 5, 486, 108)	1.11	0.44–3.33	1
monoterpenoids	AIA	(26, 1, 485, 112)	5.99	1.11–125.95	0.043
triterpenoids	AIA	(19, 3, 492, 110)	1.42	0.45–6.1	0.78
coumarins	AIA	(20, 1, 491, 112)	4.56	0.83–96.63	0.15
sesquiterpenoids	AIA	(18, 3, 493, 110)	1.34	0.42–5.79	0.78
phenolic others	AIA	(16, 3, 495, 110)	1.18	0.37–5.17	1
phenolic acids	AIA	(16, 2, 495, 111)	1.79	0.46–11.67	0.75
short aliphatic acids	AIA	(11, 7, 500, 106)	0.33	0.13–0.93	0.029
tannins	AIA	(14, 1, 497, 112)	3.15	0.55–68.05	0.33
diterpenoids	AIA	(13, 1, 498, 112)	2.92	0.5–63.36	0.48
sulfur compounds	AIA	(10, 4, 501, 109)	0.54	0.17–2.04	0.3
monoterpenoid glycosides	AIA	(12, 1, 499, 112)	2.69	0.46–58.69	0.48
steroid glycosides	AIA	(8, 3, 503, 110)	0.58	0.16–2.76	0.43
fatty acids	AIA	(7, 3, 504, 110)	0.51	0.13–2.46	0.4
phenolic acid esters	AIA	(9, 1, 502, 112)	2.01	0.32–44.8	0.7
phenylpropanoids (others) *	AIA	(8, 2, 503, 111)	0.88	0.2–6.16	1
triterpenoid glycosides	AIA	(10, 0, 501, 113)	Infinity	—	0.22

Legend.* Other than the main classes of (iso)flavonoids, e.g., coumarins, stilbenes, lignans, and hydroxycinnamic acids, hydroxycinnamic acids derivatives (such as amides or esters), cinnamic acid esters, methoxyphenols.

The analysis was limited to flavonoids to determine whether the positive association between flavonoids and AIA was mediated by a specific taste, and the result was statistically significant for bitter taste only (see the row "bitter (flavonoids only)" in Table 1). A similar computation was done for alkaloids, and no association was found between the pharmacodynamic activity and taste. The same holds for amino acids.

For saccharides, sweet taste might be conceived as the mediator of the association with the absence of AIA/ACA; however, this cannot be proven statistically, as all but one saccharide (gentiobiose) are sweet.

Pooling together chemical classes did not influence these results (Table 3).

Table 3. The correlation between anti-cancer/anti-inflammatory activity and pooled chemical classes. Legend: ACA—anti-cancer activity, AIA—anti-inflammatory activity, chemClass—pooled chemical class. Note: The third column contains the number of phytocompounds in each of the 4 cells of the 2 × 2 tables built on the model mentioned in Section 4 (used for performing Fisher's exact test): a = chemClass-yes, AIA/ACA-yes; b = chemClass-yes, AIA/ACA-no; c = chemClass-no, AIA/ACA-yes; d = chemClass-no, AIA/ACA-no. As multiple comparisons were performed, the significance level (commonly set at 0.05) was lowered according to Bonferroni correction: the corrected significance level was 0.0015 (i.e., 0.05 divided by 34, the number of comparisons). Statistically significant results are in bold type.

Pooled Chemical Class	PDA	(a, b, c, d)	Odds Ratio (OR)	95% Confidence Interval for OR	p-Value
alkaloids	AIA	(76, 34, 435, 79)	0.41	0.25–0.66	0.0003
amino acids	AIA	(25, 5, 486, 108)	1.11	0.44–3.33	1
coumarins	AIA	(22, 1, 489, 112)	5.03	0.92–106.32	0.01
diterpenoids	AIA	(16, 1, 495, 112)	3.62	0.64–77.5	0.33
fatty compounds	AIA	(16, 6, 495, 107)	0.58	0.23–1.64	0.26
flavonoids	AIA	(97, 4, 414, 109)	6.37	2.5–20.81	9×10^{-6}
monoterpenoids	AIA	(48, 3, 463, 110)	3.8	1.29–15.65	0.014
phenolic acids	AIA	(27, 3, 484, 110)	2.04	0.67–8.62	0.33
phenolic others	AIA	(19, 3, 492, 110)	1.42	0.45–6.1	0.78
phenylpropanoids	AIA	(9, 2, 502, 111)	1	0.23–6.84	1
saccharides	AIA	(16, 16, 495, 97)	0.2	0.09–0.41	2×10^{-5}
sesquiterpenoids	AIA	(18, 5, 493, 108)	0.79	0.3–2.43	0.59
short aliphatic acids	AIA	(11, 7, 500, 106)	0.33	0.13–0.93	0.029
steroids	AIA	(13, 3, 498, 110)	0.96	0.29–4.26	1
sulfur compounds	AIA	(10, 5, 501, 108)	0.43	0.15–1.42	0.16
tannins	AIA	(14, 1, 497, 112)	3.15	0.55–68.05	0.33
triterpenoids	AIA	(29, 3, 482, 110)	2.2	0.73–9.26	0.24
alkaloids	ACA	(73, 37, 388, 126)	0.64	0.41–1.01	0.056
amino acids	ACA	(9, 21, 452, 142)	0.14	0.06–0.3	3×10^{-7}
coumarins	ACA	(21, 2, 440, 161)	3.84	1.03–24.49	0.055
diterpenoids	ACA	(13, 4, 448, 159)	1.15	0.39–4.16	1
fatty compounds	ACA	(15, 7, 446, 156)	0.75	0.3–2	0.62
flavonoids	ACA	(95, 6, 366, 157)	6.78	3.08–17.41	5×10^{-8}

Table 3. Cont.

Pooled Chemical Class	PDA	(a, b, c, d)	Odds Ratio (OR)	95% Confidence Interval for OR	p-Value
monoterpenoids	ACA	(40, 11, 421, 152)	1.31	0.67–2.73	0.51
phenolic acids	ACA	(23, 7, 438, 156)	1.17	0.51–2.99	0.83
phenolic others	ACA	(19, 3, 442, 160)	2.29	0.73–9.83	0.22
phenylpropanoids	ACA	(8, 3, 453, 160)	0.94	0.25–4.44	1
saccharides	ACA	(14, 18, 447, 145)	0.25	0.12–0.52	0.0002
sesquiterpenoids	ACA	(18, 5, 443, 158)	1.28	0.49–3.93	0.81
short aliphatic acids	ACA	(9, 9, 452, 154)	0.34	0.13–0.9	0.028
steroids	ACA	(15, 1, 446, 162)	5.44	0.96–116.79	0.083
sulfur compounds	ACA	(8, 7, 453, 156)	0.39	0.14–1.16	0.078
tannins	ACA	(14, 1, 447, 162)	5.07	0.89–109.2	0.13
triterpenoids	ACA	(29, 3, 432, 160)	3.58	1.19–14.97	0.024

2.2. Correlation between Anti-Cancer and Anti-Inflammatory Activity

The statistical analysis revealed a strong correlation between ACA and AIA, which was maintained over the entire range of tastes/orosensations (Table 4) and chemical classes (Table 5), with the exception of amino acids.

Table 4. The correlation between anti-inflammatory (AIA) and anti-cancer activity (ACA) for all tastes and for each taste is taken separately. Salty and umami are absent due to the low count of corresponding phytocompounds. Note: The second column contains the number of phytocompounds in each of the 4 cells of the 2 × 2 tables built on the model mentioned in Section 4 (used for performing Fisher's exact test): a = AIA-no, ACA-no; b = AIA-yes, ACA-no; c = AIA-no, ACA-yes; d = AIA-yes, ACA-yes. As multiple comparisons were performed, the significance level (commonly set at 0.05) was lowered according to Bonferroni correction: the corrected significance level was 0.01 (i.e., 0.05 divided by 6, the number of comparisons).

Taste	(a, b, c, d)	Odds Ratio (OR)	95% Confidence Interval for OR	p-Value
All tastes	(81, 32, 82, 429)	13.16	8.25–21.32	3×10^{-30}
Astringent	(9, 1, 8, 74)	75.56	10.69–1847.1	3×10^{-7}
Bitter	(40, 21, 50, 303)	11.44	6.27–21.31	4×10^{-16}
Pungent	(8, 4, 10, 60)	11.45	2.93–51.13	0.0004
Sour	(10, 1, 9, 28)	28.62	4.05–700.41	0.0001
Sweet	(22, 5, 23, 50)	9.33	3.26–30.75	1×10^{-5}

In Table 4, all results are either extremely high (for All Tastes and for Bitter) or highly statistically significant. AIA-ACA association holds, irrespective of taste/orosensation or chemical class.

As illustrated in Table 5, the odds ratio (OR) is equal to zero for the chemical classes in which no phytocompound was devoid of both AIA and ACA (a = 0) (coumarins, diterpenoids, monoterpenoid glycosides, triterpenoid glycosides). For all these chemical classes, the vast majority of phytocompounds have both AIA and ACA (d is disproportionately higher than a, b, and c). For all the other chemical classes, OR is greater than one (and sometimes even infinite), but it does not reach the level of statistical significance due to the (very) low count of phytocompounds devoid of both AIA and ACA. The p-value is higher than the Bonferroni corrected threshold and the less-than-one inferior limit of the 95% confidence interval for OR.

Table 5. The correlation between anti-inflammatory (AIA) and anti-cancer activity (ACA) for each chemical class is taken separately. Note: The second column contains the number of phytocompounds in each of the 4 cells of the 2×2 tables built on the model mentioned in Section 4 (used for performing Fisher's exact test): a = AIA-no, ACA-no; b = AIA-yes, ACA-no; c = AIA-no, ACA-yes; d = AIA-yes, ACA-yes. Inf = infinity. As multiple comparisons were performed, the significance level (commonly set at 0.05) was lowered according to Bonferroni correction: the corrected significance level was 0.002 (i.e., 0.05 divided by 21, the number of comparisons). Statistically significant results are in bold type.

Chemical Class	(a, b, c, d)	Odds Ratio (OR)	95% Confidence Interval for OR	p-Value
alkaloids	**(24, 13, 10, 61)**	**10.93**	**3.97–32.64**	$\mathbf{2 \times 10^{-7}}$
flavonoids	(1, 1, 0, 62)	Inf	0.79–Inf	0.031
flavonoid glycosides	(2, 2, 1, 32)	25.21	0.98–1904.49	0.026
saccharides	(12, 6, 4, 10)	4.73	0.89–30.52	0.073
amino acids	(5, 16, 0, 9)	Inf	0.41-Inf	0.29
monoterpenoids	(1, 5, 0, 21)	Inf	0.09-Inf	0.22
triterpenoids	(1, 1, 2, 18)	7.55	0.08–738.06	0.26
coumarins	(0, 1, 1, 19)	0	0–770.62	1
sesquiterpenoids	(2, 1, 1, 17)	23.02	0.74–2065.5	0.041
phenolic others	(2, 1, 1, 15)	20.38	0.65–1840.77	0.051
phenolic acids	(2, 2, 0, 14)	Inf	0.75-Inf	0.039
short aliphatic acids	(6, 3, 1, 8)	13.25	1–819.63	0.05
tannins	(1, 0, 0, 14)	Inf	0.36-Inf	0.067
diterpenoids	(0, 2, 1, 11)	0	0–233.15	1
sulfur compounds	(3, 3, 1, 7)	5.99	0.33–417.16	0.24
monoterpenoid glycosides	(0, 1, 1, 11)	0	0–464.61	1
steroid glycosides	(1, 0, 2, 8)	Inf	0.07-Inf	0.27
fatty acids	(1, 1, 2, 6)	2.65	0.03–273.2	1
phenolic acid esters	(1, 2, 0, 7)	Inf	0.06-Inf	0.3
phenylpropanoids	(1, 2, 1, 6)	2.65	0.03–273.2	1
triterpenoid glycosides	(0, 1, 0, 9)	0	0-Inf	1

The most significant results are synthesized in Figure 1.

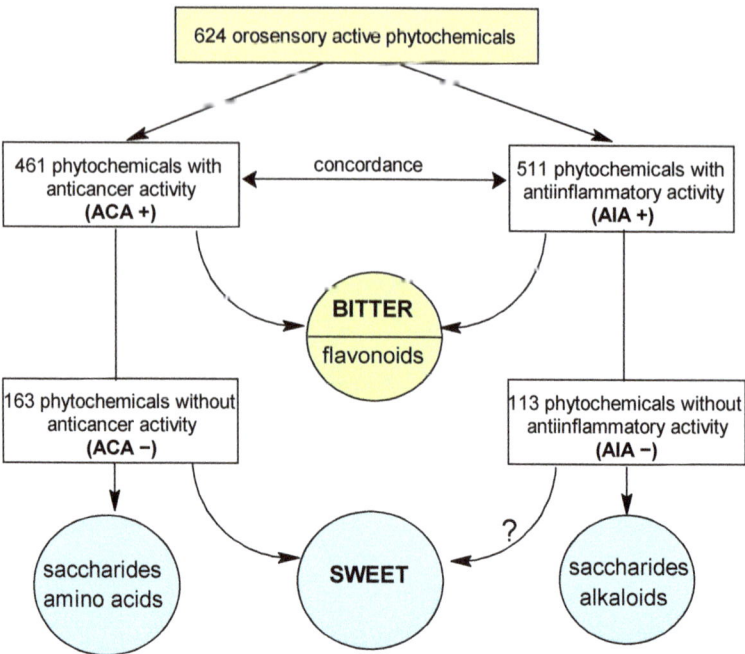

Figure 1. Flowchart showing the main statistical concordances found in the present study (Legend: ACA = anti-cancer activity, AIA = anti-inflammatory activity, (+) = present, (−) = absent): ACA(+) with AIA(+), bitter with ACA(+), bitter with AIA(+), flavonoids with ACA (+), flavonoids with AIA(+), sweet with ACA(−), saccharides with ACA(−), saccharides with AIA(−), amino acids with ACA(−), alkaloids with AIA(−). The association of sweet with AIA(+) is marginally statistically significant - this is the reason a question mark accompanies the correspondent curved arrow.

3. Discussion

From the 624 total phytotastants that met our inclusion criteria, ACA activity was present in 461 phytocompounds.

3.1. Taste as an Important Determinant of Pharmacodynamic Activity

The most relevant finding of the present study is that only bitter taste has a statistically significant positive association with both ACA and AIA. The last concordance (bitter -AIA) has already been proven in a previous study [53], performed on a smaller number of phytocompounds. The present investigation included a larger number of phytocompounds in the PMTDB because more of them met the inclusion criterion of 40 hits in PubMed. Additionally, we updated the data on the AIA of phytotastants available in the PMTDB. In line with our observation/results, there is an increasing body of evidence that supports the involvement of TAS2R agonists in alleviating the inflammatory processes [59,60] and their role as chemopreventive and/or chemotherapeutic agents [19,61]. Regarding ACA, it is relevant that the activation of various TAS2Rs subtypes (e.g., TAS2R4, TAS2R8, TAS2R13, TAS2R14, TAS2R10, and TAS2R30/47) by bitter compounds such as quinine, apigenin, noscapine, caffeine, and denatonium led to significant ACA in several cancer cell lines by multiple mechanisms: reduced cell proliferation, metabolic activity, migration, invasion, motility, metastasis and angiogenesis, increased apoptosis, and enhanced chemosensitivity to conventional anti-cancer drugs [18–20,61]. TAS2Rs also play a role in the tumor-restraining function of the fibroblasts found in the tumoral microenvironment. For instance, TAS2R9 is upregulated in cancer-associated fibroblasts, the most representative cellular type in the stroma of pancreatic ductal adenocarcinoma, and it was proposed as a novel molecular target, a candidate for the inhibition of cancer progression, by reprogramming the crosstalk between fibroblasts and cancer epithelial cells [62].

A secondary finding is that there was only one other relevant association that was identified: sweet taste is negatively correlated with both AIA and ACA. This association does not contradict the idea that taste is an important determinant of pharmacodynamic activity, which may be more important than the chemical class [54]. It is in fact the most important general idea suggested by us in our present study, as well as in our previous studies, regarding the relationship between tastes and (ethno)pharmacological activities [3,9,53,63].

3.2. Upgrade of the Previously Reported Taste—AIA Associations

Our previous study reported a negative correlation between sour taste and AIA [53], but this finding was not confirmed in the present analysis. There are several possible explanations for this discrepancy. Firstly, new studies have been published regarding the AIA of some phytochemicals, such as caproic acid [64] and cis-aconitic acid [58]. Secondly, there were different numbers of compounds that met the inclusion criteria of at least 40 hits in PubMed, such as hydroxy-α-sanshool.

3.3. The Pharmacodynamic Activity of Phytochemicals: Taste Has Predictive Primacy over Chemical Classes

Among the chemical classes, only flavonoids have a statistically significant positive association with both AIA and ACA. In contrast, saccharides and alkaloids have a negative association with AIA, while saccharides and amino acids have a negative association with ACA. The positive association between flavonoids and AIA/ACA does not contradict the primacy of bitter taste over chemical classes as the determinant of AIA/ACA, since the vast majority of flavonoids are bitter. Similarly, the negative association between saccharides and AIA/ACA can be explained by the fact that most saccharides are sweet.

3.4. Bitter—Sweet: Are They in Opposition?

Both bitter and sweet taste receptors are G-coupled protein receptors. Bitter taste receptors (TAS2R) consist of only one type of receptor and belong to the A class type receptors, while sweet taste receptors (TAS1R) are dimers formed by two different G coupled protein receptors (TAS1R2 and TAS1R3) and belong to the C class type receptors [2,65,66].

Regarding the present contrasting results between bitter and sweet associations with AIA and ACA (positive and negative associations, respectively) reported by our study, it is interesting to note that these two tastes are frequently framed in various types of opposition, from both traditional [3] and modern medical points of view [67].

For instance, in Ayurveda, bitter taste is considered to have dry and light (decreasing weight) qualities, while sweet taste is considered to have wet/oily (emollient/moisturizing) and heavy (increasing weight) qualities [3].

Modern science points to various types of bitter–sweet opposition. Structurally, the majority of bitter tastants have a smaller size than sweet compounds, as well as higher hydrophobicity [68]. Functionally, bitter taste receptor activation can produce a biological effect, such as the secretion of antimicrobial peptides in sinonasal epithelial cells that co-express both types of taste receptors. However, this effect may be suppressed by sweet taste receptor activation [69–71]. Interestingly, two drugs that have similar, well-known AIA, ibuprofen and flufenamic acid, showed contrasting results regarding the affinity for TASRs: flufenamic acid was revealed as an agonist of bitter taste receptors TAS2R14 [72], while ibuprofen was a potent inhibitor of sweet taste receptors TAS1R2/TAS1R3 [73].

Also, bitter tastants seem to have many common off-targets (e.g., cytochrome P450 enzymes, carbonic anhydrases, adenosine A3 receptor, hERG potassium channel), while sweet compounds have very few [67]. In regard to caloric value, sweet foods such as fruits and vegetables have a high nutritional value, while bitter have none, or are even anti-nutritional [74]. Bitter foods such as leafy greens and cruciferous vegetables are highly nutritious, but bitter compounds in some plants can be toxic in large amounts [75]. In terms of taste preferences, bitter is innately aversive and rapidly rejected, whereas sweet is appetitive and avidly ingested [76]. Nevertheless, the inclusion of bitter items in diet was associated with health-promoting effects [77,78], while a high-sugar diet was outlined as contributing to the pathogenesis of several diseases (e.g., obesity, metabolic syndrome, and inflammatory diseases) [79].

3.5. Anti-Inflammatory Activity- Anti-Cancer Activity Association Is Independent of Taste

Given the very strong association between AIA and ACA, any factor associated with AIA (such as bitter taste) is expected to also be associated with ACA; of course, the reciprocal is also true. Table 4 suggests that AIA-ACA association is independent of taste as it holds over the entire spectrum of tastes/orosensations. The strong (and taste-independent) AIA-ACA association is probably due to the many molecular pathways that inflammation and neoplasia share [25,43–46]. The perpetuation of regenerative processes induced by chronic inflammation frequently degenerates in cancer [29,30].

The potential role of anti-inflammatory plant-derived agents in cancer therapy has been already hypothesized by other scientists [80]. The AIA-ACA concordance was also highlighted by a previous mixed study based on field data obtained from Indian tribal healers, chemoinformatic prediction tools (PASS database, admetSAR, CLC-pred), and in vitro experiments, which concluded that the ethnopharmacological anti-inflammatory plants may have anti-cancer potential [81]. Another research showed that synthesized quinoline glycoconjugate derivatives exhibited a positive correlation between ACA and AIA [82]. One of the most anti-inflammatory compounds against COX-2, compound C8, also had the strongest cytotoxic activity against HeLa cells [82].

Our results are also in line with data proving the central role of NF-kB and COX-2/PGE2 pathways in both inflammation and cancer. NF-kB is induced by pro-inflammatory mediators, such as TNF, IL-1, and itself controls pro-inflammatory factors gene expression, such as TNF, IL-1, IL-6, COX-2 [83]. Also, NF-kB occupies a crucial role in tumor initiation and in cancer progression and spread [84], being simultaneously a facilitator of inflammation progression towards cancer [85]. Various natural inhibitors of NF-kB signaling (e.g., polyphenols, terpenoids) displayed simultaneous anti-inflammatory and anti-cancer potential [86,87]. Therefore, some of these NF-kB inhibitors, administered as monotherapy or combined therapy, were either investigated or are under current evaluation in clinical trials for both types of conditions (e.g., the effects of curcumin in rheumatoid arthritis [88], chemotherapy- or radiotherapy-induced oral mucositis [89], and oral leukoplakia [90], as well as prostate cancer [91], metastatic tumors [92], resveratrol effects in smoking-induced inflammation [93], and multiple myeloma [94]).

Interestingly, numerous studies have provided evidence that nonsteroidal anti-inflammatory drugs (NSAIDs), including aspirin, may hold promise in helping to prevent cancer. Experimental and epidemiologic studies, along with randomized clinical trials, have shown that NSAIDs may have a prophylactic effect against certain cancers [95–104]. Also, specific anti-inflammatory therapy with canakinumab, an interleukin-1β inhibitor, significantly reduced the incidence of lung cancer in patients with atherosclerosis [105]. Few studies reported opposite effects of excessive use of certain NSAIDs [106,107].

NSAIDs are known for their COX inhibitory activity [108]. COX-2 is the inducible isoform and is linked to inflammatory processes [109], as well as to cancer [110]. Overexpression of this enzyme identified in various types of cancer, including breast, colon, and prostate cancer, was associated to poor outcomes, poor prognosis, and reduced survival rates [111,112].

The effects of COX-2 on cancer progression are often mediated via the COX-2/PGE2 pathway [25]. PGE2 is a proinflammatory factor, proven to be upregulated in cancer cells [113–115] that bind to EP1, EP2, EP3, and EP4 receptors. Consequently, certain downstream signaling pathways involved in tumor growth are activated, such as the

PKA, β-catenin, NF-kB, or PI3K/AKT pathways [25]. Inhibition of the PGE2 pathway by targeting EP receptors is currently being evaluated as a new therapeutic strategy for cancer treatment [116–118].

3.6. Anti-Cancer Activity—Is Bitter Better?

The association of bitter taste with ACA is not surprising, since there is an important body of evidence showing that TAS2R agonists are able to exert ACA, and TAS2Rs might play an important role in carcinogenesis. In the majority of cases, TAS2R activation was associated with antitumor activity [16,18,20,61]. The anti-cancer effects of bitter taste receptor activation include the impact on apoptosis, proliferation, migration, invasion, viability, cycle cell arrest, and stemness of cancer cells, and the influence on tumor growth. There is a difference in TAS2R expression in neoplastic cells compared to normal cells. For example, quinine (through the activation of TAS2R4) and apigenin (through the activation of TAS2R14) significantly attenuated metastatic breast cancer cells proliferation and increased the number of cells in the early apoptotic states, whereas, in a normal breast epithelial cell line, these effects were absent [20]. As well, noscapine stimulation of TAS2R14 increased ovarian cancer cells apoptosis [18], while Carey et al. highlighted TAS2R's involvement in the apoptotic process of head and neck squamous cell carcinoma cell lines [119].

To date, numerous studies show certain types of bitter taste receptors tend to be downregulated in cancer cells compared to cancer-free cell lines (TAS2R1, TAS2R4, TAS2R8, TAS2R10, TAS2R14, TAS2R38) [17–20]. Carey et al. examined the variation in expression of bitter, sweet, and umami receptors in 45 solid tumors. They reported that TAS2R4, TAS2R5, TAS2R14, TAS2R19, TAS2R20, and TAS2R31 expression was at a lower level in neoplastic tissues compared to cancer-free tissues [120]. However, some studies indicate that there is an overexpression in some bitter taste receptors in tumors. For instance, TAS2R14, TAS2R20, and TAS2R30/31/43/45/46 have been shown to be expressed more in highly metastatic cancer cell lines (MDA-MB-231) than in normal breast cell lines (MCF-10A) [121]. Another study demonstrated that, despite the tendency for some bitter taste receptors to be downregulated in cancer tissues, TAS2R38 was often overexpressed in solid tumors, as compared to normal tissues [120].

3.7. Anti-Cancer Activity—Is Sweet Worse?

Sweet taste is negatively correlated with ACA. Notably, a higher dietary intake of sugar, which is more rapidly absorbed than other sources of carbohydrates, may increase plasma glucose and insulin levels, which are known as risk factors for carcinogenesis [122,123]. According to a systematic review and meta-analysis of observational studies, there is a statistically significant positive correlation between the incidence of breast and prostate cancer and higher intake of sugar-sweetened beverages. The study also found a positive correlation between fruit juice consumption and the risk of prostate cancer [124]. Obesity is another redoubtable risk factor for cancer [125], while the ingestion of concentrated sugars is probably the principal cause of obesity [126]. Moreover, there is mounting evidence that caloric restriction and fasting, mimicking a low-carbohydrate, low-protein diet, are beneficial in cancer prevention by reshaping metabolism and anti-cancer immunity [127,128]. Our findings may also be consistent with the results of a recent clinical trial that found an association between increased cancer risk (all cancers, prostate cancer, breast cancer, and obesity-related cancers) and the intake of artificial sweeteners, mainly aspartame and acesulfame-K [129].

3.8. Limitations of the Study

Our research has several limitations that need to be considered. Firstly, the lack of studies concerning ACA may still be caused by the absence of evidence, despite our 40 hits inclusion criteria. Secondly, studies regarding ACA/AIA were excluded from this investigation if a metabolite of a specific phytocompound showed ACA/AIA activities, but the corresponding parent phytochemical did not show such activities. For instance, gluconasturtiin itself, found in cruciferous vegetables, has no evidence-based ACA and was therefore categorized in our statistical analysis as ACA(−), while its metabolite, phenylethyl isothiocyanate (PEITC), has ACA [130,131]. Thirdly, there are contradictory data regarding the positive or negative evidence of pharmacological activities of some phytochemicals. For example, morphine has both antineoplastic and protumor effects [132–134], which makes it difficult to categorize phytochemicals in one class or the other (positive evidence or negative evidence). Fourthly, the inclusion criterion of at least 40 hits in a PubMed search is justified by two reasons: (1) to use the same methodology as the one used in our previous study; (2) to lower the probability for a specific item to be identified as not having a biological role because it is not studied enough. On the other hand, there are phytocompounds that have either AIA or ACA but do not meet the inclusion criterion of at least 40 hits in PubMed. For example, santamarin displays both AIA and ACA [135–138], but it did not meet the inclusion criterion, and therefore it was not included in our statistical analysis. Lastly, time limitations are an important factor that can change outcomes. The literature search for our study started in February 2023 and finished in June 2023. For some phytocompounds, new studies may have been published after our search ended.

Finally, our study is limited by the lack of experimental validation of our results. Simultaneous testing of AIA and ACA of a battery of phytotastants belonging to various chemical classes and looking for potential AIA-ACA or taste -ACA/AIA or chemical class-ACA/AIA concordances, or screening phytochemicals agonists of TAS2Rs for cancer cell growth inhibitory capacity and looking for potential association between their half-maximal inhibitory concentration (IC50) values and bitter taste threshold concentrations may be interesting approaches for upcoming research initiatives.

4. Materials and Methods

The study relies on the information available from PMTDB (http://plantmoleculartastedb.org accessed at 1 February 2023), a public database previously published, which contains a total of 1527 phytotastants [9].

For any given compound, AIA and ACA are two of the most, and, implicitly, two of the first, studied biological activities, only second to antimicrobial activity, according to our previous study [53].

Both ACA and AIA were considered evidence-based if they were supported by at least one correctly conducted study, irrespective of being performed in vitro or on animal or human subjects. However, among the phytochemicals with positive evidence for AIA and ACA, only those that also fulfilled the inclusion criterion were included/used in the statistical analysis.

The ACA was searched for these compounds in three international databases: PubMed, Google Scholar, and ScienceDirect.

The systematic literature research was made by using the phrases: [specific phytochemical name] AND (cancer) or [specific phytochemical name] AND (chemopreventive) or [specific phytochemical name] AND (cytotoxic) or [specific phytochemical name] AND (antiproliferative) or [specific phytochemical name] AND (tumor) or [specific phytochemical name] AND (neoplastic) or [specific phytochemical name] AND (chemotherapy).

ACA was considered when that specific phytocompound had a direct activity on cancer cells or tumors, such as antiproliferative activity, induction of apoptosis, cytotoxic activity on cancer cells, lowering the viability of the cancer cells, or diminishing the tumor volume or growth. The effects on metastasis potential or the effects on invasion capability were not taken into account. Also, the effects on cancer vessels and the effects of increasing the outcome of potentiating some chemotherapy treatment or reversing chemoresistance were not considered. The effects of phytocompounds as chemosensitizers was also overlooked.

The eligible studies for our work were those using only single phytotastants. Studies using plant extracts, a combination of a phytocompound with a chemotherapeutic agent, or mixtures of two or more phytocompounds were excluded in the present research. Also, studies were excluded from this research if a metabolite of a specific phytocompound showed ACA, but that parent phytochemical did not show any anti-cancer effect. The exclusion of the phytochemical's metabolite was necessary to evaluate the impact of taste category on the pharmacodynamic activity of the phytochemical, as differences in taste between the two could affect the results.

In case of AIA, we updated the data available in the PMTDB, performing again the search for the phytotastants recorded as having negative evidence in the PMTDB and the previous study, using the same keywords as before [53].

Taking into account that lack of AIA or ACA is difficult to identify by searching the literature, we considered as "negative evidence for AIA/ACA" the fulfilment of two criteria, a rule already used in our previous study [53]: (1) lack of any positive evidence related to the respective pharmacological activity (AIA or ACA); and (2) the PubMed search using the name of the phytotastant as a keyword produced at least 40 articles, meaning that the phytocompound has been the object of a sufficient research/number of studies for the respective pharmacological activity (AIA or ACA) to be identified, and that the lack of positive evidence is not caused by a deficiency of studies.

Only 624 phytotastants (either with negative or positive evidence of AIA/ACA) out of 1527 in the PMTDB fulfilled the inclusion criterion and were therefore included in the statistical analysis (Figure 2).

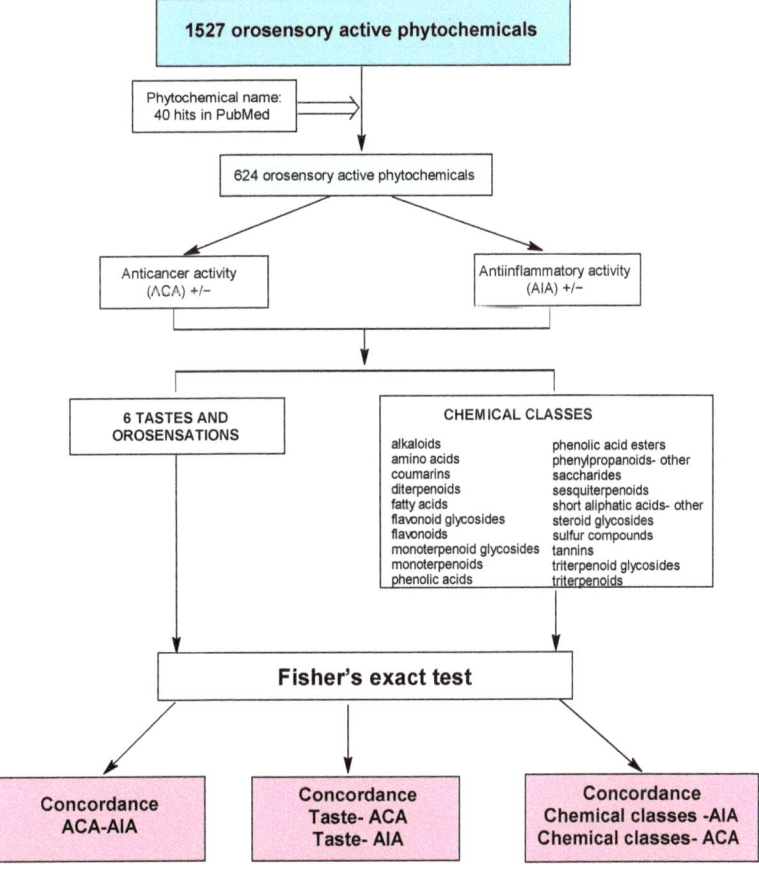

Figure 2. Flowchart outlining the steps of data preparation and statistical analysis (www.plantmoleculartastedb.org, accessed on 1 February 2023).

The correlations between two categorical parameters (such as taste and AIA/ACA or chemical class and AIA/ACA) were analyzed by means of Fisher's exact test, performed on 2 × 2 contingency tables built on the model in Table 6. Fisher's exact test was employed (instead of the more commonly used Chi-squared test) because, in many instances, the number of cells in these contingency tables, especially a, b, and/or c, are quite small, which result in small (<5) corresponding expected values, precluding the employment of the Chi-squared test. Moreover, Fisher's exact test is always preferable to the Chi-squared test, as it computes the probability directly and exactly, while the Chi-squared test only approximates the probability, yielding results that are close to the true probability only when the number of cells in the contingency table are (relatively) large.

Table 6. The 2 × 2 contingency table used for performing Fisher's exact test (AIA/ACA = anti-inflammatory/anti-cancer activity).

	No AIA/ACA	AIA/ACA
No Taste/Chemical class	a	b
Taste/Chemical class	c	d

The results were considered statistically significant if the p-value was below the generally accepted threshold of 0.05. When multiple comparisons were performed, the significance level (commonly set at 0.05) was lowered according to Bonferroni correction: the corrected significance level was 0.05 divided by the number of comparisons. The rationale for employing Bonferroni correction is that whenever large number of comparisons are performed, there is a high probability that some results (about 1 in 20, should a threshold of 0.05 be used for p-value) appear significant by sheer chance, without reflecting a truth about the real world. For example, if two comparisons are performed and a threshold of 0.05 is employed, the probability that each of the comparisons yields a falsely significant result is 0.05, but the probability that at least one of the two comparisons yields such a result is 0.05 + 0.05 = 0.1, so the 0.05 threshold for p-value is no longer observed. However, if the threshold for the p-value is lowered o 0.025 (i.e., 0.0.5 divided by 2), then the probability that at least one of the two comparisons yields a falsely significant result is 0.025 + 0.025 = 0.05, so the generally accepted threshold of 0.05 is observed.

Odds ratio (OR) was used to estimate the odds that, say, a bitter phytocompound (if we look at Table 1) has, for example, ACA. An OR of 1 means that there is no relation between the bitter compound and ACA. An OR larger/smaller than 1 means that a bitter compound has a higher/lower probability to have ACA than a non-bitter phytocompound (1.92 in Table 1). In order to estimate the value in the real world, the 95% confidence interval for OR is also provided, signifying that there is a 95% probability that the value in the real world is somewhere between 1.32 and 2.77.

All the statistical calculations were performed using the R language and environment for statistical computing and graphics, version 4.0.3 (copyrighted by The R Foundation for Statistical Computing).

The chemical classes were chosen so as to be as disjunct as possible, i.e., each compound fell in one, and only one, chemical class. In other words, the phytocompounds were classified in mutually exclusive chemical classes. About two thirds of these classes (monoterpenes, lignans, organic acids, carotenoids, cyanogen glycoside, fatty aldehydes, steroids, diterpenoid glycosides, phenolic glycosides, polyketides, proteins, alkaloid glycosides, alkylamides, amides, anthraquinones, aromatic aldehydes, aromatic ketones, chromones, coumarin glycosides, fatty acid esters, fatty alcohols, high aliphatic acids, high aliphatic alcohols, lactones, medium aliphatic acids, naphthofurans, phenolic acid glycosides, sesquiterpene, vitamins, amines, anthraquinone glycosides, aromatic esters, carboxylic acids, cardenolides, cyclic polyols, guanidines, indoles, lignan glycosides, low aliphatic alcohols, monoterpene, monoterpene alcohols, organic acids esters, phenolic acid amides, phenylpropanoid glycosides, polyol phosphates, and sulfur compound glycosides) were too sparsely populated (less than 10 phytocompounds each) to be included in the statistical analysis. Those included in the statistical analysis are listed in the first column of Table 2. In order not to miss some important associations, some of these classes were then pooled together (alkaloids = alkaloids + alkaloid glycosides, anthraquinones = anthraquinones + anthraquinone glycosides, coumarins = coumarins + coumarin glycosides, cyanogen = cyanogen + cyanogen glycosides, diterpenoids = diterpenoids + diterpenoid glycosides, fatty compounds = fatty acids + fatty acid esters + fatty aldehydes + fatty alcohols + high aliphatic acids + high aliphatic alcohols, flavonoids = flavonoids + flavonoids glycosides, lignans = lignans + lignan glycosides, monoterpenoids = monoterpenoids + monoterpenoids glycosides + monoterpene + monoterpene alcohols + monoterpenes, phenolic acids = phenolic acids + phenolic acid glycosides + phenolic acids esters + phenolic acid amides, phenolic others = phenolic others + phenolic glycosides, phenylpropanoids (others) = phenylpropanoids (others) + phenylpropanoid (other) glycosides, polyols = polyols + polyol phosphates, sesquiterpenoids = sesquiterpenoids + sesquiterpene, steroids = steroids + steroids glycosides + cardenolides, sulfur compounds = sulfur compounds + sulfur compound glycosides, triterpenoids = triterpenoids + triterpenoids glycosides). Still, more than half of the resultant classes (lignans, organic acids, cyanogen, carotenoids, proteins, polyketides, anthraquinones, vitamins, naphthofurans, medium aliphatic acids, lactones, chromones, aromatic ketones, aromatic aldehydes, amides, alkylamides, polyols, phenolic acid esters, organic acids esters, low aliphatic alcohols, indoles, guanidines, cyclic polyols, carboxylic acids, aromatic esters, and amines) included less than 10 phytocompounds and were consequently eliminated from the statistical analysis.

The classes that were pooled together were: alkaloids, flavonoids, monoterpenoids, triterpenoids, saccharides, phenolic acids, amino acids, sesquiterpenoids, coumarins, phenolic others, fatty compounds, short aliphatic acids, diterpenoids, steroids, tannins, sulfur compounds, and phenylpropanoids (others).

5. Conclusions

The present study demonstrates a strong association between ACA and AIA in phytocompounds. In other words, an anti-inflammatory phytocompound is more likely to also have ACA. This outcome supports the idea that targeting inflammation processes may represent a useful chemopreventive, and even chemotherapeutic, strategy.

Bitter phytotastants showed a higher probability to exert both AIA and ACA, while sweet ones had a negative correlation with both AIA and ACA. This result suggests a potential beneficial implication of bitter taste receptor agonists and sweet taste receptor antagonists in slowing down the progression of inflammation to cancer. TAS2Rs, for example, are seen as promising targets in treating inflammation [14,60] and as potential targets in cancer prevention and treatment [16]. Among chemical classes, only flavonoids, which are most frequently bitter, had a positive association with both anti-inflammatory and anti-cancer activities, confirming the predictive primacy of taste over chemical classes. Experimental studies and clinical trials are necessary to confirm these results in the future.

Author Contributions: Conceptualization, M.G. and T.-C.G.; Methodology, T.-C.G., D.D. and M.G.; Validation A.V. and M.G.; Statistical Analysis, D.D.; Resources, T.-C.G.; Data Curation, D.D. and T.-C.G.; Writing—Original Draft Preparation, T.-C.G., D.D. and M.G.; Writing—Review and Editing, A.V., D.D. and M.G.; Supervision, D.D., A.V. and M.G.; Study Coordination, M.G. All authors have read and agreed to the published version of the manuscript.

Funding: This research received no external funding.

Informed Consent Statement: No human (or animal) subjects were involved in performing this research; therefore, no informed consent was necessary.

Data Availability Statement: The data used in this study are freely available in PMTDB (http://plantmoleculartastedb.org, accessed on 1 February 2023), PubMed, ScienceDirect, Google Scholar.

Conflicts of Interest: The authors declare no conflict of interest.

Abbreviations

ACA	anti-cancer activity
AIA	anti-inflammatory activity
chemClass	chemical class
PMTDB	PlantMolecularTasteDB
PDA	pharmacodynamic activity
TASRs	taste receptors

References

1. Behrens, M.; Lang, T. Extra-Oral Taste Receptors-Function, Disease, and Perspectives. *Front. Nutr.* **2022**, *9*, 881177. [CrossRef]
2. Sanematsu, K.; Yoshida, R.; Shigemura, N.; Ninomiya, Y. Structure, function, and signaling of taste G-protein-coupled receptors. *Curr. Pharm. Biotechnol.* **2014**, *15*, 951–961. [CrossRef]
3. Gilca, M.; Dragos, D. Extraoral Taste Receptor Discovery: New Light on Ayurvedic Pharmacology. *Evid. -Based Complement. Altern. Med.* **2017**, *2017*, 5435831. [CrossRef] [PubMed]
4. Roper, S.D. TRPs in taste and chemesthesis. *Handb. Exp. Pharmacol.* **2014**, *223*, 827–871. [CrossRef]
5. Lu, P.; Zhang, C.-H.; Lifshitz, L.M.; ZhuGe, R. Extraoral bitter taste receptors in health and disease. *J. Gen. Physiol.* **2017**, *149*, 181–197. [CrossRef]
6. Laffitte, A.; Neiers, F.; Briand, L. Functional roles of the sweet taste receptor in oral and extraoral tissues. *Curr. Opin. Clin. Nutr. Metab. Care* **2014**, *17*, 379–385. [CrossRef] [PubMed]
7. Behrens, M.; Meyerhof, W. Gustatory and extragustatory functions of mammalian taste receptors. *Physiol. Behav.* **2011**, *105*, 4–13. [CrossRef]
8. Ziegler, F.; Steuer, A.; Di Pizio, A.; Behrens, M. Physiological activation of human and mouse bitter taste receptors by bile acids. *Commun. Biol.* **2023**, *6*, 612. [CrossRef]
9. Gradinaru, T.-C.; Petran, M.; Dragos, D.; Gilca, M. Plant Molecular Taste DB: A Database of Taste Active Phytochemicals. *Front. Pharmacol.* **2022**, *12*, 751712. [CrossRef]
10. Behrens, M.; Somoza, V. Gastrointestinal taste receptors: Could tastants become drugs? *Curr. Opin. Endocrinol. Diabetes Obes.* **2020**, *27*, 110–114. [CrossRef] [PubMed]
11. Di Pizio, A.; Behrens, M.; Krautwurst, D. Beyond the Flavour: The Potential Druggability of Chemosensory G Protein-Coupled Receptors. *Int. J. Mol. Sci.* **2019**, *20*, 1402. [CrossRef] [PubMed]
12. D'Urso, O.; Drago, F. Pharmacological significance of extra-oral taste receptors. *Eur. J. Pharmacol.* **2021**, *910*, 174480. [CrossRef] [PubMed]
13. Zhou, Z.; Xi, R.; Liu, J.; Peng, X.; Zhao, L.; Zhou, X.; Li, J.; Zheng, X.; Xu, X. TAS2R16 Activation Suppresses LPS-Induced Cytokine Expression in Human Gingival Fibroblasts. *Front. Immunol.* **2021**, *12*, 726546. [CrossRef]
14. Tiroch, J.; Sterneder, S.; Di Pizio, A.; Lieder, B.; Hoelz, K.; Holik, A.-K.; Pignitter, M.; Behrens, M.; Somoza, M.; Ley, J.P.; et al. Bitter Sensing TAS2R50 Mediates the trans-Resveratrol-Induced Anti-inflammatory Effect on Interleukin 6 Release in HGF-1 Cells in Culture. *J. Agric. Food Chem.* **2021**, *69*, 13339–13349. [CrossRef]
15. Costa, A.R.; Duarte, A.C.; Costa-Brito, A.R.; Gonçalves, I.; Santos, C.R.A. Bitter taste signaling in cancer. *Life Sci.* **2023**, *315*, 121363. [CrossRef] [PubMed]
16. Zehentner, S.; Reiner, A.T.; Grimm, C.; Somoza, V. The role of bitter taste receptors in cancer: A systematic review. *Cancers* **2021**, *13*, 5891. [CrossRef]
17. Singh, N.; Chakraborty, R.; Bhullar, R.P.; Chelikani, P. Differential expression of bitter taste receptors in non-cancerous breast epithelial and breast cancer cells. *Biochem. Biophys. Res. Commun.* **2014**, *446*, 499–503. [CrossRef]
18. Martin, L.T.P.; Nachtigal, M.W.; Selman, T.; Nguyen, E.; Salsman, J.; Dellaire, G.; Dupré, D.J. Bitter taste receptors are expressed in human epithelial ovarian and prostate cancers cells and noscapine stimulation impacts cell survival. *Mol. Cell. Biochem.* **2019**, *454*, 203–214. [CrossRef]
19. Seo, Y.; Kim, Y.-S.; Lee, K.E.; Park, T.H.; Kim, Y. Anti-cancer stemness and anti-invasive activity of bitter taste receptors, TAS2R8 and TAS2R10, in human neuroblastoma cells. *PLoS ONE* **2017**, *12*, e0176851. [CrossRef]
20. Singh, N.; Shaik, F.A.; Myal, Y.; Chelikani, P. Chemosensory bitter taste receptors T2R4 and T2R14 activation attenuates proliferation and migration of breast cancer cells. *Mol. Cell. Biochem.* **2020**, *465*, 199–214. [CrossRef]
21. Ferlay, J.; Colombet, M.; Soerjomataram, I.; Parkin, D.M.; Piñeros, M.; Znaor, A.; Bray, F. Cancer statistics for the year 2020: An overview. *Int. J. Cancer* **2021**, *149*, 778–789. [CrossRef]
22. Askeland, E.J.; Newton, M.R.; O'Donnell, M.A.; Luo, Y. Bladder Cancer Immunotherapy: BCG and Beyond. *Adv. Urol.* **2012**, *2012*, 181987. [CrossRef] [PubMed]
23. Yamaguchi, Y.; Miyahara, E.; Ohshita, A.; Kawabuchi, Y.; Ohta, K.; Shimizu, K.; Minami, K.; Hihara, J.; Sawamura, A.; Toge, T. Locoregional immunotherapy of malignant effusion from colorectal cancer using the streptococcal preparation OK-432 plus interleukin-2: Induction of autologous tumor-reactive CD4+ Th1 killer lymphocytes. *Br. J. Cancer* **2003**, *89*, 1876–1884. [CrossRef]
24. Munn, L.L. Cancer and inflammation. *Wiley Interdiscip. Rev. Syst. Biol. Med.* **2017**, *9*, e1370. [CrossRef] [PubMed]

25. Jin, K.; Qian, C.; Lin, J.; Liu, B. Cyclooxygenase-2-Prostaglandin E2 pathway: A key player in tumor-associated immune cells. *Front. Oncol.* **2023**, *13*, 1099811. [CrossRef] [PubMed]
26. Greten, F.R.; Grivennikov, S.I. Inflammation and Cancer: Triggers, Mechanisms, and Consequences. *Immunity* **2019**, *51*, 27–41. [CrossRef]
27. Korniluk, A.; Koper, O.; Kemona, H.; Dymicka-Piekarska, V. From inflammation to cancer. *Ir. J. Med. Sci.* **2017**, *186*, 57–62. [CrossRef]
28. Palli, D.; Masala, G.; Del Giudice, G.; Plebani, M.; Basso, D.; Berti, D.; Numans, M.E.; Ceroti, M.; Peeters, P.H.M.; Bueno de Mesquita, H.B.; et al. CagA+ Helicobacter pylori infection and gastric cancer risk in the EPIC-EURGAST study. *Int. J. Cancer* **2007**, *120*, 859–867. [CrossRef]
29. Balkwill, F.R.; Mantovani, A. Cancer-related inflammation: Common themes and therapeutic opportunities. *Semin. Cancer Biol.* **2012**, *22*, 33–40. [CrossRef]
30. Crusz, S.M.; Balkwill, F.R. Inflammation and cancer: Advances and new agents. *Nat. Rev. Clin. Oncol.* **2015**, *12*, 584–596. [CrossRef]
31. Song, C.; Lv, J.; Liu, Y.; Chen, J.G.; Ge, Z.; Zhu, J.; Dai, J.; Du, L.-B.; Yu, C.; Guo, Y.; et al. Associations Between Hepatitis B Virus Infection and Risk of All Cancer Types. *JAMA Netw. Open* **2019**, *2*, e195718. [CrossRef] [PubMed]
32. Yang, Y.; Jiang, Z.; Wu, W.; Ruan, L.; Yu, C.; Xi, Y.; Wang, L.; Wang, K.; Mo, J.; Zhao, S. Chronic Hepatitis Virus Infection Are Associated With High Risk of Gastric Cancer: A Systematic Review and Cumulative Analysis. *Front. Oncol.* **2021**, *11*, 703558. [CrossRef] [PubMed]
33. Khan, G. Epstein-Barr virus, cytokines, and inflammation: A cocktail for the pathogenesis of Hodgkin's lymphoma? *Exp. Hematol.* **2006**, *34*, 399–406. [CrossRef] [PubMed]
34. Fernandes, J.V.; DE Medeiros Fernandes, T.A.A.; DE Azevedo, J.C.V.; Cobucci, R.N.O.; DE Carvalho, M.G.F.; Andrade, V.S.; DE Araújo, J.M.G. Link between chronic inflammation and human papillomavirus-induced carcinogenesis (Review). *Oncol. Lett.* **2015**, *9*, 1015–1026. [CrossRef] [PubMed]
35. Ito, N.; Tsujimoto, H.; Ueno, H.; Xie, Q.; Shinomiya, N. Helicobacter pylori-Mediated Immunity and Signaling Transduction in Gastric Cancer. *J. Clin. Med.* **2020**, *9*, 3699. [CrossRef] [PubMed]
36. Axelrad, J.E.; Lichtiger, S.; Yajnik, V. Inflammatory bowel disease and cancer: The role of inflammation, immunosuppression, and cancer treatment. *World J. Gastroenterol.* **2016**, *22*, 4794–4801. [CrossRef]
37. Deng, T.; Lyon, C.J.; Bergin, S.; Caligiuri, M.A.; Hsueh, W.A. Obesity, Inflammation, and Cancer. *Annu. Rev. Pathol.* **2016**, *11*, 421–449. [CrossRef]
38. Zolondick, A.A.; Gaudino, G.; Xue, J.; Pass, H.I.; Carbone, M.; Yang, H. Asbestos-induced chronic inflammation in malignant pleural mesothelioma and related therapeutic approaches—A narrative review. *Precis. Cancer Med.* **2021**, *4*, 27. [CrossRef] [PubMed]
39. Kouokam, J.C.; Meaza, I.; Wise, J.P.S. Inflammatory effects of hexavalent chromium in the lung: A comprehensive review. *Toxicol. Appl. Pharmacol.* **2022**, *455*, 116265. [CrossRef]
40. Hanahan, D. Hallmarks of Cancer: New Dimensions. *Cancer Discov.* **2022**, *12*, 31–46. [CrossRef] [PubMed]
41. Hanahan, D.; Weinberg, R.A. Hallmarks of cancer: The next generation. *Cell* **2011**, *144*, 646–674. [CrossRef]
42. Huang, X.; Le, Q.-T.; Giaccia, A.J. MiR-210—Micromanager of the hypoxia pathway. *Trends Mol. Med.* **2010**, *16*, 230–237. [CrossRef]
43. Qiao, Y.; He, H.; Jonsson, P.; Sinha, I.; Zhao, C.; Dahlman-Wright, K. AP-1 Is a Key Regulator of Proinflammatory Cytokine TNFα-mediated Triple-negative Breast Cancer Progression. *J. Biol. Chem.* **2016**, *291*, 5068–5079. [CrossRef]
44. Elinav, E.; Nowarski, R.; Thaiss, C.A.; Hu, B.; Jin, C.; Flavell, R.A. Inflammation-induced cancer: Crosstalk between tumours, immune cells and microorganisms. *Nat. Rev. Cancer* **2013**, *13*, 759–771. [CrossRef]
45. Xia, Y.; Shen, S.; Verma, I.M. NF-κB, an active player in human cancers. *Cancer Immunol. Res.* **2014**, *2*, 823–830. [CrossRef] [PubMed]
46. Reader, J.; Holt, D.; Fulton, A. Prostaglandin E 2 EP receptors as therapeutic targets in breast cancer. *Cancer Metastasis Rev.* **2011**, *30*, 449–463. [CrossRef] [PubMed]
47. Iqbal, J.; Abbasi, B.A.; Mahmood, T.; Kanwal, S.; Ali, B.; Shah, S.A.; Khalil, A.T. Plant-derived anticancer agents: A green anticancer approach. *Asian Pac. J. Trop. Biomed.* **2017**, *7*, 1129–1150. [CrossRef]
48. Kim, M.-K.; Kim, K.; Han, J.Y.; Lim, J.M.; Song, Y.S. Modulation of inflammatory signaling pathways by phytochemicals in ovarian cancer. *Genes Nutr.* **2011**, *6*, 109–115. [CrossRef] [PubMed]
49. Almatroudi, A.; Allemailem, K.S.; Alwanian, W.M.; Alharbi, B.F.; Alrumaihi, F.; Khan, A.A.; Almatroodi, S.A.; Rahmani, A.H. Effects and Mechanisms of Kaempferol in the Management of Cancers through Modulation of Inflammation and Signal Transduction Pathways. *Int. J. Mol. Sci.* **2023**, *24*, 8630. [CrossRef] [PubMed]
50. Honari, M.; Shafabakhsh, R.; Reiter, R.J.; Mirzaei, H.; Asemi, Z. Resveratrol is a promising agent for colorectal cancer prevention and treatment: Focus on molecular mechanisms. *Cancer Cell Int.* **2019**, *19*, 180. [CrossRef]
51. Giordano, A.; Tommonaro, G. Curcumin and Cancer. *Nutrients* **2019**, *11*, 2376. [CrossRef] [PubMed]
52. Madka, V.; Rao, C.V. Anti-inflammatory phytochemicals for chemoprevention of colon cancer. *Curr. Cancer Drug Targets* **2013**, *13*, 542–557. [CrossRef] [PubMed]
53. Dragoș, D.; Petran, M.; Gradinaru, T.-C.; Gilca, M. Phytochemicals and Inflammation: Is Bitter Better? *Plants* **2022**, *11*, 2991. [CrossRef]

54. Dragos, D.; Gilca, M. Taste of phytocompounds: A better predictor for ethnopharmacological activities of medicinal plants than the phytochemical class? *J. Ethnopharmacol.* **2018**, *220*, 129–146. [CrossRef] [PubMed]
55. Kou, X.; Shi, P.; Gao, C.; Ma, P.; Xing, H.; Ke, Q.; Zhang, D. Data-Driven Elucidation of Flavor Chemistry. *J. Agric. Food Chem.* **2023**, *71*, 6789–6802. [CrossRef]
56. Rojas, C.; Ballabio, D.; Pacheco Sarmiento, K.; Pacheco Jaramillo, E.; Mendoza, M.; García, F. ChemTastesDB: A curated database of molecular tastants. *Food Chem. Mol. Sci.* **2022**, *4*, 100090. [CrossRef] [PubMed]
57. Guan, S.; Sun, L.; Wang, X.; Huang, X.; Luo, T. Isoschaftoside Inhibits Lipopolysaccharide-Induced Inflammation in Microglia through Regulation of HIF-1α-Mediated Metabolic Reprogramming. *Evid.-Based Complement Altern. Med.* **2022**, *2022*, 5227335. [CrossRef] [PubMed]
58. de Oliveira, D.P.; de Garcia, E.F.; de Oliveira, M.A.; Candido, L.C.M.; Coelho, F.M.; Costa, V.V.; Batista, N.V.; Queiroz-Junior, C.M.; Brito, L.F.; Sousa, L.P.; et al. cis-Aconitic Acid, a Constituent of Echinodorus grandiflorus Leaves, Inhibits Antigen Induced Arthritis and Gout in Mice. *Planta Med.* **2022**, *88*, 1123–1131. [CrossRef]
59. Sharma, P.; Yi, R.; Nayak, A.P.; Wang, N.; Tang, F.; Knight, M.J.; Pan, S.; Oliver, B.; Deshpande, D.A. Bitter Taste Receptor Agonists Mitigate Features of Allergic Asthma in Mice. *Sci. Rep.* **2017**, *7*, 46166. [CrossRef]
60. Grassin-Delyle, S.; Salvator, H.; Mantov, N.; Abrial, C.; Brollo, M.; Faisy, C.; Naline, E.; Couderc, L.J.; Devillier, P. Bitter Taste Receptors (TAS2Rs) in Human Lung Macrophages: Receptor Expression and Inhibitory Effects of TAS2R Agonists. *Front. Physiol.* **2019**, *10*, 1267. [CrossRef]
61. Salvestrini, V.; Ciciarello, M.; Pensato, V.; Simonetti, G.; Laginestra, M.A.; Bruno, S.; Pazzaglia, M.; De Marchi, E.; Forte, D.; Orecchioni, S.; et al. Denatonium as a Bitter Taste Receptor Agonist Modifies Transcriptomic Profile and Functions of Acute Myeloid Leukemia Cells. *Front. Oncol.* **2020**, *10*, 1225. [CrossRef]
62. Hung, J.; Perez, S.M.; Dasa, S.S.K.; Hall, S.P.; Heckert, D.B.; Murphy, B.P.; Crawford, H.C.; Kelly, K.A.; Brinton, L.T. A Bitter Taste Receptor as a Novel Molecular Target on Cancer-Associated Fibroblasts in Pancreatic Ductal Adenocarcinoma. *Pharmaceuticals* **2023**, *16*, 389. [CrossRef]
63. Gilca, M.; Barbulescu, A. Taste of medicinal plants: A potential tool in predicting ethnopharmacological activities? *J. Ethnopharmacol.* **2015**, *174*, 464–473. [CrossRef] [PubMed]
64. El-Far, M.; Durand, M.; Turcotte, I.; Larouche-Anctil, E.; Sylla, M.; Zaidan, S.; Chartrand-Lefebvre, C.; Bunet, R.; Ramani, H.; Sadouni, M. Upregulated IL-32 expression and reduced gut short chain fatty acid caproic acid in people living with HIV with subclinical atherosclerosis. *Front. Immunol.* **2021**, *12*, 664371. [CrossRef]
65. Lee, A.A.; Owyang, C. Sugars, Sweet Taste Receptors, and Brain Responses. *Nutrients* **2017**, *9*, 653. [CrossRef]
66. Smith, N.J.; Grant, J.N.; Moon, J.I.; So, S.S.; Finch, A.M. Critically evaluating sweet taste receptor expression and signaling through a molecular pharmacology lens. *FEBS J.* **2021**, *288*, 2660–2672. [CrossRef]
67. Di Pizio, A.; Ben Shoshan-Galeczki, Y.; Hayes, J.E.; Niv, M.Y. Bitter and sweet tasting molecules: It's complicated. *Neurosci. Lett.* **2019**, *700*, 56–63. [CrossRef]
68. Dagan-Wiener, A.; Nissim, I.; Ben Abu, N.; Borgonovo, G.; Bassoli, A.; Niv, M.Y. Bitter or not? BitterPredict, a tool for predicting taste from chemical structure. *Sci. Rep.* **2017**, *7*, 12074. [CrossRef] [PubMed]
69. Lee, R.J.; Kofonow, J.M.; Rosen, P.L.; Siebert, A.P.; Chen, B.; Doghramji, L.; Xiong, G.; Adappa, N.D.; Palmer, J.N.; Kennedy, D.W.; et al. Bitter and sweet taste receptors regulate human upper respiratory innate immunity. *J. Clin. Invest.* **2014**, *124*, 1393–1405. [CrossRef] [PubMed]
70. Maina, I.W.; Workman, A.D.; Cohen, N.A. The role of bitter and sweet taste receptors in upper airway innate immunity: Recent advances and future directions. *World J. Otorhinolaryngol.-Head Neck Surg.* **2018**, *4*, 200–208. [CrossRef]
71. Lee, R.J.; Cohen, N.A. Taste receptors in innate immunity. *Cell. Mol. Life Sci.* **2015**, *72*, 217–236. [CrossRef]
72. Di Pizio, A.; Waterloo, L.A.W.; Brox, R.; Löber, S.; Weikert, D.; Behrens, M.; Gmeiner, P.; Niv, M.Y. Rational design of agonists for bitter taste receptor TAS2R14: From modeling to bench and back. *Cell. Mol. Life Sci.* **2020**, *77*, 531–542. [CrossRef]
73. Nakagita, T.; Taketani, C.; Narukawa, M.; Hirokawa, T.; Kobayashi, T.; Misaka, T. Ibuprofen, a Nonsteroidal Anti-Inflammatory Drug, is a Potent Inhibitor of the Human Sweet Taste Receptor. *Chem. Senses* **2020**, *45*, 667–673. [CrossRef]
74. Cardenas, P.D.; Sonawane, P.D.; Heinig, U.; Bocobza, S.E.; Burdman, S.; Aharoni, A. The bitter side of the nightshades: Genomics drives discovery in Solanaceae steroidal alkaloid metabolism. *Phytochemistry* **2015**, *113*, 24–32. [CrossRef] [PubMed]
75. Liem, D.G.; Russell, C.G. The Influence of Taste Liking on the Consumption of Nutrient Rich and Nutrient Poor Foods. *Front. Nutr.* **2019**, *6*, 174. [CrossRef] [PubMed]
76. Gutierrez, R.; Simon, S.A. Physiology of Taste Processing in the Tongue, Gut, and Brain. *Compr. Physiol.* **2021**, *11*, 2489–2523. [CrossRef]
77. Cavallo, C.; Cicia, G.; Del Giudice, T.; Sacchi, R.; Vecchio, R. Consumers' Perceptions and Preferences for Bitterness in Vegetable Foods: The Case of Extra-Virgin Olive Oil and Brassicaceae-A Narrative Review. *Nutrients* **2019**, *11*, 1164. [CrossRef]
78. Beckett, E.L.; Martin, C.; Yates, Z.; Veysey, M.; Duesing, K.; Lucock, M. Bitter taste genetics—The relationship to tasting, liking, consumption and health. *Food Funct.* **2014**, *5*, 3040–3054. [CrossRef]
79. Freeman, C.R.; Zehra, A.; Ramirez, V.; Wiers, C.E.; Volkow, N.D.; Wang, G.J. Impact of sugar on the body brain and behavior. *Front. Biosci.* **2018**, *23*, 4704. [CrossRef]
80. Aravindaram, K.; Yang, N.-S. Anti-inflammatory plant natural products for cancer therapy. *Planta Med.* **2010**, *76*, 1103–1117. [CrossRef]

81. Chinnasamy, P.; Arumugam, R. In silico prediction of anticarcinogenic bioactivities of traditional anti-inflammatory plants used by tribal healers in Sathyamangalam wildlife Sanctuary, India. *Egypt. J. Basic Appl. Sci.* **2018**, *5*, 265–279. [CrossRef]
82. Pallavi, B.; Sharma, P.; Baig, N.; Kumar Madduluri, V.; Sah, A.K.; Saumya, U.; Dubey, U.S.; Shukla, P. Quinoline Glycoconjugates as Potentially Anticancer and Anti-Inflammatory Agents: An Investigation Involving Synthesis, Biological Screening, and Docking. *ChemistrySelect* **2020**, *5*, 9878–9882. [CrossRef]
83. Taniguchi, K.; Karin, M. NF-κB, inflammation, immunity and cancer: Coming of age. *Nat. Rev. Immunol.* **2018**, *18*, 309–324. [CrossRef]
84. Xia, L.; Tan, S.; Zhou, Y.; Lin, J.; Wang, H.; Oyang, L.; Tian, Y.; Liu, L.; Su, M.; Wang, H.; et al. Role of the NFκB-signaling pathway in cancer. *Onco Targets Ther.* **2018**, *11*, 2063–2073. [CrossRef] [PubMed]
85. DiDonato, J.A.; Mercurio, F.; Karin, M. NF-κB and the link between inflammation and cancer. *Immunol. Rev.* **2012**, *246*, 379–400. [CrossRef] [PubMed]
86. Salminen, A.; Lehtonen, M.; Suuronen, T.; Kaarniranta, K.; Huuskonen, J. Terpenoids: Natural inhibitors of NF-κB signaling with anti-inflammatory and anticancer potential. *Cell. Mol. Life Sci.* **2008**, *65*, 2979–2999. [CrossRef] [PubMed]
87. Liu, H.-M.; Cheng, M.-Y.; Xun, M.-H.; Zhao, Z.-W.; Zhang, Y.; Tang, W.; Cheng, J.; Ni, J.; Wang, W. Possible Mechanisms of Oxidative Stress-Induced Skin Cellular Senescence, Inflammation, and Cancer and the Therapeutic Potential of Plant Polyphenols. *Int. J. Mol. Sci.* **2023**, *24*, 3755. [CrossRef]
88. Pourhabibi-Zarandi, F.; Rafraf, M.; Zayeni, H.; Asghari-Jafarabadi, M.; Ebrahimi, A.-A. Effects of curcumin supplementation on metabolic parameters, inflammatory factors and obesity values in women with rheumatoid arthritis: A randomized, double-blind, placebo-controlled clinical trial. *Phytother. Res.* **2022**, *36*, 1797–1806. [CrossRef]
89. Ramezani, V.; Ghadirian, S.; Shabani, M.; Boroumand, M.A.; Daneshvar, R.; Saghafi, F. Efficacy of curcumin for amelioration of radiotherapy-induced oral mucositis: A preliminary randomized controlled clinical trial. *BMC Cancer* **2023**, *23*, 354. [CrossRef]
90. Kuriakose, M.A.; Ramdas, K.; Dey, B.; Iyer, S.; Rajan, G.; Elango, K.K.; Suresh, A.; Ravindran, D.; Kumar, R.R.; R, P.; et al. A Randomized Double-Blind Placebo-Controlled Phase IIB Trial of Curcumin in Oral Leukoplakia. *Cancer Prev. Res.* **2016**, *9*, 683–691. [CrossRef]
91. Choi, Y.H.; Han, D.H.; Kim, S.-W.; Kim, M.-J.; Sung, H.H.; Jeon, H.G.; Jeong, B.C.; Seo, S., II; Jeon, S.S.; Lee, H.M.; et al. A randomized, double-blind, placebo-controlled trial to evaluate the role of curcumin in prostate cancer patients with intermittent androgen deprivation. *Prostate* **2019**, *79*, 614–621. [CrossRef] [PubMed]
92. Greil, R.; Greil-Ressler, S.; Weiss, L.; Schönlieb, C.; Magnes, T.; Radl, B.; Bolger, G.T.; Vcelar, B.; Sordillo, P.P. A phase 1 dose-escalation study on the safety, tolerability and activity of liposomal curcumin (Lipocurc^{TM})) in patients with locally advanced or metastatic cancer. *Cancer Chemother. Pharmacol.* **2018**, *82*, 695–706. [CrossRef]
93. Bo, S.; Ciccone, G.; Castiglione, A.; Gambino, R.; De Michieli, F.; Villois, P.; Durazzo, M.; Cavallo-Perin, P.; Cassader, M. Anti-inflammatory and antioxidant effects of resveratrol in healthy smokers a randomized, double-blind, placebo-controlled, cross-over trial. *Curr. Med. Chem.* **2013**, *20*, 1323–1331. [CrossRef] [PubMed]
94. Popat, R.; Plesner, T.; Davies, F.; Cook, G.; Cook, M.; Elliott, P.; Jacobson, E.; Gumbleton, T.; Oakervee, H.; Cavenagh, J. A phase 2 study of SRT501 (resveratrol) with bortezomib for patients with relapsed and or refractory multiple myeloma. *Br. J. Haematol.* **2013**, *160*, 714–717. [CrossRef] [PubMed]
95. Zappavigna, S.; Cossu, A.M.; Grimaldi, A.; Bocchetti, M.; Ferraro, G.A.; Nicoletti, G.F.; Filosa, R.; Caraglia, M. Anti-Inflammatory Drugs as Anticancer Agents. *Int. J. Mol. Sci.* **2020**, *21*, 2605. [CrossRef]
96. Drew, D.A.; Cao, Y.; Chan, A.T. Aspirin and colorectal cancer: The promise of precision chemoprevention. *Nat. Rev. Cancer* **2016**, *16*, 173–186. [CrossRef]
97. Elwood, P.; Protty, M.; Morgan, G.; Pickering, J.; Delon, C.; Watkins, J. Aspirin and cancer: Biological mechanisms and clinical outcomes. *Open Biol.* **2022**, *12*, 220124. [CrossRef] [PubMed]
98. Burn, J.; Sheth, H.; Elliott, F.; Reed, L.; Macrae, F.; Mecklin, J.-P.; Möslein, G.; McRonald, F.E.; Bertario, L.; Evans, D.G.; et al. Cancer prevention with aspirin in hereditary colorectal cancer (Lynch syndrome), 10-year follow-up and registry-based 20-year data in the CAPP2 study: A double-blind, randomised, placebo-controlled trial. *Lancet* **2020**, *395*, 1855–1863. [CrossRef]
99. Qiao, Y.; Yang, T.; Gan, Y.; Li, W.; Wang, C.; Gong, Y.; Lu, Z. Associations between aspirin use and the risk of cancers: A meta-analysis of observational studies. *BMC Cancer* **2018**, *18*, 288. [CrossRef]
100. Sebastian, N.T.; Stokes, W.A.; Behera, M.; Jiang, R.; Gutman, D.A.; Huang, Z.; Burns, A.; Sukhatme, V.; Lowe, M.C.; Ramalingam, S.S.; et al. The Association of Improved Overall Survival with NSAIDs in Non-Small Cell Lung Cancer Patients Receiving Immune Checkpoint Inhibitors. *Clin. Lung Cancer* **2023**, *24*, 287–294. [CrossRef]
101. Rahme, E.; Ghosn, J.; Dasgupta, K.; Rajan, R.; Hudson, M. Association between frequent use of nonsteroidal anti-inflammatory drugs and breast cancer. *BMC Cancer* **2005**, *5*, 159. [CrossRef]
102. Liu, Y.; Ren, T.; Xu, X.; Jin, J. Association of aspirin and nonaspirin NSAIDs therapy with the incidence risk of hepatocellular carcinoma: A systematic review and meta-analysis on cohort studies. *Eur. J. Cancer Prev.* **2022**, *31*, 35–43. [CrossRef]
103. Majidi, A.; Na, R.; Jordan, S.J.; DeFazio, A.; Obermair, A.; Friedlander, M.; Grant, P.; Webb, P.M. Common analgesics and ovarian cancer survival: The Ovarian cancer Prognosis And Lifestyle (OPAL) Study. *J. Natl. Cancer Inst.* **2023**, *115*, 570–577. [CrossRef]
104. Sasamoto, N.; Babic, A.; Vitonis, A.F.; Titus, L.; Cramer, D.W.; Trabert, B.; Tworoger, S.S.; Terry, K.L. Common Analgesic Use for Menstrual Pain and Ovarian Cancer Risk. *Cancer Prev. Res.* **2021**, *14*, 795–802. [CrossRef] [PubMed]

105. Ridker, P.M.; MacFadyen, J.G.; Thuren, T.; Everett, B.M.; Libby, P.; Glynn, R.J. Effect of interleukin-1β inhibition with canakinumab on incident lung cancer in patients with atherosclerosis: Exploratory results from a randomised, double-blind, placebo-controlled trial. *Lancet* **2017**, *390*, 1833–1842. [CrossRef] [PubMed]
106. Cho, E.; Curhan, G.; Hankinson, S.E.; Kantoff, P.; Atkins, M.B.; Stampfer, M.; Choueiri, T.K. Prospective evaluation of analgesic use and risk of renal cell cancer. *Arch. Intern. Med.* **2011**, *171*, 1487–1493. [CrossRef] [PubMed]
107. Trabert, B.; Poole, E.M.; White, E.; Visvanathan, K.; Adami, H.-O.; Anderson, G.L.; Brasky, T.M.; Brinton, L.A.; Fortner, R.T.; Gaudet, M.; et al. Analgesic Use and Ovarian Cancer Risk: An Analysis in the Ovarian Cancer Cohort Consortium. *J. Natl. Cancer Inst.* **2019**, *111*, 137–145. [CrossRef]
108. Cryer, B.; Feldman, M. Cyclooxygenase-1 and Cyclooxygenase-2 Selectivity of Widely Used Nonsteroidal Anti-Inflammatory Drugs. *Am. J. Med.* **1998**, *104*, 413–421. [CrossRef]
109. Simon, L.S. Role and regulation of cyclooxygenase-2 during inflammation. *Am. J. Med.* **1999**, *106*, 37S–42S. [CrossRef]
110. Hashemi Goradel, N.; Najafi, M.; Salehi, E.; Farhood, B.; Mortezaee, K. Cyclooxygenase-2 in cancer: A review. *J. Cell. Physiol.* **2019**, *234*, 5683–5699. [CrossRef]
111. Zhu, Y.; Shi, C.; Zeng, L.; Liu, G.; Jiang, W.; Zhang, X.; Chen, S.; Guo, J.; Jian, X.; Ouyang, J.; et al. High COX-2 expression in cancer-associated fibroblasts contributes to poor survival and promotes migration and invasiveness in nasopharyngeal carcinoma. *Mol. Carcinog.* **2020**, *59*, 265–280. [CrossRef]
112. Du, J.; Feng, J.; Luo, D.; Peng, L. Prognostic and Clinical Significance of COX-2 Overexpression in Laryngeal Cancer: A Meta-Analysis. *Front. Oncol.* **2022**, *12*, 854946. [CrossRef]
113. Rigas, B.; Goldman, I.S.; Levine, L. Altered eicosanoid levels in human colon cancer. *J. Lab. Clin. Med.* **1993**, *122*, 518–523.
114. McLemore, T.L.; Hubbard, W.C.; Litterst, C.L.; Liu, M.C.; Miller, S.; McMahon, N.A.; Eggleston, J.C.; Boyd, M.R. Profiles of prostaglandin biosynthesis in normal lung and tumor tissue from lung cancer patients. *Cancer Res.* **1988**, *48*, 3140–3147. [PubMed]
115. Schrey, M.P.; Patel, K. V Prostaglandin E2 production and metabolism in human breast cancer cells and breast fibroblasts. Regulation by inflammatory mediators. *Br. J. Cancer* **1995**, *72*, 1412–1419. [CrossRef]
116. Hong, D.S.; Parikh, A.; Shapiro, G.I.; Varga, A.; Naing, A.; Meric-Bernstam, F.; Ataman, Ö.; Reyderman, L.; Binder, T.A.; Ren, M.; et al. First-in-human phase I study of immunomodulatory E7046, an antagonist of PGE 2 -receptor E-type 4 (EP4), in patients with advanced cancers. *J. Immunother. Cancer* **2020**, *8*, e000222. [CrossRef] [PubMed]
117. Ching, M.M.; Reader, J.; Fulton, A.M. Eicosanoids in Cancer: Prostaglandin E(2) Receptor 4 in Cancer Therapeutics and Immunotherapy. *Front. Pharmacol.* **2020**, *11*, 819. [CrossRef] [PubMed]
118. Take, Y.; Koizumi, S.; Nagahisa, A. Prostaglandin E Receptor 4 Antagonist in Cancer Immunotherapy: Mechanisms of Action. *Front. Immunol.* **2020**, *11*, 324. [CrossRef]
119. Carey, R.M.; McMahon, D.B.; Miller, Z.A.; Kim, T.; Rajasekaran, K.; Gopallawa, I.; Newman, J.G.; Basu, D.; Nead, K.T.; White, E.A.; et al. T2R bitter taste receptors regulate apoptosis and may be associated with survival in head and neck squamous cell carcinoma. *Mol. Oncol.* **2022**, *16*, 1474–1492. [CrossRef]
120. Carey, R.M.; Kim, T.; Cohen, N.A.; Lee, R.J.; Nead, K.T. Impact of sweet, umami, and bitter taste receptor (TAS1R and TAS2R) genomic and expression alterations in solid tumors on survival. *Sci. Rep.* **2022**, *12*, 8937. [CrossRef]
121. Jaggupilli, A.; Singh, N.; Upadhyaya, J.; Sikarwar, A.S.; Arakawa, M.; Dakshinamurti, S.; Bhullar, R.P.; Duan, K.; Chelikani, P. Analysis of the expression of human bitter taste receptors in extraoral tissues. *Mol. Cell. Biochem.* **2017**, *426*, 137–147. [CrossRef]
122. Hopkins, B.D.; Pauli, C.; Du, X.; Wang, D.G.; Li, X.; Wu, D.; Amadiume, S.C.; Goncalves, M.D.; Hodakoski, C.; Lundquist, M.R.; et al. Suppression of insulin feedback enhances the efficacy of PI3K inhibitors. *Nature* **2018**, *560*, 499–503. [CrossRef]
123. Dong, H.; Kong, X.; Wang, X.; Liu, Q.; Fang, Y.; Wang, J. The Causal Effect of Dietary Composition on the Risk of Breast Cancer: A Mendelian Randomization Study. *Nutrients* **2023**, *15*, 2586. [CrossRef]
124. Llaha, F.; Gil-Lespinard, M.; Unal, P.; de Villasante, I.; Castañeda, J.; Zamora-Ros, R. Consumption of Sweet Beverages and Cancer Risk. A Systematic Review and Meta-Analysis of Observational Studies. *Nutrients* **2021**, *13*, 516. [CrossRef]
125. Pati, S.; Irfan, W.; Jameel, A.; Ahmed, S.; Shahid, R.K. Obesity and Cancer: A Current Overview of Epidemiology, Pathogenesis, Outcomes, and Management. *Cancers* **2023**, *15*, 485. [CrossRef] [PubMed]
126. Faruque, S.; Tong, J.; Lacmanovic, V.; Agbonghae, C.; Minaya, D.M.; Czaja, K. The Dose Makes the Poison: Sugar and Obesity in the United States—A Review. *Polish J. food Nutr. Sci.* **2019**, *69*, 219–233. [CrossRef]
127. Vidoni, C.; Ferraresi, A.; Esposito, A.; Maheshwari, C.; Dhanasekaran, D.N.; Mollace, V.; Isidoro, C. Calorie Restriction for Cancer Prevention and Therapy: Mechanisms, Expectations, and Efficacy. *J. Cancer Prev.* **2021**, *26*, 224–236. [CrossRef] [PubMed]
128. Vernieri, C.; Fucà, G.; Ligorio, F.; Huber, V.; Vingiani, A.; Iannelli, F.; Raimondi, A.; Rinchai, D.; Frigè, G.; Belfiore, A.; et al. Fasting-Mimicking Diet Is Safe and Reshapes Metabolism and Antitumor Immunity in Patients with Cancer. *Cancer Discov.* **2022**, *12*, 90–107. [CrossRef] [PubMed]
129. Debras, C.; Chazelas, E.; Srour, B.; Druesne-Pecollo, N.; Esseddik, Y.; Szabo de Edelenyi, F.; Agaësse, C.; De Sa, A.; Lutchia, R.; Gigandet, S.; et al. Artificial sweeteners and cancer risk: Results from the NutriNet-Santé population-based cohort study. *PLOS Med.* **2022**, *19*, e1003950. [CrossRef]
130. Hwang, E.-S.; Lee, H.J. Effects of phenylethyl isothiocyanate and its metabolite on cell-cycle arrest and apoptosis in LNCaP human prostate cancer cells. *Int. J. Food Sci. Nutr.* **2010**, *61*, 324–336. [CrossRef]
131. Gupta, P.; Wright, S.E.; Kim, S.-H.; Srivastava, S.K. Phenethyl isothiocyanate: A comprehensive review of anti-cancer mechanisms. *Biochim. Biophys. Acta* **2014**, *1846*, 405–424. [CrossRef]

132. Gach, K.; Wyrębska, A.; Fichna, J.; Janecka, A. The role of morphine in regulation of cancer cell growth. *Naunyn. Schmiedebergs. Arch. Pharmacol.* **2011**, *384*, 221–230. [CrossRef]
133. Liu, X.; Yang, J.; Yang, C.; Huang, X.; Han, M.; Kang, F.; Li, J. Morphine promotes the malignant biological behavior of non-small cell lung cancer cells through the MOR/Src/mTOR pathway. *Cancer Cell Int.* **2021**, *21*, 622. [CrossRef]
134. Li, C.; Li, L.; Qin, Y.; Jiang, Y.; Wei, Y.; Chen, J.; Xie, Y. Exogenous morphine inhibits the growth of human gastric tumor in vivo. *Ann. Transl. Med.* **2020**, *8*, 385. [CrossRef] [PubMed]
135. Mehmood, T.; Maryam, A.; Tian, X.; Khan, M.; Ma, T. Santamarine Inhibits NF-κB and STAT3 Activation and Induces Apoptosis in HepG2 Liver Cancer Cells via Oxidative Stress. *J. Cancer* **2017**, *8*, 3707–3717. [CrossRef]
136. Wu, X.; Zhu, H.; Yan, J.; Khan, M.; Yu, X. Santamarine Inhibits NF-κB Activation and Induces Mitochondrial Apoptosis in A549 Lung Adenocarcinoma Cells via Oxidative Stress. *Biomed Res. Int.* **2017**, *2017*, 4734127. [CrossRef] [PubMed]
137. Al-Attas, A.A.M.; El-Shaer, N.S.; Mohamed, G.A.; Ibrahim, S.R.M.; Esmat, A. Anti-inflammatory sesquiterpenes from Costus speciosus rhizomes. *J. Ethnopharmacol.* **2015**, *176*, 365–374. [CrossRef]
138. Choi, H.-G.; Lee, D.-S.; Li, B.; Choi, Y.H.; Lee, S.-H.; Kim, Y.-C. Santamarin, a sesquiterpene lactone isolated from Saussurea lappa, represses LPS-induced inflammatory responses via expression of heme oxygenase-1 in murine macrophage cells. *Int. Immunopharmacol.* **2012**, *13*, 271–279. [CrossRef] [PubMed]

Disclaimer/Publisher's Note: The statements, opinions and data contained in all publications are solely those of the individual author(s) and contributor(s) and not of MDPI and/or the editor(s). MDPI and/or the editor(s) disclaim responsibility for any injury to people or property resulting from any ideas, methods, instructions or products referred to in the content.

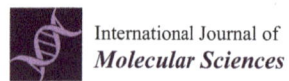

Article

Tea Polyphenols Protects Tracheal Epithelial Tight Junctions in Lung during *Actinobacillus pleuropneumoniae* Infection via Suppressing TLR-4/MAPK/PKC-MLCK Signaling

Xiaoyue Li [1,2,3], Zewen Liu [4], Ting Gao [4], Wei Liu [4], Keli Yang [4], Rui Guo [4], Chang Li [4], Yongxiang Tian [4], Ningning Wang [1], Danna Zhou [4], Weicheng Bei [1,2,3,*] and Fangyan Yuan [4,*]

[1] National Key Laboratory of Agricultural Microbiology, College of Veterinary Medicine, Huazhong Agricultural University, Wuhan 430070, China; lixiaoyue1208@webmail.hzau.edu.cn (X.L.); aningaha0802@163.com (N.W.)
[2] Cooperative Innovation Center of Sustainable Pig Production, Wuhan 430070, China
[3] Hubei Hongshan Laboratory, Wuhan 430070, China
[4] Key Laboratory of Prevention and Control Agents for Animal Bacteriosis (Ministry of Agriculture and Rural Affairs), Hubei Provincial Key Laboratory of Animal Pathogenic Microbiology, Institute of Animal Husbandry and Veterinary, Hubei Academy of Agricultural Sciences, Wuhan 430064, China; liuzwen2004@sina.com (Z.L.); gaotingyefeiyeziyu@163.com (T.G.); liuwei85@126.com (W.L.); keliy6@126.com (K.Y.); hlguorui@163.com (R.G.); lichang1113@hbaas.com (C.L.); tyxanbit@163.com (Y.T.); zdn_66@126.com (D.Z.)
* Correspondence: beiwc@hzau.edu.cn (W.B.); fyyuan@hbaas.com (F.Y.)

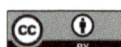

Abstract: *Actinobacillus pleuropneumoniae* (APP) is the causative pathogen of porcine pleuropneumonia, a highly contagious respiratory disease in the pig industry. The increasingly severe antimicrobial resistance in APP urgently requires novel antibacterial alternatives for the treatment of APP infection. In this study, we investigated the effect of tea polyphenols (TP) against APP. MIC and MBC of TP showed significant inhibitory effects on bacteria growth and caused cellular damage to APP. Furthermore, TP decreased adherent activity of APP to the newborn pig tracheal epithelial cells (NPTr) and the destruction of the tight adherence junction proteins β-catenin and occludin. Moreover, TP improved the survival rate of APP infected mice but also attenuated the release of the inflammation-related cytokines IL-6, IL-8, and TNF-α. TP inhibited activation of the TLR/MAPK/PKC-MLCK signaling for down-regulated TLR-2, TLR4, p-JNK, p-p38, p-PKC-α, and MLCK in cells triggered by APP. Collectively, our data suggest that TP represents a promising therapeutic agent in the treatment of APP infection.

Keywords: tea polyphenols; *Actinobacillus pleuropneumoniae*; epithelial barrier; TLR-4/MAPK/PKC-MLCK signaling

1. Introduction

Tea is a popular beverage consumed worldwide. It is made from the leaves of the plant *Camellia sinensis*, which originated in ancient China [1,2]. Tea polyphenols (TP) are a specific bioactive ingredient of tea, and have various health promoting properties [3], including antioxidant, antimutagenic, immuno-regulatory, hypocholesterolemic, antibacterial, and anticancer activities [4,5]. If TP reach sufficient concentrations after drinking tea for a long time, they are absorbed and retained and exert their desired effects in plasma and tissues [1]. Supplementation with TP mainly alters the gut microbiome composition and can benefit bone health [6], which can control obesity and related metabolic disorders [3,7]. TP have protective effects on high glucose-induced cell proliferation and senescence in human glomerular mesangial cells (HGMCs) [8]. In addition, several studies have shown that natural polyphenols not only have antibacterial effects, but also show low toxicity and great bioavailability [9,10]. TP show great promise as antibiotic alternatives with good antibacterial effects. Previous studies have shown that TP can lower the secretion of pro-inflammatory cytokines and reduce the inflammatory response to *Fusobacterium nucleatum* [11], inhibit the virulence of *Pseudomonas aeruginosa* [12], and protect against *Haemophilus parasuis* challenge [13]. However, the effects of TP on *Actinobacillus pleuropneumoniae* infection are not completely understood.

Actinobacillus pleuropneumoniae (APP) is one of the most common bacterial pathogens causing porcine respiratory infections. It is an etiological agent for porcine pleuropneumonia, which is characterized by acute hemorrhagic, purulent, and fibrous pleuropneumonia symptoms [14]. APP can infect pigs of all ages, colonize the upper respiratory tract, and breach the epithelial barrier to cause local or systemic infection [15]. The morbidity of the resulting disease can be as high as 100%, but generally varies between 30–50% [16], and causes considerable economic losses in the swine rearing industry [17]. It comprises two biotypes based on their dependence on nicotinamide adenine dinucleotide (NAD) (biotype 1, biotype 2) [18]. At present, 19 different serotypes of APP have been recognized based on their polysaccharide compositions [19], with serovars 1, 5, 9, and 11 considered the most virulent [20]. Serotypes 1, 3, 4, 5, and 7 are typically isolated in China [21]. The varieties and prevalence of the serotypes vary between most regions of China. Owing to the diversity of serotypes and differences in their regional prevalence, there is currently no satisfactory vaccine to control outbreaks of APP infection and antibiotics remain the most effective means of control in most regions [22]. For pigs, APP infections are often treated with macrolides, β-lactams, fluoroquinolones, and/or florfenicol in the swine industry [23–25]. From 2002 to 2013, a total of 71 APP isolates from pig farms in Australia showed a high frequency of resistance to erythromycin and tetracycline [26]. Among 162 APP strains collected from pigs in Spain from 2017 to 2019, a highly antibiotic resistance to doxycycline was discovered [23]. However, some APP strains have begun to show varying degrees of antibiotic resistance, and this presents problems in controlling outbreaks of porcine pleuropneumonia [27–29], leading to an urgent need for alternatives to antibiotics.

Infection with APP can damage the porcine respiratory epithelial barrier [30]. Tracheal epithelial cells play a defensive role in the epithelial barrier [31]. The epithelium is composed of adherent cells, which are polarized and have an apical domain and a basolateral domain [32]. It forms a physical barrier between the internal and external environment, protecting against environmental contaminants and pathogens [33,34]. The epithelial cells are tightly joined by a set of intercellular junctions composed of gap junctions, desmosomes, tight junctions (TJs), and adherence junctions (AJs) [32,35]. Epithelial tight junctions are located at the apicolateral boundary of the epithelial cells and form the paracellular barrier. This barrier regulates epithelial permeability and the intramembrane barrier, which separates the membrane components [32,36]. They are composed of at least three membrane proteins, including zonula occludens-1 (ZO-1), claudins, and occludin [37,38]. Claudins and occludin are polytopic membrane proteins with four transmembrane domains. The consensus is that claudins mainly modify the pore pathways, and that ZO-1, occludin, and tricellulin regulate the leak pathways [36,39]. Adherence junctions are located directly beneath the TJs and provide intercellular adhesion to maintain epithelial integrity [40,41]. They are composed of E-cadherin, nectin, and α and β-catenin, which have diverse functions, including the maintenance of actin binding, cells polarization, and signal transduction-related transcriptional regulation [42–44]. The formation, dismantling, and maintenance of TJs are regulated, in part, by phosphorylation and dephosphorylation of TJ proteins as well as some signaling pathways, including protein kinase C (PKC), myosin light chain kinase (MLCK), and mitogen-activated protein kinases (MAPK) [45–48].

Pleuropneumonia infection causes substantial economic losses to the swine rearing industry worldwide, and its various strains exhibit varying degrees of antibiotic resistance, causing an urgent need for alternatives to antibiotics in combatting APP infection [27–29]. Despite the aforementioned antimicrobial potential of TP, their effectiveness against APP infection remains to be elucidated. Other studies report that infection with APP can damage the porcine respiratory epithelial barrier [30], although data regarding the effects of TP on the respiratory epithelium remain limited. This study investigated the possible mechanisms by which the application of TP might affect the growth and virulence of APP and its effect on the epithelial barrier in order to provide a new strategy for preventing APP infection in pigs.

2. Results

2.1. TP Inhibit the Growth of APP In Vitro

The results of the micro-broth dilution assay showed that TP exhibited antibacterial activity against APP (Table 1). The MIC and MBC values of TP were 0.625 mg/mL and 1.25 mg/mL, respectively. The growth properties of APP strains and TP (0 MIC, 0.5 MIC, 1 MIC, and 2 MIC) when co-cultured for 0, 1, 2, 3, 4, and 5 h were investigated. Cultures were serially diluted with PBS and plated onto TSA, and the number of bacteria were counted. The growth curves of the APP strains showed that TP exhibited a dose-dependent bactericidal effect on APP. The growth of APP was significantly inhibited after co-culture with TP (1 MIC) for 5 h ($p < 0.001$) (Figure 1A). The MIC and MBC values of florfenicol were 1 µg/mL and 2 µg/mL, respectively. The addition of florfenicol to bacteria was used as a control (Figure 1A).

Table 1. Minimal inhibitory concentration (MIC) and minimal bactericidal concentration (MBC) values of TP for APP.

Medium	Compound	MIC (mg/mL)	MBC (mg/mL)
TSB	TP	0.625	1.25

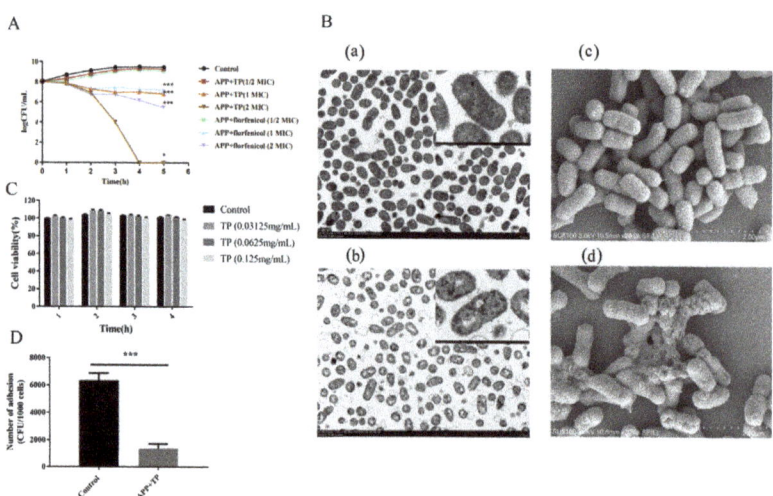

Figure 1. (**A**): Kinetics of the antimicrobial effects of TP on APP. APP and TP (0 MIC, 1/2 MIC, 1 MIC, and 2 MIC) were co-cultured for 0, 1, 2, 3, 4, and 5 h. The number of colonies was counted, and kinetics curves were constructed. (**B**): Transmission electron microscope and scanning electron microscopy analysis of APP. (**a**): Control untreated bacteria via TEM, the bar at the bottom right means 5.0 µm. High-magnification image of area indicated in upper right corner, the bar at the bottom right means 500 nm. (**b**): Bacteria treated with TP via TEM, the bar at the bottom right means 5.0 µm. High-magnification image of area indicated in upper right corner, the bar at the bottom right means 500 nm. (**c**): Untreated bacteria control analysis via SEM, the bar at the bottom right means 2.0 µm. (**d**): Bacteria treated with TP analysis via SEM, the bar at the bottom right means 2.0 µm. (**C**): The cell viability of NPTr cells of TP treatment. (**D**): The adherent ability of APP to NPTr cells or NPTr cells pretreatment with TP. Statistical analysis was performed by Student's t-test. $n = 3$ in each group. Results are expressed as the mean ± SD of three independent experiments. * $p < 0.05$, *** $p < 0.001$.

2.2. TP Affect the Cellular Integrity of APP

The effect of TP on the cell integrity of APP was observed using a TEM and an SEM. APP cells treated with TP (0.625 mg/mL) showed obvious damage when compared with the control cells (Figure 1B). The treated cells showed instances of cell wall damage and ruptured membranes, accompanied by the leakage of cytoplasmic contents.

2.3. TP Effect on the Adhesion of APP Bacteria

Figure 1C shows the results of LDH release from NPTr cells treated with different concentrations of TP. Different concentrations of TP had little effect on the toxicity of NPTr cells. As shown in Figure 1D, pretreatment with TP affected the capacity of APP strains to adhere to NPTr cells. TP inhibited the ability of APP to adhere to NPTr cells.

2.4. Effect of TP on Pro-Inflammatory Cytokine Secretion and the mRNA Level of TLR2 and TLR4 in NPTr Cells

TP influenced the secretion of pro-inflammatory factors in NPTr cells infected by APP. As shown in Figure 2A–C, secretion of IL-6, IL-8, and TNF-α pro-inflammatory factors in NPTr cells infected by APP was significantly higher than in the control group. However, pretreatment with TP for 3 h reduced the secretion of IL-6, IL-8, and TNF-α inflammatory factors in NPTr cells.

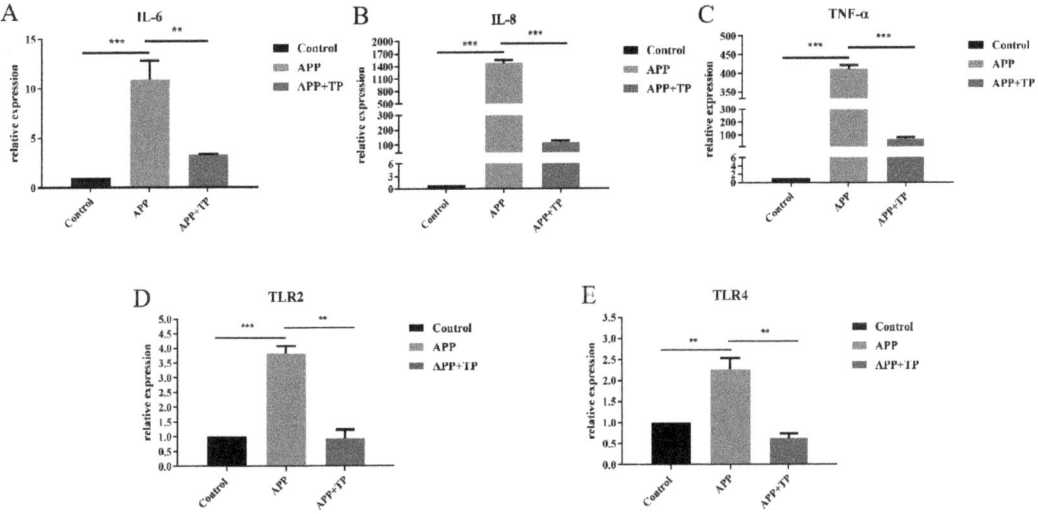

Figure 2. (**A–C**): Effect of APP on the Secretion of Inflammatory Factors in NPTr Cells or NPTr Cells Pretreated with TP. (**D,E**): The mRNA levels of TLR2 and TLR4 in NPTr cells and TP pretreatment cells infection with APP. Statistical analysis was performed by Student's t-test. $n = 3$ in each group, ** $p < 0.01$, *** $p < 0.001$.

TP influenced the mRNA level of TLR2 and TLR4 in NPTr cells infected by APP. As shown in Figure 2D,E, the secretion of TLR2 and TLR4 in NPTr cells stimulated by APP was significantly than in the control groups. However, the secretion of TLR2 and TLR4 in cells pretreated with TP was significantly lower than in cells treated with APP alone (Figure 2D,E). These results suggest that TP could inhibit the secretion of TLR2 and TLR4 in NPTr cells infected by APP.

2.5. TP Decrease the Disruption of Cellular Junctions in NPTr Cells

The effect of TP on the integrity of the epithelial barriers infected by APP was further evidenced by the β-catenin and occluding levels of the two important TJ and AJ proteins.

The localization of immunofluorescence of ß-catenin and occluding was observed by microscope. As shown in Figure 3, there was a destructive effect on the NPTr cell TJs infected by APP when compared with the control cells, and β-catenin and occludin expression was downregulated. However, when NPTr cells were pretreated with TP, the downregulation of these expressions was inhibited. This result was confirmed by immunoblotting. As shown in Figure 4B, protein expression levels of β-catenin and occludin were significantly decreased post-infection by APP in contrast to those of uninfected control cells. Following pretreatment of NPTr cells with TP, the protein expression levels of β-catenin and occludin were higher than those in untreated cells stimulated by APP. These results showed that pretreatment of cells with TP can inhibit the destruction of the β-catenin and occludin proteins, respectively, by APP.

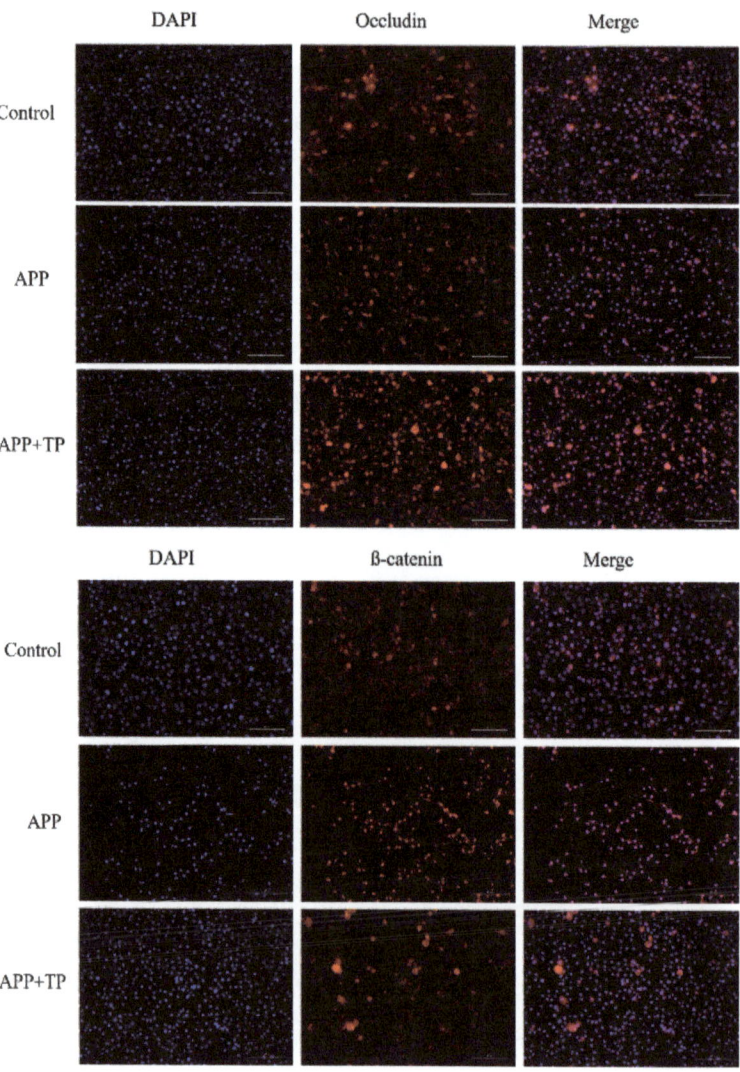

Figure 3. Immunofluorescence localization of occluding and β-catenin in NPTr cells. Scale bar indicated 100 μm.

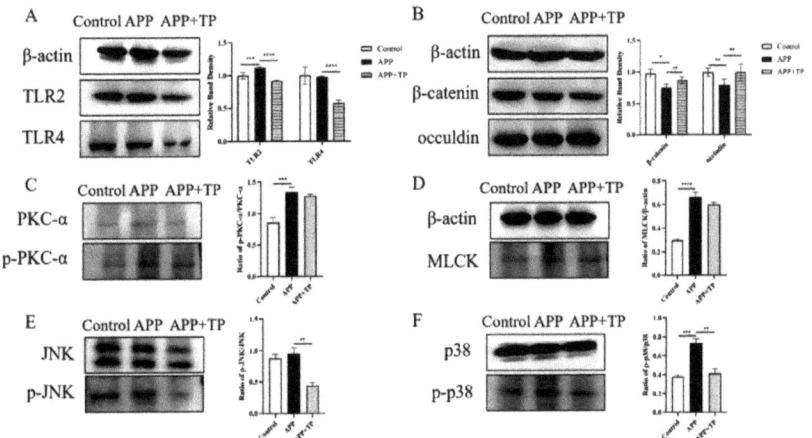

Figure 4. (**A,B**): The protein levels of TLR2, TLR4, ß-catenin, and occludin in NPTr cells and TP pretreatment cells infection with APP. GAPDH in whole cell lysates was detected as the loading control. (**C**): the ratio of p-PKC-α/PKC-α, (**D**): the ratio of MLCK: Effects of TP on PKC and MLCK pathways in NPTrs activated by APP. (**E**): the ratio of p-JNK/JNK, (**F**): the ratio of p-p38/p38: Effect of TP on phospho-JNK, and -p38 and total -JNK, and -p38 expression in NPTrs by Western blotting. (mean ± SD, n = 3).* $p < 0.05$, ** $p < 0.01$, *** $p < 0.001$, **** $p < 0.0001$.

2.6. The Effect of TP on the Expression of Toll-like Receptor-Related Proteins in NPTr Cells

TP influenced the proteins expression level of TLR2 and TLR4 in NPTr cells infected by APP. As shown in Figure 4A, the expression level of TLR2 protein in NPTr cells stimulated by APP was significantly lower than that in the control groups. However, the protein expression levels of TLR2 in cells pretreated with TP was significantly lower than in cells treated with APP alone. For the pretreatment of NPTr cells with TP, the protein expression levels of TLR4 were significantly lower than those in treated cells stimulated by APP. These results suggest that TP could inhibit the upregulation of TLR2 and TLR4 protein expression in NPTr cells infected by APP.

2.7. Effects of TP on PKC-α and MLCK Signaling Pathway Activated by APP

The protection mechanisms of TP on TJ of APP infected NPTr cells were determined by measuring related protein expressions using Western blot assays. The phosphorylation level of PKC-α was significantly increased under APP infection ($p < 0.001$). TP could downregulate the expression of p-PKC-α induced by APP (Figure 4C). The MLCK protein was significantly increased in the NPTrs in APP group when compared to control group ($p < 0.0001$). TP could inhibit the expression of MLCK protein (Figure 4D).

2.8. Effect of TP on the MAPK Signaling Pathway Activated by APP

We investigated the effect of APP on activation of the MAPK signaling pathway in NPTr cells using Western blot analysis. The NPTr cells were infected with APP, and phosphorylation of MAPK was measured using phospho-specific Abs. The data showed that APP promoted the phosphorylation of JNK and p38 when compared with that in the control condition (Figure 4E), whereas the phosphorylation of JNK and p38 in NPTr cells challenged with APP was inhibited by TP (Figure 4F).

2.9. Protective Effect of TP on Mice Infected by APP

In a mouse model, the protective effect of TP was assessed by instillation of TP prior to infection with APP. The results showed that the mice treated with TP suffered reduced inflammation and had higher survival rates when compared with untreated mice infected with APP. TP were demonstrated to confer protective effects against a lethal dose of APP (Figure 5A). We analyzed pathological samples of lung tissues of mice in the different groups and collected serum to detect pro-inflammatory factors. The levels of serum pro-inflammatory factors in the mice showed that the secretion of IL-1β, IL-6, and TNF-α inflammatory factors significantly increased in mice infected APP. Pretreatment with TP reduced the secretion of IL-1β, IL-6, IL-8, and TNF-α inflammatory factors, though the differences do not seem to be significant (Figure 5B). As shown in Figure 5C, the tissues of mice infected with APP showed abnormal lung tissue structure, partial alveolar atrophy, alveolar wall thickening, and some protein fluid and inflammatory cell infiltration when compared with the control group. However, symptoms were reduced in the lung tissues of mice treated with TP.

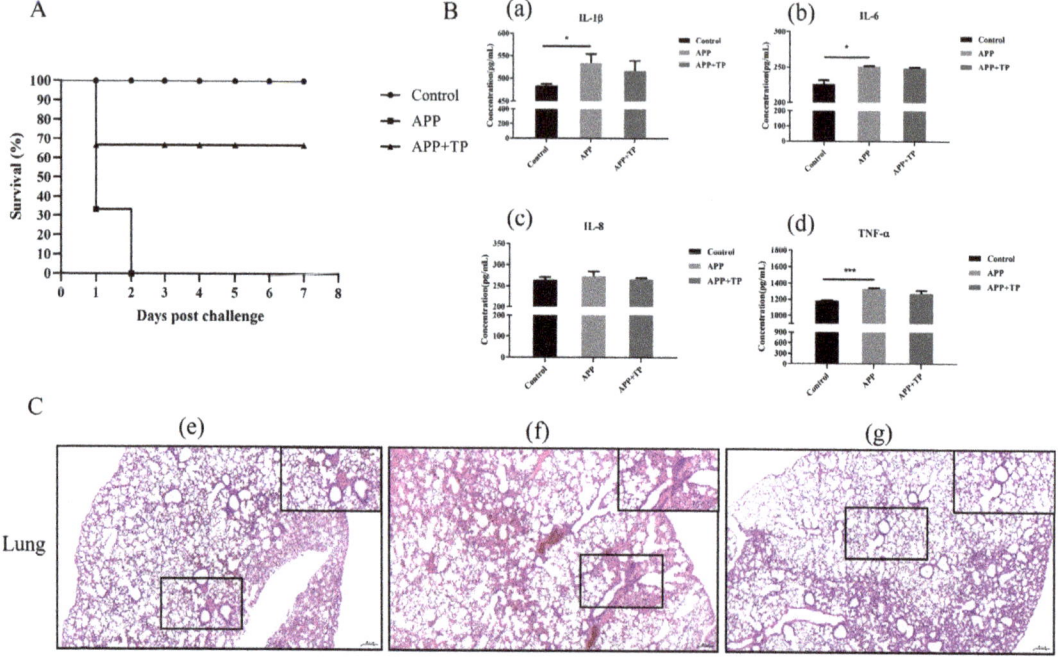

Figure 5. (**A**): Survival curves for mice in infection experiment. (**B**): Secretion of IL-1β, IL-6, IL-8, and TNF-α in the serum of mice infected with APP, as measured by ELISA. * $p < 0.05$, *** $p < 0.001$. (**a**): IL-1β production in serum of APP-infected mice affected by TP. (**b**): IL-6 production in serum of APP-infected mice affected by TP. (**c**): IL-8 production in serum of APP-infected mice affected by TP. (**d**): TNF-α production in serum of APP-infected mice afected by TP. (**C**): Histopathology of representative lung tissues from BALB/c mice and TP pretreatment mice infected with APP. (**e**): control group. (**f**): mice with APP infection group. (**g**): mice administered with TP. The black band at the bottom left of each picture indicates the scale bar (200 μm).

3. Discussion

Porcine pleuropneumonia is a common respiratory disease caused by APP infection. There are 19 different serotypes of APP, and the current vaccines does not cover all the serotypes. Antibiotic treatment remains an effective measure, but some strains have begun to show varying degrees of antibiotic resistance. Antibiotic resistance is a major global problem and there is an urgent need to develop new therapeutics. Considerable interest has been shown in the potential of botanical medicines to prevent and alleviate diseases, and these show great promise as antibiotic alternatives.

Tea is one of the most frequently consumed beverages in the world and has a long and rich history of medicinal benefits [49]. While there are multiple factors of tea influencing the effective biological properties, tea polyphenols are the most significant and valuable components [50]. Previous research has shown that TP have strong antibacterial properties and show significant promise as antibacterial agents in combating bacterial diseases [10,13,51]. TP is a kind of pure natural biological active substance extracted from green tea; the content is 98% in certificate of analysis. TP consist of different sorts of compounds. There are four major tea catechins, including epigallocatechin gallate (EGCG, 31.12%), epicatechin gallate (ECG, 20.31%), epicatechin (EC, 7.83%), and epigallocatechin (EGC, 6.02%), in accord with compounds about tea catechins shown in previous studies [50]. This provides some theoretical basis for achieving the observed biological effect. In this study, TP extracted from green tea exhibits antimicrobial activity towards APP. The determination of MIC, MBC, and the growth curves of APP strains showed that TP had a dose-dependent bactericidal effect on APP. The influence of TP on the integrity of APP cells was observed using a TEM, which confirmed that APP cells treated with TP showed obvious damage, in accord with those of previous studies [10,13,51,52]. In this study, we used a mouse model to examine the influence of APP on lung tissues. APP associated lung damage was reduced, and the survival rate was higher in mice fed TP when compared with untreated mice. The levels of serum pro-inflammatory factors detected in mice showed that pretreatment with TP reduced the secretion of IL-6, IL-8, and TNF-α inflammatory factors (Figure 5B). These results suggest that TP confer protection against APP infection and may provide a new means of disease prevention and treatment. Previous studies have used NPTr as a cellular model to study the role of pathogens in porcine respiratory diseases [53–55]. In this study, pretreatment of NPTr cells with TP showed that they inhibited the ability of APP to adhere to NPTr cells, in concurrence with previous studies [11,52,56].

Tracheal epithelial cells play a significant role in airway defense under multiple pathogen attacks [31]. TJs regulate the passage of ions and molecules through paracellular pathways in epithelial and endothelial cells [47]. TJ and AJ proteins have multiple functions and play important roles in maintaining epithelial barrier integrity [32,36,40,41]. However, there are little data available on how TJ and AJ changes under APP infection and their interaction mechanism. To explore the effect of TP on the integrity of the epithelial barrier against APP infection, we examined the levels of two important TJ and AJ proteins, β-catenin and occludin. Immunofluorescence analysis showed that APP infection altered the localization of β-catenin and occludin in epithelial cells and disrupted the TJ and AJ of NPTr cells. The distributions of occludin and β-catenin protein of APP infected NPTr cells were significantly disrupted. These data provide evidence that APP infection can alter the AJ and TJ and damage the epithelial barrier. The damage to junction proteins was alleviated when we pretreated the cells with TP, showing that TP can prevent the abnormalities caused by APP. This is in accordance with the results of previous studies that show that TP promote the expression of connexins, thereby protecting them from pathogens, a process largely prevented by TP supplementation [52,57–59].

It has been shown that PKCs can regulate the epithelial and endothelial barriers through their regulatory effects as intracellular signaling molecules [48]. Activation of PKC will increase cell permeability, which plays an important role in the regulation of tight junctions [48]. This study confirmed the changes of PKC-α protein in NPTr cells infected with APP. Compared with the control group, the expression of phosphorylation of PKC-α of APP-infected was significantly increased. TP can attenuate the phosphorylation of PKC-α. The results suggest that the protection effect of TP of tight junction abnormalities may relate directly to inhibition of PKC and/or the downstream signaling pathways such as MLCK.

Myosin light chain kinase (MLCK) is a key signaling node in physiological and pathophysiological regulation of epithelial tight junctions [60]. MLCK has been demonstrated to be the most important factor that influence TJ during inflammation. Increased MLCK is an indicator of TJ barrier disruption and can be triggered by pro-inflammatory cytokines, including TNF-α, IL-1β, and several related molecules [60]. Our results showed that the MLCK protein was significantly increased in APP challenged NPTr cells, suggesting that APP infection could cause TJ barrier disruption. However, TP inhibited the protein levels of MLCK induced by APP. The results indicate that the protective effects of TP on TJ may derive from inhibiting the MLCK pathway. In order to comprehend the protective effect of TP on epithelial barrier, further studies must be conducted.

An increasing number of cytokines have recently been confirmed to influence TJ barrier function, and to be associated with intrinsic TJ proteins [61]. Previous research has shown that IL-1β is the hallmark innate cytokine that plays a key role in the initiation of inflammatory immune responses and has been associated with inflammatory cell migration and osteoclastogenesis [62,63]. IL-6 is rapidly and transiently produced in response to infections and tissue injuries, and is implicated in inflammation, hematopoiesis, and immune responses [64]. IL-8 is a chemokine mainly produced by monocytes and epithelial cells, and mediates the chemotaxis of neutrophils during acute phase of inflammation [65]. TNF-α is a multi-function cytokine and an important mediator of inflammatory responses, produced by many types of immune cells including mucosal cells (such as epithelial cells) [66]. It regulates a number of inflammatory signaling pathways in macrophages [67]. Previous studies have demonstrated that APP can induce breakdown of the integrity of the porcine tracheal epithelial barrier, allowing tracheal epithelial cells to secrete various cytokines [30]. In this study, porcine tracheal epithelial cells also produced IL-6, IL-8, and TNF-α following exposure to APP, a result consistent with previous studies [30,53]. However, pretreatment with TP decreased the secretion of inflammatory factors IL-6, IL-8, and TNF-α in porcine tracheal epithelial cells.

Activation of the MAPK pathway can lead to TJ and AJ opening or assembly. To our knowledge, this is the first report showing TP inhibiting inflammatory responses inhibiting p38 MAPK signaling and the TLR signaling pathway in tracheal epithelial cells (Figure 6). JNK play an important role in regulating cell viability [68]. It has been reported that activation of inflammatory signaling pathways, including JNK and p38, induces secretion of cytokines [69]. In our study, TP decreased the secretion of inflammatory factors IL-6, IL-8, and TNF-α. APP activated the inflammatory signaling molecules JNK and p38 in NPTr cells. TP treatment significantly reduced APP-induced JNK and p38 phosphorylation expression. It is suggested that TP potentially mediates activation of the p-p38 MAPK pathway induced by APP. These data suggest that TP modulate the inflammatory immune response to fight infection and improve healing.

Toll-like receptors (TLRs) are transmembrane pattern recognition receptors (PRRs) that play a key role in microbial recognition, systemic bacterial infection, and control of adaptive immune responses [70,71]. Toll-like receptor 2 (TLR2), one member of the TLR family, recognizes conserved molecular patterns related to both Gram-negative and Gram-positive bacteria, such as lipoteichoic acid (LTA), lipoarabinomannan, lipoproteins, and peptidoglycan (PGN) [72,73]. Toll-like receptor 4 (TLR4) plays a crucial role in the infective inflammation caused by Gram-negative bacteria [74,75]. Related research shows that Toll-like receptor 4 plays a key role in mediating the innate immune response to pneumonia infection [75,76]. A previous study demonstrated that Emodin inhibits influenza viral pneumonia by inhibiting IAV-induced activation of TLR4, MAPK, and NF-kB pathways [77]. Ugonin M might exert efficacy on LPS-induced lung infection and inhibit not only NF-kB and MAPK activation but also TLR4 protein expression [78]. In the present study, mRNA levels of TLR2 and TLR4 in NPTr cells infected with APP were higher than those in control cells. When NPTr cells were pretreated with TP, a similar result was obtained and the TLR2 and TLR4 mRNA level of NPTr cells infected with APP were suppressed and the protein expression levels of TLR2 and TLR4 were significantly lower than those in treated cells stimulated by APP.

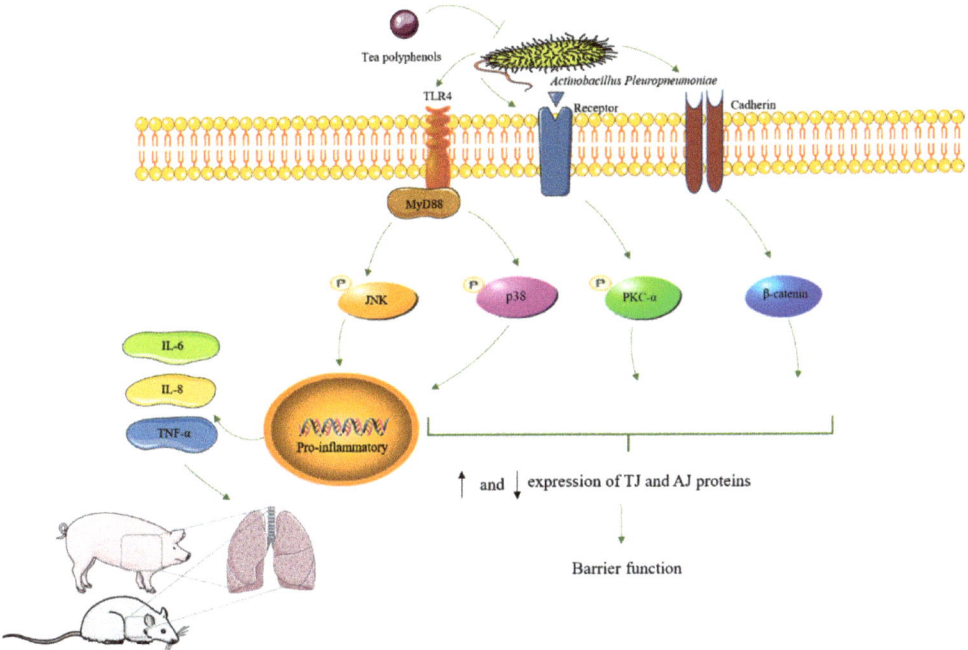

Figure 6. Schematic representation of TP in APP invasion of tracheal epithelial cells. "P" indicate phosphorylation. arrows ("↑" indicate increasing, "↓" indicate decreasing).

4. Materials and Methods

4.1. Cell Culture, Bacterial Culture, and TP

Newborn pig tracheal epithelial cells (NPTr) were cultured in Dulbecco's modified eagle medium (DMEM, high-glucose; Cytiva, Washington, DC, USA) supplemented with 10% fetal bovine serum (Gibco, New York, NY, USA), 100 U/mL penicillin, and 100 U/mL streptomycin (Solarbio, Beijing, China) at 37 °C with 5% CO_2. APP serotype 5b was obtained from the State Key Laboratory of Agricultural Microbiology (Huazhong Agricultural University, Wuhan, China). The bacterial strains were cultivated in BD™ tryptic soy broth (TSB) and tryptic soy agar (TSA) or Mueller–Hinton (Beckton Dickson, New York, NY, USA) supplemented with sterile newborn calf serum (10%, v/v, AusGeneX, Brisbane, Australia) and 10 µg/mL nicotinamide adenine dinucleotide (NAD) at 37 °C. TP (purity: 98%, molecular weight: 281.36) were bought from the Nanjing Tianrun Biotechnology Co., Ltd. (Nanjing, China). This product is a kind of pure natural biological active substance extracted from tea; its main components are epigallocatechin gallate (EGCG), epigallocatechin (EGC), epicatechin gallate (ECG), and epicatechin (EC).

Determination of minimum inhibitory concentration (MIC) and minimum bactericidal concentration (MBC).

The determination of MIC and MBC values of TP against APP were tested using a modified broth micro-dilution assay as described by the Clinical and Laboratory Standards Institute, CLSI 2015 [12]. Serial two-fold dilutions of TP (from 160 mg/mL) in culture medium were placed in 96-well micro-titer plates, 100 µL per well. Each well was seeded with APP at a final concentration of 5×10^5 CFU/mL. Medium samples without bacteria or TP were placed in wells as controls. The MIC value was the lowest concentration of TP at which no bacterial growth was observed after 12 h at 37 °C. Samples of 10 µL aliquots per well were spread onto TSA plates and left for 24 h at 37 °C, and the lowest concentration in which no APP colony formed was taken as the tea polyphenol MBC.

4.2. TP and APP Co-Cultivation Affects Bacteria Growth

The effect of TP on APP growth was explored as previously described [5], with minor modifications. In summary, APP (1×10^8 CFU/mL) and TP (0 MIC, 1/2 MIC, 1 MIC, and 2 MIC) were co-cultured for 0, 1, 2, 3, 4, and 5 h. At each hourly point, cultures were diluted, seeded onto TSA plates, and incubated for 24 h at 37 °C. The bactericidal effects of TP against APP were defined by measuring the CFUs of each culture by counting the number of APP colonies. The log10 CFU/mL vs. time over a 5 h period was plotted to visualize the APP growth curves.

Transmission electron microscope (TEM) and Scanning electron microscope (SEM) analysis of APP cellular integrity.

The damage caused to APP cells by TP was detected using TEM and SEM as previously described [79], with modifications. APP was grown in TSB until OD_{600} to 0.6, then bacteria were incubated with TP (0.625 mg/mL) at 37 °C for 3 h, and then fixed with electron microscope fixative (2.5% glutaraldehyde) at 4 °C overnight. The bacteria samples were post-fixed in 1% osmic acid for 2 h at room temperature, and ethanol and acetone were then added in turn for dehydration. Finally, ultra-thin sections were embedded and dyed with uranium and lead double staining. The morphology of the cells was observed under a TEM (Hitachi, HT7700, Tokyo, Japan), or the dried samples were observed via a SEM (Hitachi, SU8010, Tokyo, Japan); images were collected for analysis.

4.3. Cytotoxicity Detection Assay

In the cytotoxicity detection assay, NPTr cells were seeded into 96-well plates, with 10^6 cells per well. Different concentrations of TP were added to the cells as treatment groups, and cells without added TP were used as negative controls. The viability of the NPTr cells under different conditions were detected by measuring the amount of lactose dehydrogenase (LDH) using an LDH assay kit (Beyotime, Shanghai, China) according to the manufacturer's protocols. The LDH viability in the supernatant was measured using a microplate reader (Molecular Devices, Sunnyvale, CA, USA) at 490 nm.

4.4. Adherence Assay

In the adherence assay, NPTr cells were seeded into 24-well culture plates, with 10^6 cells per well. After incubation overnight, control cells were not pretreated, and treatment group cells were pretreated with TP (0.0625 mg/mL) for 3 h. Cells were then infected with APP at a multiplicity of infection (MOI; bacterial cells per cell) of 10:1. Plates were incubated for 2 h at 37 °C in 5% CO_2 and washed three times with PBS to remove unadhered bacteria. The cells with adherence bacteria were lysed with 0.025% Triton X-100 (Sinopharm Chemical Reagent Co., Ltd., Shanghai, China) on ice for 15 min. The number of bacteria adhering to NPTr cells were calculated.

4.5. Analysis of Cytokine, TLR2 and TLR4 mRNA Expression Using qRT-PCR

For analysis, 10^6 NPTr cells per well were seeded into 12-well plates. NPTr cells were treated and infected as described above, with untreated cells serving as controls. One group of cells were pretreated with TP (0.0625 mg/mL) for 3 h, and the other groups were not pretreated. Cells were then infected with APP at a multiplicity of infection (MOI; bacterial cells per cell) of 10:1. Plates were incubated at 37 °C in 5% CO_2. After 2 h, the total RNA of NPTr cells was extracted using Trizol reagent (Invitrogen, Burlington, ON, Canada) according to the manufacturer's protocols. The cDNA was amplified using reverse transcriptase (Vazyme, Nanjing, China) and qRT-PCR with a SYBY Green qPCR Kit (Vazyme, Nanjing, China) and were performed in triplicate. Expression of every gene was normalized to glyceraldehyde 3-phosphate dehydrogenase (GAPDH). The sequences of primers used for the qRT-PCR analyses are listed in Table 2.

Table 2. Primers used for qRT-PCR.

Gene	Nucleotide Sequence (5'-3')	Tm (°C)
GAPDH	GGCTGCCCAGAACATCATCC GACGCCTGCTTCACCACCTTCTTG	60
IL-6	GGAACGCCTGGAAGAAGATG ATCCACTCGTTCTGTGACTG	58
IL-8	TTTCTGCAGCTCTCTGTGAGG CTGCTGTTGTTGTTGCTTCTC	58
TNF-α	CGCATCGCCGTCTCCTACCA GACGCCTGCTTCACCACCTTCTTG	60
TLR-2	ACGGACTGTGGTGCATGAAG GGACACGAAAGCGTCATAGC	58
TLR-4	CATACAGAGCCGATGGTG CCTGCTGAGAAGGCGATA	58

4.6. Immunofluorescence Assay

NPTr cells were treated and infected as described above. Untreated cells were used as controls. One group of cells were pretreated with TP (0.0625 mg/mL) for 3 h; the other group was not pretreated. Cells were then infected with APP at a multiplicity of infection (MOI; bacterial cells per cell) of 10:1. Plates were incubated for 2 h at 37 °C in 5% CO_2. The cells were fixed in 4% paraformaldehyde and blocked in 5% BSA in PBS-Tween 20 (PBS containing 0.1% Tween 20) for 2 h at 37 °C. The cells were then labelled with antibodies against β-catenin (Proteintech, Chicago, IL, USA) and occludin (Proteintech, Chicago, IL, USA) at 4 °C overnight. After washing, cells were treated with a secondary antibody (CyTM3 AffiniPure Goat Anti-Mouse IgG (H + L)) (Jackson, PA, USA) and incubated for 1 h at room temperature. They were then washed with PBS three times, and the cell nuclei were counterstained with DAPI staining solution. The slides were then sealed with a coverslip using nail polish and kept in the dark until used. TJ and AJ proteins were visualized using a Nikon Eclipse CI fluorescence microscope and Nikon DS-U3 imaging (Nikon, Tokyo, Japan).

4.7. Western Blotting

NPTr cells were treated and infected as described above. Untreated cells were used as controls; one group of cells were pretreated with TP (0.0625 mg/mL) for 3 h and the other groups were not pretreated. Cells were then infected with APP at a multiplicity of infection (MOI; bacterial cells per cell) of 10:1. Plates were incubated at 37 °C for 2 h in 5% CO_2. After 2 h, cells were lysed with RIPA lysis buffer (Beyotime, Shanghai, China) with added protease inhibitors. The protein concentrations were measured with a BCA protein assay kit (Beyotime, Shanghai, China). After SDS-PAGE separation, the protein samples were transferred to PVDF membranes and blocked in Tris-buffered saline/Tween 20 (TBST) containing 5% skim milk (Beckton Dickson, New York, NY, USA). The PVDF membranes were incubated overnight with the corresponding antibodies (Occludin Monoclonal antibody, Beta Catenin Monoclonal antibody, HRP-conjugated βeta actin antibody, TLR2 Monoclonal antibody, TLR4 Monoclonal antibody, MLCK Polyclonal antibody, JNK Monoclonal antibody, Phospho-JNK (Tyr185) Recombinant antibody, p38 MAPK Monoclonal antibody, and Phospho-p38 MAPK (Thr180/Tyr182) Polyclonal antibody, Proteintech, Chicago, IL, USA; PKC alpha Antibody, Phospho-PKC alpha (Ser657) Antibody, Affinity Biosciences, Cincinnati, OH, USA) at 4 °C. Then, the PVDF membranes were washed with TBST and incubated with HRP-conjugated secondary antibodies (HRP-conjugated Affinipure Goat Anti-Mouse IgG (H + L), HRP-conjugated Affinipure Goat Anti-Rabbit IgG (H + L), Proteintech, Chicago, IL, USA) for 1 h at room temperature and visualized with ECL solution (Vazyme, Nanjing, China). Finally, the PVDF membranes were observed using the ChemoDoc™ Touch Imaging System (Bio-Rad, Watford, UK).

4.8. Animal Assay

A total of 18 female BALB/c mice (6-weeks-old) were purchased from the Center for Disease Control of Hubei Province (Hubei CDC, Wuhan, China). All animal experiments followed the recommendations of the Laboratory Animal Monitoring Committee of Huazhong Agricultural University. The mice were randomly divided into three groups (six per group). One group was treated with TP (100 mg/kg) by oral gavage for 5 days. The two other groups were treated with equivalent distilled water. The group pretreated with TP and one of distilled water group were infected with APP (1.46×10^8 CFU) by intraperitoneal injection. The other group were treated with normal saline by intraperitoneal injection, as a control group. Blood and lungs were obtained from the mice. Lung tissues were fixed in 4% para-formaldehyde and used for histopathological analysis. The amounts of inflammatory factors, including IL-1β, IL-6, IL-8, and TNF-α, in the serum of the mice were determined using an ELISA Kit (ml063132-J, ml063159, ml063162, ml063162, mlbio, Shanghai, China) according to the manufacturer's protocols.

4.9. Statistical Analysis

The results were analyzed using various statistical tests in GraphPad Prism version 8 (GraphPad Software, San Diego, CA, USA). Student's *t*-test was used to analyze differences between groups; '*' indicates statistical significance at $p < 0.05$, '**' indicates statistical significance at $p < 0.01$, '***' indicates statistical significance at $p < 0.001$, and '****' indicates statistical significance at $p < 0.0001$.

5. Conclusions

In summary, our results demonstrated that TP inhibited the growth of APP, disrupting the integrity of APP cells. In a mouse model, TP reduced damage due to APP and gave protection against APP exposure. In addition, it was found that TP inhibited the ability of APP to adhere to NPTr cells. TP promoted the expression of junction proteins to conserve the epithelial barrier integrity. It is possible that the protective effects of TP on TJ are closely related to the inhibition of the activation of PKC and MLCK pathways. Our results suggested that APP induces MAPK signaling pathway activation and TP inhibits the MAPK signaling pathway via regulation of the inflammatory immune response. Our results suggest that TP were demonstrated to confer protective effects against a lethal dose of APP, and that they can be used as a replacement for antibiotics to provide a new strategy for preventing APP infection in pigs.

Author Contributions: X.L., Z.L., Y.T., D.Z., W.B. and F.Y. designed research; X.L. and Z.L. performed research; T.G., K.Y. and R.G. contributed investigation and data curation; W.L., N.W. and C.L. contributed analyzed data; and X.L., Z.L., D.Z., W.B. and F.Y. wrote the paper. All authors have read and agreed to the published version of the manuscript.

Funding: This research was funded by the Technical Innovation Project of Hubei Province (2022ABA002; 2022BBA0055), the Hubei Province Natural Science Foundation for Innovative Research Groups (2021CFA019), the Hubei Province Innovation Center of Agricultural Sciences and Technology (2021-620-000-001-017), the National Key R&D Plan (2022YFD1800905). The funders had no role in the study design, data collection, and analysis, decision to publish, or preparation of the manuscript.

Institutional Review Board Statement: All animal studies were conducted in strict accordance with the guidelines of animal welfare of World Organization for Animal Health. All mice used in this study were purchased from the Wuhan Institute of Biological Products Co., Ltd. (Wuhan, China). The animal study protocol was approved by the Ethics Committee of Huazhong Agricultural University (Wuhan, China) and conducted in accordance with the Hubei Province Laboratory Animal Management Regulations of 2005. All efforts were made to minimize animal suffering.

Informed Consent Statement: Not applicable.

Data Availability Statement: The datasets generated and analyzed during the current study are available from the corresponding author on reasonable request.

Acknowledgments: We appreciated Hongbo Zhou at Huazhong Agricultural University for providing NPTr cells.

Conflicts of Interest: The authors declare no conflict of interest.

References

1. Caruana, M.; Vassallo, N. Tea Polyphenols in Parkinson's Disease. *Adv. Exp. Med. Biol.* **2015**, *863*, 117–137. [PubMed]
2. Guo, Y.J.; Sun, L.Q.; Yu, B.Y.; Qi, J. An integrated antioxidant activity fingerprint for commercial teas based on their capacities to scavenge reactive oxygen species. *Food Chem.* **2017**, *237*, 645–653. [CrossRef] [PubMed]
3. Li, Y.; Gao, X.; Lou, Y. Interactions of tea polyphenols with intestinal microbiota and their implication for cellular signal conditioning mechanism. *J. Food Biochem.* **2019**, *43*, e12953. [CrossRef] [PubMed]
4. Zou, L.-Q.; Liu, W.; Liu, W.-L.; Liang, R.-H.; Li, T.; Liu, C.-M.; Cao, Y.-L.; Niu, J.; Liu, Z. Characterization and Bioavailability of Tea Polyphenol Nanoliposome Prepared by Combining an Ethanol Injection Method with Dynamic High-Pressure Microfluidization. *J. Agric. Food Chem.* **2014**, *62*, 934–941. [CrossRef]
5. Xu, X.; Zhou, X.D.; Wu, C.D. The tea catechin epigallocatechin gallate suppresses cariogenic virulence factors of Streptococcus mutans. *Antimicrob. Agents Chemother.* **2011**, *55*, 1229–1236. [CrossRef]
6. Elmassry, M.M.; Chung, E.; Cao, J.J.; Hamood, A.N.; Shen, C.L. Osteoprotective effect of green tea polyphenols and annatto-extracted tocotrienol in obese mice is associated with enhanced microbiome vitamin K2 biosynthetic pathways. *J. Nutr. Biochem.* **2020**, *86*, 108492. [CrossRef]
7. Zhao, Y.; Zhang, X. Interactions of tea polyphenols with intestinal microbiota and their implication for anti-obesity. *J. Sci. Food Agric.* **2020**, *100*, 897–903. [CrossRef]
8. Cao, D.; Zhao, M.; Wan, C.; Zhang, Q.; Tang, T.; Liu, J.; Shao, Q.; Yang, B.; He, J.; Jiang, C. Role of tea polyphenols in delaying hyperglycemia-induced senescence in human glomerular mesangial cells via miR-126/Akt-p53-p21 pathways. *Int. Urol. Nephrol.* **2019**, *51*, 1071–1078. [CrossRef] [PubMed]
9. Ogawa, M.; Shimojima, M.; Saijo, M.; Fukasawa, M. Several catechins and flavonols from green tea inhibit severe fever with thrombocytopenia syndrome virus infection in vitro. *J. Infect. Chemother.* **2021**, *27*, 32–39. [CrossRef]
10. Reygaert, W.C. The antimicrobial possibilities of green tea. *Front. Microbiol.* **2014**, *5*, 434. [CrossRef]
11. Lagha, A.B.; Grenier, D. Tea polyphenols inhibit the activation of NF-kappaB and the secretion of cytokines and matrix metalloproteinases by macrophages stimulated with Fusobacterium nucleatum. *Sci. Rep.* **2016**, *6*, 34520. [CrossRef]
12. Yin, H.; Deng, Y.; Wang, H.; Liu, W.; Zhuang, X.; Chu, W. Tea polyphenols as an antivirulence compound Disrupt Quorum-Sensing Regulated Pathogenicity of Pseudomonas aeruginosa. *Sci. Rep.* **2015**, *5*, 16158. [CrossRef]
13. Guo, L.; Guo, J.; Liu, H.; Zhang, J.; Chen, X.; Qiu, Y.; Fu, S. Tea polyphenols suppress growth and virulence-related factors of Haemophilus parasuis. *J. Vet. Med. Sci.* **2018**, *80*, 1047–1053. [CrossRef]
14. Ma, X.; Zheng, B.; Wang, J.; Li, G.; Cao, S.; Wen, Y.; Huang, X.; Zuo, Z.; Zhong, Z.; Gu, Y. Quinolone Resistance of Actinobacillus pleuropneumoniae Revealed through Genome and Transcriptome Analyses. *Int. J Mol. Sci.* **2021**, *22*, 10036. [CrossRef]
15. Opriessnig, T.; Gimenez-Lirola, L.G.; Halbur, P.G. Polymicrobial respiratory disease in pigs. *Anim. Health Res. Rev* **2011**, *12*, 133–148. [CrossRef]
16. Hoflack, G.; Maes, D.; Mateusen, B.; Verdonck, M.; de Kruif, A. Efficacy of tilmicosin phosphate (Pulmotil premix) in feed for the treatment of a clinical outbreak of Actinobacillus pleuropneumoniae infection in growing-finishing pigs. *J. Vet. Med. B Infect. Dis. Vet. Public. Health* **2001**, *48*, 655–664. [CrossRef]
17. Chiers, K.; De Waele, T.; Pasmans, F.; Ducatelle, R.; Haesebrouck, F. Virulence factors of Actinobacillus pleuropneumoniae involved in colonization, persistence and induction of lesions in its porcine host. *Vet. Res.* **2010**, *41*, 65. [CrossRef]
18. Bosse, J.T.; Janson, H.; Sheehan, B.J.; Beddek, A.J.; Rycroft, A.N.; Kroll, J.S.; Langford, P.R. Actinobacillus pleuropneumoniae: Pathobiology and pathogenesis of infection. *Microbes Infect.* **2002**, *4*, 225–235. [CrossRef]
19. Stringer, O.W.; Bosse, J.T.; Lacouture, S.; Gottschalk, M.; Fodor, L.; Angen, O.; Velazquez, E.; Penny, P.; Lei, L.; Langford, P.R.; et al. Proposal of Actinobacillus pleuropneumoniae serovar 19, and reformulation of previous multiplex PCRs for capsule-specific typing of all known serovars. *Vet. Microbiol.* **2021**, *255*, 109021. [CrossRef]
20. Bosse, J.T.; Li, Y.; Sarkozi, R.; Fodor, L.; Lacouture, S.; Gottschalk, M.; Casas Amoribieta, M.; Angen, O.; Nedbalcova, K.; Holden, M.T.G.; et al. Proposal of serovars 17 and 18 of Actinobacillus pleuropneumoniae based on serological and genotypic analysis. *Vet. Microbiol.* **2018**, *217*, 1–6. [CrossRef]
21. Xu, Z.; Zhou, Y.; Li, L.; Zhou, R.; Xiao, S.; Wan, Y.; Zhang, S.; Wang, K.; Li, W.; Li, L.; et al. Genome biology of Actinobacillus pleuropneumoniae JL03, an isolate of serotype 3 prevalent in China. *PLoS ONE* **2008**, *3*, e1450. [CrossRef] [PubMed]
22. Bosse, J.T.; Li, Y.; Walker, S.; Atherton, T.; Fernandez Crespo, R.; Williamson, S.M.; Rogers, J.; Chaudhuri, R.R.; Weinert, L.A.; Oshota, O.; et al. Identification of dfrA14 in two distinct plasmids conferring trimethoprim resistance in Actinobacillus pleuropneumoniae. *J. Antimicrob. Chemother.* **2015**, *70*, 2217–2222. [CrossRef] [PubMed]
23. Vilaro, A.; Novell, E.; Enrique-Tarancon, V.; Balielles, J.; Vilalta, C.; Martinez, S.; Fraile Sauce, L.J. Antimicrobial Susceptibility Pattern of Porcine Respiratory Bacteria in Spain. *Antibiotics* **2020**, *9*, 402. [CrossRef] [PubMed]

24. Vanni, M.; Merenda, M.; Barigazzi, G.; Garbarino, C.; Luppi, A.; Tognetti, R.; Intorre, L. Antimicrobial resistance of Actinobacillus pleuropneumoniae isolated from swine. *Vet. Microbiol.* **2012**, *156*, 172–177. [CrossRef] [PubMed]
25. Dayao, D.; Gibson, J.S.; Blackall, P.J.; Turni, C. Antimicrobial resistance genes in Actinobacillus pleuropneumoniae, Haemophilus parasuis and Pasteurella multocida isolated from Australian pigs. *Aust. Vet. J.* **2016**, *94*, 227–231. [CrossRef]
26. Dayao, D.; Gibson, J.S.; Blackall, P.J.; Turni, C. Antimicrobial resistance in bacteria associated with porcine respiratory disease in Australia. *Vet. Microbiol.* **2014**, *171*, 232–235. [CrossRef]
27. Wang, Y.C.; Chan, J.P.; Yeh, K.S.; Chang, C.C.; Hsuan, S.L.; Hsieh, Y.M.; Chang, Y.C.; Lai, T.C.; Lin, W.H.; Chen, T.H. Molecular characterization of enrofloxacin resistant Actinobacillus pleuropneumoniae isolates. *Vet. Microbiol.* **2010**, *142*, 309–312. [CrossRef]
28. Kucerova, Z.; Hradecka, H.; Nechvatalova, K.; Nedbalcova, K. Antimicrobial susceptibility of Actinobacillus pleuropneumoniae isolates from clinical outbreaks of porcine respiratory diseases. *Vet. Microbiol.* **2011**, *150*, 203–206. [CrossRef]
29. Pridmore, A.; Burch, D.; Lees, P. Determination of minimum inhibitory and minimum bactericidal concentrations of tiamulin against field isolates of Actinobacillus pleuropneumoniae. *Vet. Microbiol.* **2011**, *151*, 409–412. [CrossRef]
30. Bercier, P.; Gottschalk, M.; Grenier, D. Effects of Actinobacillus pleuropneumoniae on barrier function and inflammatory response of pig tracheal epithelial cells. *Pathog. Dis.* **2019**, *77*, fty079. [CrossRef]
31. Gon, Y.; Hashimoto, S. Role of airway epithelial barrier dysfunction in pathogenesis of asthma. *Allergol. Int.* **2018**, *67*, 12–17. [CrossRef]
32. Matter, K.; Balda, M.S. Signalling to and from tight junctions. *Nat. Rev. Mol. Cell Biol.* **2003**, *4*, 225–236. [CrossRef]
33. Pohunek, P. Development, structure and function of the upper airways. *Paediatr. Respir. Rev.* **2004**, *5*, 2–8. [CrossRef]
34. Ganz, T. Epithelia: Not just physical barriers. *Proc. Natl. Acad. Sci. USA* **2002**, *99*, 3357–3358. [CrossRef]
35. Jiao, J.; Wang, C.; Zhang, L. Epithelial physical barrier defects in chronic rhinosinusitis. *Expert. Rev. Clin. Immunol.* **2019**, *15*, 679–688. [CrossRef]
36. Zihni, C.; Mills, C.; Matter, K.; Balda, M.S. Tight junctions: From simple barriers to multifunctional molecular gates. *Nat. Rev. Mol. Cell Biol.* **2016**, *17*, 564–580. [CrossRef]
37. Shen, L.; Weber, C.R.; Raleigh, D.R.; Yu, D.; Turner, J.R. Tight junction pore and leak pathways: A dynamic duo. *Annu. Rev. Physiol.* **2011**, *73*, 283–309. [CrossRef]
38. Weber, C.R. Dynamic properties of the tight junction barrier. *Ann. N. Y. Acad. Sci.* **2012**, *1257*, 77–84. [CrossRef]
39. Pearce, S.C.; Al-Jawadi, A.; Kishida, K.; Yu, S.; Hu, M.; Fritzky, L.F.; Edelblum, K.L.; Gao, N.; Ferraris, R.P. Marked differences in tight junction composition and macromolecular permeability among different intestinal cell types. *BMC Biol.* **2018**, *16*, 19. [CrossRef]
40. Yuksel, H.; Turkeli, A. Airway epithelial barrier dysfunction in the pathogenesis and prognosis of respiratory tract diseases in childhood and adulthood. *Tissue Barriers* **2017**, *5*, e1367458. [CrossRef]
41. Schleimer, R.P. Immunopathogenesis of Chronic Rhinosinusitis and Nasal Polyposis. *Annu. Rev. Pathol.* **2017**, *12*, 331–357. [CrossRef] [PubMed]
42. Bruser, L.; Bogdan, S. Adherens Junctions on the Move-Membrane Trafficking of E-Cadherin. *Cold Spring Harb. Perspect. Biol.* **2017**, *9*, a029140. [CrossRef] [PubMed]
43. Coopman, P.; Djiane, A. Adherens Junction and E-Cadherin complex regulation by epithelial polarity. *Cell Mol. Life Sci.* **2016**, *73*, 3535–3553. [CrossRef] [PubMed]
44. De Benedetto, A.; Rafaels, N.M.; McGirt, L.Y.; Ivanov, A.I.; Georas, S.N.; Cheadle, C.; Berger, A.E.; Zhang, K.; Vidyasagar, S.; Yoshida, T.; et al. Tight junction defects in patients with atopic dermatitis. *J. Allergy Clin. Immunol.* **2011**, *127*, 773–786.e7. [CrossRef] [PubMed]
45. Clarke, H.; Marano, C.W.; Peralta Soler, A.; Mullin, J.M. Modification of tight junction function by protein kinase C isoforms. *Adv. Drug Deliv. Rev.* **2000**, *41*, 283–301. [CrossRef] [PubMed]
46. Zhou, H.Y.; Zhu, H.; Yao, X.M.; Qian, J.P.; Yang, J.; Pan, X.D.; Chen, X.D. Metformin regulates tight junction of intestinal epithelial cells via MLCK-MLC signaling pathway. *Eur. Rev. Med. Pharmacol. Sci.* **2017**, *21*, 5239–5246. [CrossRef]
47. Gonzalez-Mariscal, L.; Tapia, R.; Chamorro, D. Crosstalk of tight junction components with signaling pathways. *Biochim. Biophys. Acta* **2008**, *1778*, 729–756. [CrossRef]
48. Cong, X.; Kong, W. Endothelial tight junctions and their regulatory signaling pathways in vascular homeostasis and disease. *Cell. Signal.* **2020**, *66*, 109485. [CrossRef]
49. Yang, C.S.; Chen, G.; Wu, Q. Recent scientific studies of a traditional chinese medicine, tea, on prevention of chronic diseases. *J. Tradit. Complement. Med.* **2014**, *4*, 17–23. [CrossRef]
50. Li, S.; Zhang, L.; Wan, X.; Zhan, J.; Ho, C.-T. Focusing on the recent progress of tea polyphenol chemistry and perspectives. *Food Sci. Hum. Wellness* **2022**, *11*, 437–444. [CrossRef]
51. Bansal, S.; Choudhary, S.; Sharma, M.; Kumar, S.S.; Lohan, S.; Bhardwaj, V.; Syan, N.; Jyoti, S. Tea: A native source of antimicrobial agents. *Food Res. Int.* **2013**, *53*, 568–584. [CrossRef]
52. Ma, T.; Peng, W.; Liu, Z.; Gao, T.; Liu, W.; Zhou, D.; Yang, K.; Guo, R.; Duan, Z.; Liang, W.; et al. Tea polyphenols inhibit the growth and virulence of ETEC K88. *Microb. Pathog.* **2021**, *152*, 104640. [CrossRef]

53. Auger, E.; Deslandes, V.; Ramjeet, M.; Contreras, I.; Nash, J.H.; Harel, J.; Gottschalk, M.; Olivier, M.; Jacques, M. Host-pathogen interactions of Actinobacillus pleuropneumoniae with porcine lung and tracheal epithelial cells. *Infect. Immun.* **2009**, *77*, 1426–1441. [CrossRef]
54. Delgado-Ortega, M.; Olivier, M.; Sizaret, P.Y.; Simon, G.; Meurens, F. Newborn pig trachea cell line cultured in air-liquid interface conditions allows a partial in vitro representation of the porcine upper airway tissue. *BMC Cell Biol.* **2014**, *15*, 14. [CrossRef]
55. Cao, Q.; Wei, W.; Wang, H.; Wang, Z.; Lv, Y.; Dai, M.; Tan, C.; Chen, H.; Wang, X. Cleavage of E-cadherin by porcine respiratory bacterial pathogens facilitates airway epithelial barrier disruption and bacterial paracellular transmigration. *Virulence* **2021**, *12*, 2296–2313. [CrossRef]
56. Fournier-Larente, J.; Morin, M.P.; Grenier, D. Green tea catechins potentiate the effect of antibiotics and modulate adherence and gene expression in Porphyromonas gingivalis. *Arch. Oral Biol.* **2016**, *65*, 35–43. [CrossRef]
57. Lagha, A.B.; Groeger, S.; Meyle, J.; Grenier, D. Green tea polyphenols enhance gingival keratinocyte integrity and protect against invasion by Porphyromonas gingivalis. *Pathog. Dis.* **2018**, *76*, fty030. [CrossRef]
58. Liu, X.; Wang, Z.; Wang, P.; Yu, B.; Liu, Y.; Xue, Y. Green tea polyphenols alleviate early BBB damage during experimental focal cerebral ischemia through regulating tight junctions and PKCalpha signaling. *BMC Complement. Altern. Med.* **2013**, *13*, 187. [CrossRef]
59. Li, J.; Ye, L.; Wang, X.; Liu, J.; Wang, Y.; Zhou, Y.; Ho, W. (-)-Epigallocatechin gallate inhibits endotoxin-induced expression of inflammatory cytokines in human cerebral microvascular endothelial cells. *J. Neuroinflamm.* **2012**, *9*, 161. [CrossRef]
60. He, W.Q.; Wang, J.; Sheng, J.Y.; Zha, J.M.; Graham, W.V.; Turner, J.R. Contributions of Myosin Light Chain Kinase to Regulation of Epithelial Paracellular Permeability and Mucosal Homeostasis. *Int. J. Mol. Sci.* **2020**, *21*, 993. [CrossRef]
61. Walsh, S. Modulation of tight junction structure and function by cytokines. *Adv. Drug Deliv. Rev.* **2000**, *41*, 303–313. [CrossRef] [PubMed]
62. Lo, Y.J.; Liu, C.M.; Wong, M.Y.; Hou, L.T.; Chang, W.K. Interleukin 1beta-secreting cells in inflamed gingival tissue of adult periodontitis patients. *Cytokine* **1999**, *11*, 626–633. [CrossRef] [PubMed]
63. Bloemen, V.; Schoenmaker, T.; de Vries, T.J.; Everts, V. IL-1beta favors osteoclastogenesis via supporting human periodontal ligament fibroblasts. *J. Cell Biochem.* **2011**, *112*, 1890–1897. [CrossRef] [PubMed]
64. Tanaka, T.; Narazaki, M.; Kishimoto, T. IL-6 in inflammation, immunity, and disease. *Cold Spring Harb. Perspect. Biol.* **2014**, *6*, a016295. [CrossRef] [PubMed]
65. Kosmopoulos, M.; Christofides, A.; Drekolias, D.; Zavras, P.D.; Gargalionis, A.N.; Piperi, C. Critical Role of IL-8 Targeting in Gliomas. *Curr. Med. Chem.* **2018**, *25*, 1954–1967. [CrossRef]
66. Sedger, L.M.; McDermott, M.F. TNF and TNF-receptors: From mediators of cell death and inflammation to therapeutic giants—Past, present and future. *Cytokine Growth Factor. Rev.* **2014**, *25*, 453–472. [CrossRef]
67. Lagha, A.B.; Grenier, D. Tea polyphenols protect gingival keratinocytes against TNF-alpha-induced tight junction barrier dysfunction and attenuate the inflammatory response of monocytes/macrophages. *Cytokine* **2019**, *115*, 64–75. [CrossRef]
68. Himes, S.R.; Sester, D.P.; Ravasi, T.; Cronau, S.L.; Sasmono, T.; Hume, D.A. The JNK are important for development and survival of macrophages. *J. Immunol.* **2006**, *176*, 2219–2228. [CrossRef]
69. He, W.; Hu, S.; Du, X.; Wen, Q.; Zhong, X.P.; Zhou, X.; Zhou, C.; Xiong, W.; Gao, Y.; Zhang, S.; et al. Vitamin B5 Reduces Bacterial Growth via Regulating Innate Immunity and Adaptive Immunity in Mice Infected with Mycobacterium tuberculosis. *Front. Immunol.* **2018**, *9*, 365. [CrossRef]
70. Cario, E. Bacterial interactions with cells of the intestinal mucosa: Toll-like receptors and NOD2. *Gut* **2005**, *54*, 1182–1193. [CrossRef]
71. Cario, E.; Gerken, G.; Podolsky, D.K. Toll-like receptor 2 controls mucosal inflammation by regulating epithelial barrier function. *Gastroenterology* **2007**, *132*, 1359–1374. [CrossRef]
72. Cario, E. Barrier-protective function of intestinal epithelial Toll-like receptor 2. *Mucosal Immunol.* **2008**, *1* (Suppl. S1), S62–S66. [CrossRef]
73. Gu, M.J.; Song, S.K.; Lee, I.K.; Ko, S.; Han, S.E.; Bae, S.; Ji, S.Y.; Park, B.C.; Song, K.D.; Lee, H.K.; et al. Barrier protection via Toll-like receptor 2 signaling in porcine intestinal epithelial cells damaged by deoxynivalenol. *Vet. Res.* **2016**, *47*, 25. [CrossRef]
74. Xu, C.; Chen, G.; Yang, W.; Xu, Y.; Xu, Y.; Huang, X.; Liu, J.; Feng, Y.; Xu, Y.; Liu, B. Hyaluronan ameliorates LPS-induced acute lung injury in mice via Toll-like receptor (TLR) 4-dependent signaling pathways. *Int. Immunopharmacol.* **2015**, *28*, 1050–1058. [CrossRef]
75. Ding, J.; Liu, Q. Toll-like receptor 4: A promising therapeutic target for pneumonia caused by Gram-negative bacteria. *J. Cell Mol. Med.* **2019**, *23*, 5868–5875. [CrossRef]
76. Sender, V.; Stamme, C. Lung cell-specific modulation of LPS-induced TLR4 receptor and adaptor localization. *Commun. Integr. Biol.* **2014**, *7*, e29053. [CrossRef]
77. Dai, J.P.; Wang, Q.W.; Su, Y.; Gu, L.M.; Zhao, Y.; Chen, X.X.; Chen, C.; Li, W.Z.; Wang, G.F.; Li, K.S. Emodin Inhibition of Influenza A Virus Replication and Influenza Viral Pneumonia via the Nrf2, TLR4, p38/JNK and NF-kappaB Pathways. *Molecules* **2017**, *22*, 1754. [CrossRef]

78. Wu, K.C.; Huang, S.S.; Kuo, Y.H.; Ho, Y.L.; Yang, C.S.; Chang, Y.S.; Huang, G.J. Ugonin M, a Helminthostachys zeylanica Constituent, Prevents LPS-Induced Acute Lung Injury through TLR4-Mediated MAPK and NF-kappaB Signaling Pathways. *Molecules* **2017**, *22*, 573. [CrossRef]
79. Morin, M.P.; Bedran, T.B.; Fournier-Larente, J.; Haas, B.; Azelmat, J.; Grenier, D. Green tea extract and its major constituent epigallocatechin-3-gallate inhibit growth and halitosis-related properties of *Solobacterium moorei*. *BMC Complement. Altern. Med.* **2015**, *15*, 40. [CrossRef]

Disclaimer/Publisher's Note: The statements, opinions and data contained in all publications are solely those of the individual author(s) and contributor(s) and not of MDPI and/or the editor(s). MDPI and/or the editor(s) disclaim responsibility for any injury to people or property resulting from any ideas, methods, instructions or products referred to in the content.

Article

Luteolin Enhances Transepithelial Sodium Transport in the Lung Alveolar Model: Integrating Network Pharmacology and Mechanism Study

Lei Chen [1], Tong Yu [2], Yiman Zhai [2], Hongguang Nie [2], Xin Li [3,4,5,*] and Yan Ding [2,*]

1. Department of Pharmacology, School of Pharmacy, China Medical University, Shenyang 110122, China; lchen@cmu.edu.cn
2. Department of Stem Cells and Regenerative Medicine, College of Basic Medical Science, China Medical University, Shenyang 110122, China
3. Department of Chemistry, School of Forensic Medicine, China Medical University, Shenyang 110122, China
4. Liaoning Province Key Laboratory of Forensic Bio-Evidence Sciences, Shenyang 110122, China
5. Center of Forensic Investigation, China Medical University, Shenyang 110122, China
* Correspondence: 20071029@cmu.edu.cn (X.L.); yding@cmu.edu.cn (Y.D.)

Abstract: Luteolin (Lut), a natural flavonoid compound existing in *Perilla frutescens* (L.) Britton, has been proven to play a protective role in the following biological aspects: inflammatory, viral, oxidant, and tumor-related. Lut can alleviate acute lung injury (ALI), manifested mainly by preventing the accumulation of inflammation-rich edematous fluid, while the protective actions of Lut on transepithelial ion transport in ALI were seldom researched. We found that Lut could improve the lung appearance/pathological structure in lipopolysaccharide (LPS)-induced mouse ALI models and reduce the wet/dry weight ratio, bronchoalveolar protein, and inflammatory cytokines. Meanwhile, Lut upregulated the expression level of the epithelial sodium channel (ENaC) in both the primary alveolar epithelial type 2 (AT2) cells and three-dimensional (3D) alveolar epithelial organoid model that recapitulated essential structural and functional aspects of the lung. Finally, by analyzing the 84 interaction genes between Lut and ALI/acute respiratory distress syndrome using GO and KEGG enrichment of network pharmacology, we found that the JAK/STAT signaling pathway might be involved in the network. Experimental data by knocking down STAT3 proved that Lut could reduce the phosphorylation of JAK/STAT and enhance the level of SOCS3, which abrogated the inhibition of ENaC expression induced by LPS accordingly. The evidence supported that Lut could attenuate inflammation-related ALI by enhancing transepithelial sodium transport, at least partially, via the JAK/STAT pathway, which may offer a promising therapeutic strategy for edematous lung diseases.

Keywords: phytochemicals; network pharmacology; acute lung injury; 3D alveolar epithelial organoid; epithelial sodium channel; JAK/STAT pathway

1. Introduction

In acute lung injury (ALI), the injury to the cells of alveolar epithelium may lead to an inflammatory storm and progressive diseases. Pathological specimens from patients with ALI or its severe form—acute respiratory distress syndrome (ARDS)—often show diffuse alveolus damage, with an accumulation of inflammatory edema fluid; thus, the effective clearance of superabundant fluid is necessary for restoring the gas exchange in the alveoli [1,2]. Alveolar epithelial cells are composed mainly of alveolar epithelial type (AT) 1 and 2 cells, the latter of which are involved in the effect of secretion and regeneration to maintain lung homeostasis [3,4]. Bearing the potential of self-renewal and differentiation into AT1 cells, AT2 cells can maintain alveolar function and are identified to be the facultative progenitor cells in lung tissue repair during ALI [5]. The epithelial sodium channel (ENaC) consists mainly of $\alpha/\beta/\gamma$ subunits and is responsible for transporting Na$^+$

from the apical to the basolateral side, thus regulating the water reabsorption of alveolar epithelial cells [6].

Lipopolysaccharide (LPS), a major biologically active component of the Gram-negative bacterial cell wall, can induce the features of acute inflammation in lung epithelium and facilitate extensive tissue damage in the organs, such as kidney, heart, and liver [7–9]. In LPS-induced ALI, ENaC expressed in AT2 cells can regulate the transepithelial sodium transport, ensuring the fluid clearance in edematous alveoli [2,10]. However, despite several important advances in ALI treatment during the last few decades, the specific mechanisms of ENaC-involved regulation are still undetermined. Therefore, discovering new drugs and therapeutic targets remains an urgent priority.

Organoids are three-dimensional (3D) structures derived from stem or progenitor cells, the extracellular matrix of which possesses the fundamental composition and function of multiple organs [11]. The aforementioned attributes render them a promising candidate for both fundamental research and clinical diagnosis/treatment. At present, the lung alveolar organoid has been a new pathological model for studying cell communication and host–pathogen interactions and is a powerful platform for simulating lung diseases, which can replace some animal experiments and, thus, minimize the use of animals in respiratory research [12].

Luteolin (Lut) (3', 4', 5, 7-tetrahydroxyflavonoids), a bioactive polyphenolic compound, can be extracted from many medicinal plants and some common vegetables/fruits, including *Perilla frutescens* (L.) Britton [13]. According to the Chinese medical system, *P. frutescens* can be used ethnically to treat respiratory problems, such as cold, fever, nasal congestion, and cough [14]. Fifteen types of compounds, including Lut, apigenin, rosmarinic acid, and caffeic acid, were separated and extracted from the *P. frutescens* leaves [15]. Among them, Lut is a flavonoid compound, which possesses numerous beneficial pharmacological actions, including anti-inflammatory, anti-oxidant, anti-viral, anti-tumor, and other biological properties [16–18]. Previous studies on ALI caused by sepsis or cecal ligation puncture have shown that Lut has protective therapeutic effects [19,20]. The mechanisms of Lut treatment in ALI have been uncovered to be related to inhibit the inflammatory reaction, including reducing the pulmonary reactive oxygen sepsis, whereas the actions of Lut on transepithelial ion transport in pneumonedema were seldom researched [21].

Network pharmacology is an innovation in elucidating the intricate progress of pathophysiology by evaluating the interactions among herbs, components, targets genes, and diseases. It is helpful in understanding the instinctive laws of formulas and revealing various targets for traditional Chinese medicine actions [22]. In this research, we confirmed the actions of Lut on the expression level of ENaC in primary AT2 cells, as well as constructed a molecular docking model to study the potential mechanism in ALI treatment. Of note, we established a lung alveolar model using a 3D alveolar epithelial organoid that was similar to the actual in vivo state in order to explore a new strategy of Lut treatment in edematous lung diseases.

2. Results

2.1. Lut Increased the Expression Level of ENaC in Primary AT2 Cells

The molecular structure of Lut is shown in Figure 1A. Firstly, we evaluated the effect of Lut on primary AT2 cell viability by CCK8 assay, and the results showed that 5, 10, and 20 μM Lut could promote the proliferation of AT2 cells treated without or with LPS (Figure 1B, $p < 0.05$ vs. 0 μM group, $p < 0.001$ vs. LPS group). Notably, 10 μM of Lut showed the highest protective effect, which was used as the optimal treatment concentration for the subsequent cell experiments. However, with the further increases in concentration, 20 and 40 μM seemed to show lesser cell viability upon treatment with LPS, possibly due to the cytotoxicity, which may counteract the visibly proliferative effects.

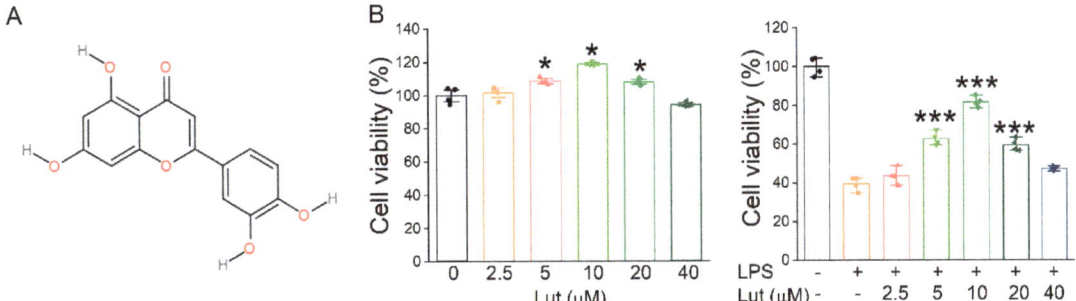

Figure 1. Effects of Lut on cell proliferation inhibited by LPS. (**A**) The molecular structure of Lut. (**B**) Left panel: Cell viability was detected after incubation with Lut (0, 2.5, 5, 10, 20, and 40 μM). * $p < 0.05$, compared with 0 μM group, $n = 4$. Mann–Whitney U test was used to analyze the difference of the means for significance. Right panel: Lut induced LPS-inhibited primary AT2 cell proliferation. *** $p < 0.001$, compared with LPS group, $n = 4$. One-way ANOVA followed by Bonferroni's test was used to analyze the difference of the means for significance.

As shown in Figure 2A, LPS reduced the quantity of α/γ-ENaC protein in AT2 cells compared with the Control group ($p < 0.01\sim0.05$), which was prominently alleviated after the Lut administration ($p < 0.001\sim0.05$ vs. LPS group). β-ENaC expression was not checked due to the lack of a suitable commercial antibody. Real-time polymerase chain reaction (PCR) assay showed that Lut eliminated the decrease in α/β/γ-ENaC mRNA induced by LPS (Figure 2B, $p < 0.05$ vs. LPS group), indicating that Lut may attenuate ALI by upregulating the expression of ENaC to improve transepithelial sodium transport. Consistently, the real-time PCR assay showed that LPS significantly increased the expression levels of inflammatory cytokines (Figure 2C, $p < 0.001\sim0.05$ vs. Control group), which were inhibited by Lut ($p < 0.01\sim0.05$ vs. LPS group).

2.2. Lut Suppressed Inflammatory Pulmonary Edema in ALI Mice

Through the prediction website pkCSM [23], we determined that the pharmacokinetic parameters for the logarithmic ratio of the partition coefficient (LogP), volume of distribution (VD_{ss} Log L/kg), total clearance (CL_{tot} Log mL/min/kg), and oral acute toxicity (LD_{50} mol/kg) were 2.2824, 1.153, 0.495, and 2.455, respectively. The results showed that Lut is a small molecule with good pharmacokinetic properties, exhibiting high intestinal absorption (>80%) and extensive distribution. Additionally, it serves as a substrate of P-glycoprotein and exhibits poor distribution in the brain. The in silico evaluation indicated that Lut has the potential to be developed as a pharmacological agent with suitable intestinal absorption and low toxicity.

To confirm the possible therapeutic action of Lut on ALI mice caused by LPS, we observed the appearance of the lungs and performed H&E for morphological research to evaluate the changes in histology. As expected, the photographs of LPS-treated lungs showed punctate hemorrhage and decreased surface smoothness, which were improved after the Lut administration (Figure 3A). Moreover, Lut significantly eliminated the LPS-induced increase in the lung wet/dry weight (W/D) ratio (Figure 3B, $p < 0.05$ vs. LPS group), which further implied that Lut could relieve the degree of pulmonary edema in ALI mice. Lung tissues in LPS group were significantly damaged, which were characterized by hemorrhage, inflammatory cell infiltration, and increased alveolar wall thickness and which were evidenced by an increased lung injury score (Figure 3C,D, $p < 0.05$ vs. Control group). As expected, Lut alleviated the histopathology changes in LPS-induced ALI mice ($p < 0.05$ vs. LPS group).

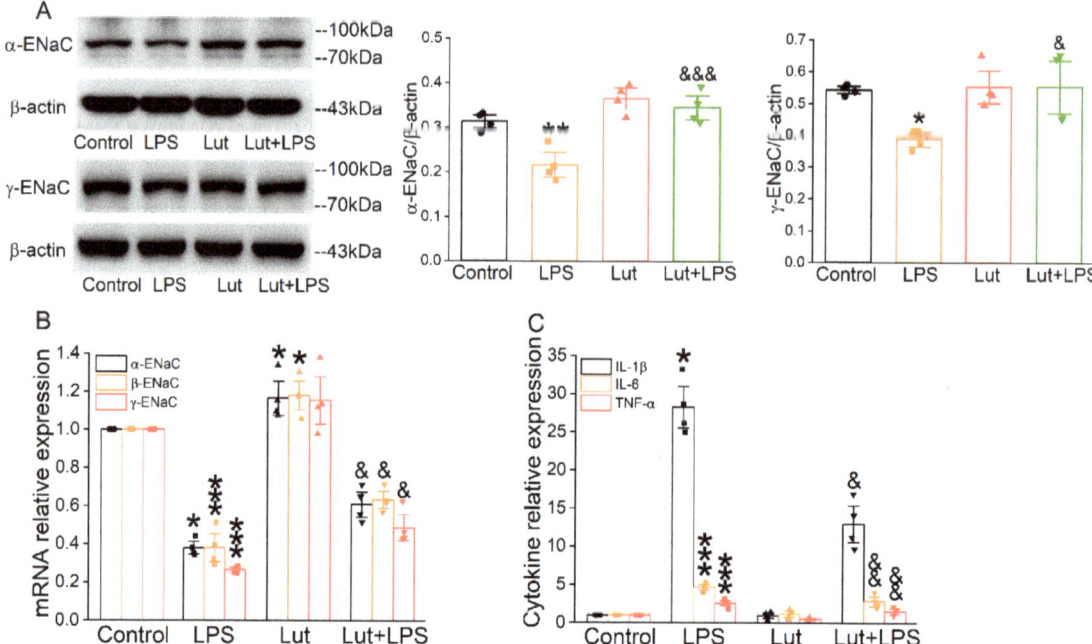

Figure 2. Lut increased the expression levels of ENaC and inhibited inflammation in primary AT2 cells. Cells were treated with Lut (10 µM, 24 h), co-presence or absence of LPS (10 µg/mL, 12 h). (**A**) Representative Western blot and corresponding graphical representation of data obtained from Western blot assays for α/γ-ENaC in primary AT2 cells, where bands were quantified using gray analysis (α, γ-ENaC/β-actin). * $p < 0.05$, ** $p < 0.01$, compared with Control group. & $p < 0.05$, &&& $p < 0.001$, compared with LPS group, $n = 4$. One-way ANOVA followed by Bonferroni's test was used to analyze the difference of the α-ENaC means for significance. Mann–Whitney U test was used to analyze the difference of the γ-ENaC means for significance. (**B**) The expression levels of α/β/γ-ENaC mRNA were examined by real-time PCR with GAPDH set as the internal standard. * $p < 0.05$, *** $p < 0.001$, compared with Control group. & $p < 0.05$, compared with LPS group, $n = 4$. Mann–Whitney U test was used to analyze the difference of the α/γ-ENaC means for significance. One-way ANOVA followed by Bonferroni's test was used to analyze the difference of the β-ENaC means for significance. (**C**) IL-1β, IL-6, and TNF-α levels in primary AT2 cells. * $p < 0.05$, *** $p < 0.001$, compared with Control group. & $p < 0.05$, && $p < 0.01$, compared with LPS group, $n = 4$–5. Mann–Whitney U test was used to analyze the difference of the IL-1β means for significance. One-way ANOVA followed by Bonferroni's test was used to analyze the difference of the IL-6/TNF-α means for significance.

Alteration of the alveolar–capillary barrier was evaluated by bronchoalveolar lavage fluid (BALF) protein concentration, which was reduced significantly by Lut (Figure 3E, $p < 0.001$ vs. LPS group). Meanwhile, Lut could reverse the LPS-increased inflammatory cytokines (Figure 3F, $p < 0.01$ vs. LPS group), supporting that inflammation reaction existed in the LPS-induced ALI model and that one of the beneficial effects of Lut may be associated with inflammation-related edema formation.

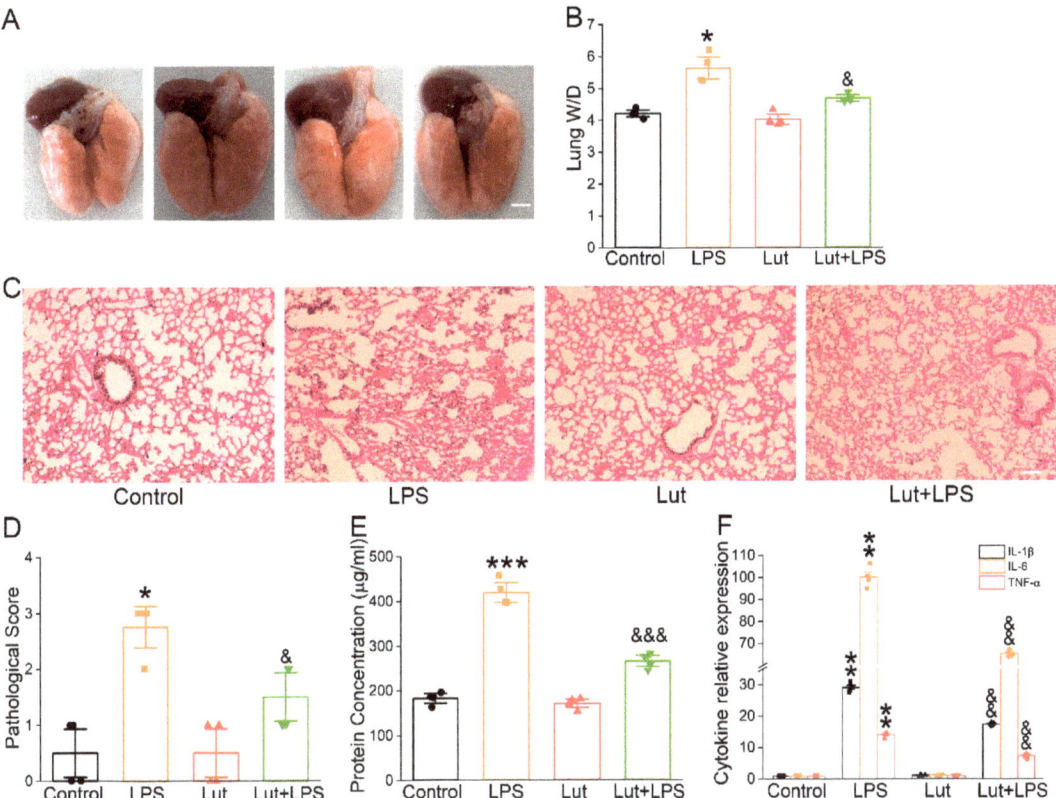

Figure 3. Effect of Lut on morphological structure and inflammation in LPS-induced ALI. Lut (20 mg/kg) was administered intraperitoneally to BALB/c mice 12 h before and after LPS (5 mg/kg) stimulation. (**A**) Representative photographs of whole lungs from all the experimental groups. Scale bar = 0.5 cm. (**B**) The lung W/D ratio was calculated as wet weight/dry weight. * $p < 0.05$, compared with Control group; $^{\&}$ $p < 0.05$, compared with LPS group, $n = 4$. Mann–Whitney U test was used to analyze the difference of the means for significance. (**C**) The effect of Lut was assessed by H&E staining. Scale bar = 200 μm. (**D**) Quantifying lung injury scores in the lungs. * $p < 0.05$, compared with Control group. $^{\&}$ $p < 0.05$, compared with LPS group, $n = 4$. Mann–Whitney U test was used to analyze the difference of the means for significance. (**E**) Protein content in BALF of mouse lung. *** $p < 0.001$, compared with Control group. $^{\&\&\&}$ $p < 0.001$, compared with LPS group $n = 4$. One-way ANOVA followed by Bonferroni's test was used to analyze the difference of the means for significance. (**F**) IL-1β, IL-6, and TNF-α levels in BALF of LPS-induced ALI. ** $p < 0.01$, compared with Control group. $^{\&\&}$ $p < 0.01$, compared with LPS group, $n = 6$. Mann–Whitney U test was used to analyze the difference of the means for significance.

2.3. Establishment of the 3D Alveolar Epithelial Organoids

The flow cytometry data showed that the purity of primary mouse AT2 cells was 81.33 ± 5.02% (Figure 4A), available for future co-culture with mouse lung fibroblasts. The 3D organoid cultures could be visualized between Days 4 and 12, and the number/size gradually increased over the culture time (Figure 4B). To better identify the 3D structure of alveolar epithelial organoids, we stained them with H&E and AT1 (PDPN)/AT2 (SP-C) markers, respectively. As shown in Figure 4C,D, monolayer-like alveolar epithelial cells were formed, and the confocal tomography identified that both AT1 and AT2 cell markers were expressed, suggesting that the lung alveolar model was successfully established.

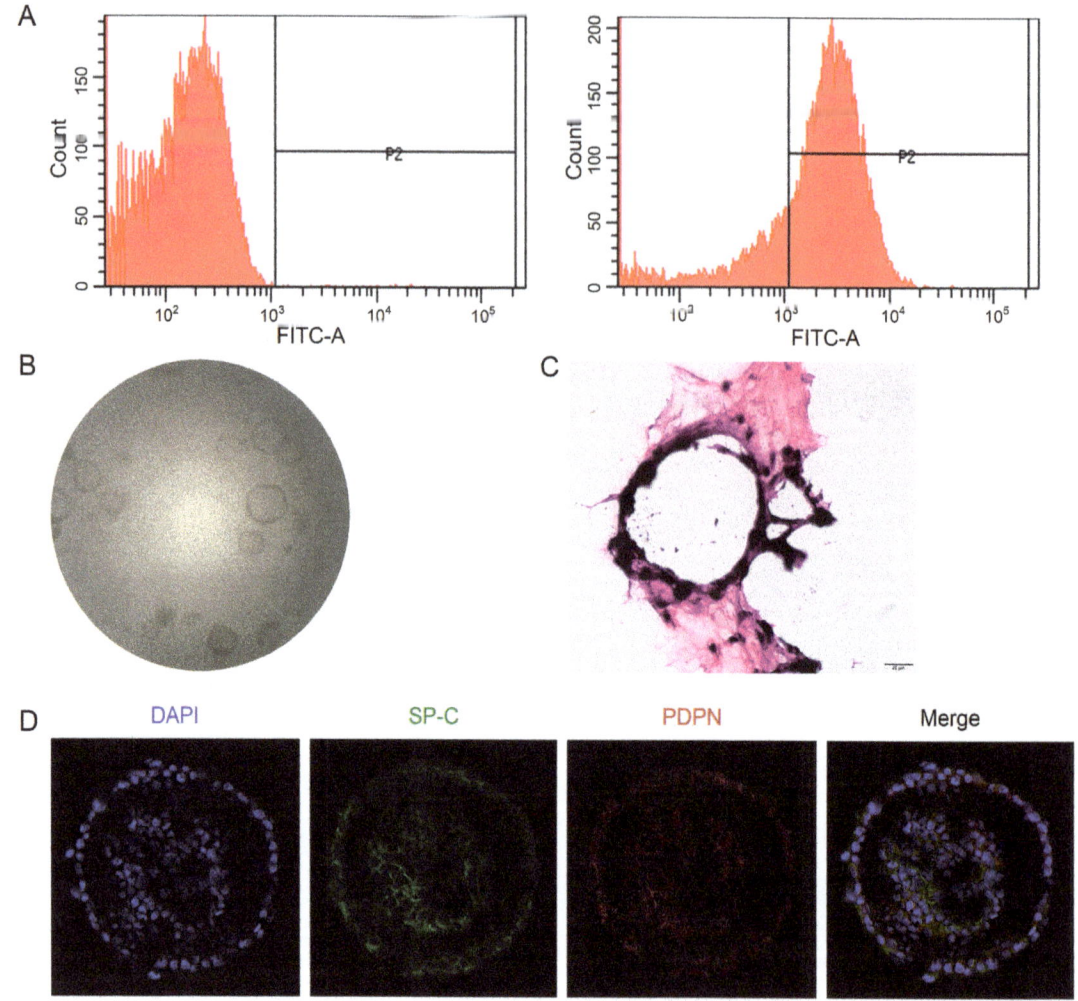

Figure 4. Establishment of 3D alveolar epithelial organoid model. (**A**) Representative data of flow cytometry for the purity of primary mouse AT2 cells (81.33 ± 5.02%), $n = 3$. (**B**) Representative DIC images of 3D organoid cultured for 8 days (40×). (**C**) H&E staining of 3D organoid culture. Scale bar, 20 μm. (**D**) Representative images of confocal images for 3D organoid stained with AT1 (PDPN)/AT2 (SP-C) markers. Scale bar, 50 μm.

2.4. Lut Elevated the Expression of ENaC in the Lung Alveolar Model

To verify the influence of Lut on the transepithelial sodium transport close to the in vivo ALI state, we used 3D alveolar epithelial organoid immunofluorescence assay to detect the ENaC protein expression level. The green fluorescence intensity of α/γ-ENaC in the LPS group was significantly lower than that in Control group (Figure 5A–C, $p < 0.001$~0.05), which was enhanced after the Lut administration ($p < 0.01$~0.05 vs. LPS group), identifying that Lut could strengthen the salt water absorption in LPS-induced ALI. Moreover, Lut reversed the LPS-reduced α/β/γ-ENaC mRNA expression in the alveolar model (Figure 5D, $p < 0.001$~0.05 vs. LPS group).

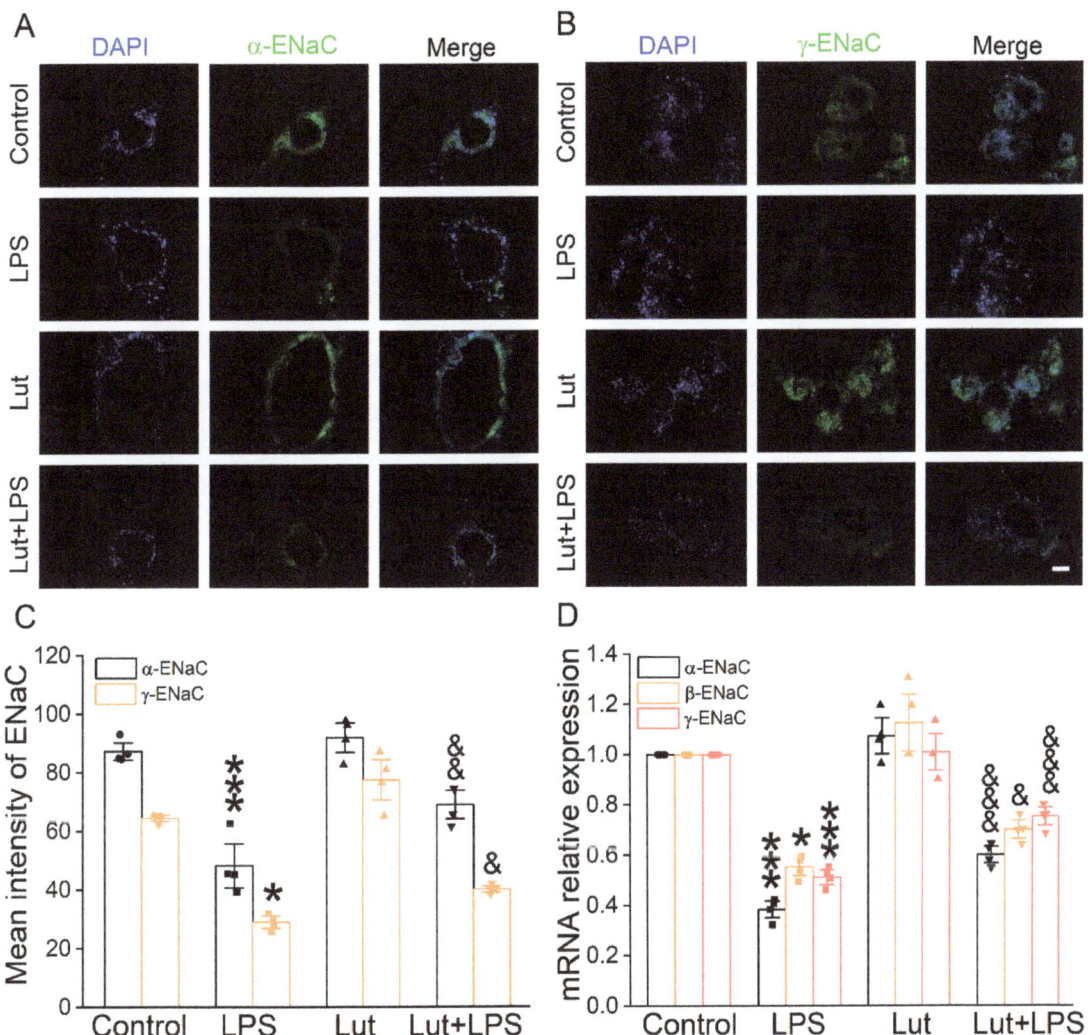

Figure 5. Effect of Lut on ENaC expression in 3D organoid culture. (**A,B**) Immunofluorescence staining showed the effect of LPS and Lut on the expression of α/γ-ENaC in 3D organoid culture. Scale bar, 50 μm. (**C**) Statistical diagram of α/γ-ENaC protein expression. * $p < 0.05$, *** $p < 0.001$, compared with Control group. & $p < 0.05$, && $p < 0.01$, compared with LPS group, $n = 4$. One-way ANOVA followed by Bonferroni's test was used to analyze the difference of the α-ENaC means for significance. Mann–Whitney U test was used to analyze the difference of the γ-ENaC means for significance. (**D**) The expression levels of α/β/γ-ENaC mRNA were examined by real-time PCR in 3D organoid culture. * $p < 0.05$, *** $p < 0.001$, compared with Control group. & $p < 0.05$, &&& $p < 0.001$, compared with LPS group, $n = 4$. One-way ANOVA followed by Bonferroni's test was used to analyze the difference of the α/γ-ENaC means for significance. Mann–Whitney U test was used to analyze the difference of the β-ENaC means for significance.

2.5. Target Identification and Protein–Protein Interaction Analysis

A total of 412 putative gene targets and 1980/1935 disease gene targets related to Lut and ALI/ARDS, respectively, were obtained, and the duplicates were removed. The protein targets were transformed to gene targets by the UniProt database. The intersection of putative Lut and ALI/ARDS disease targets resulted in 84 overlapping genes (Figure 6A), which were related to the Lut involvement of ALI/ARDS.

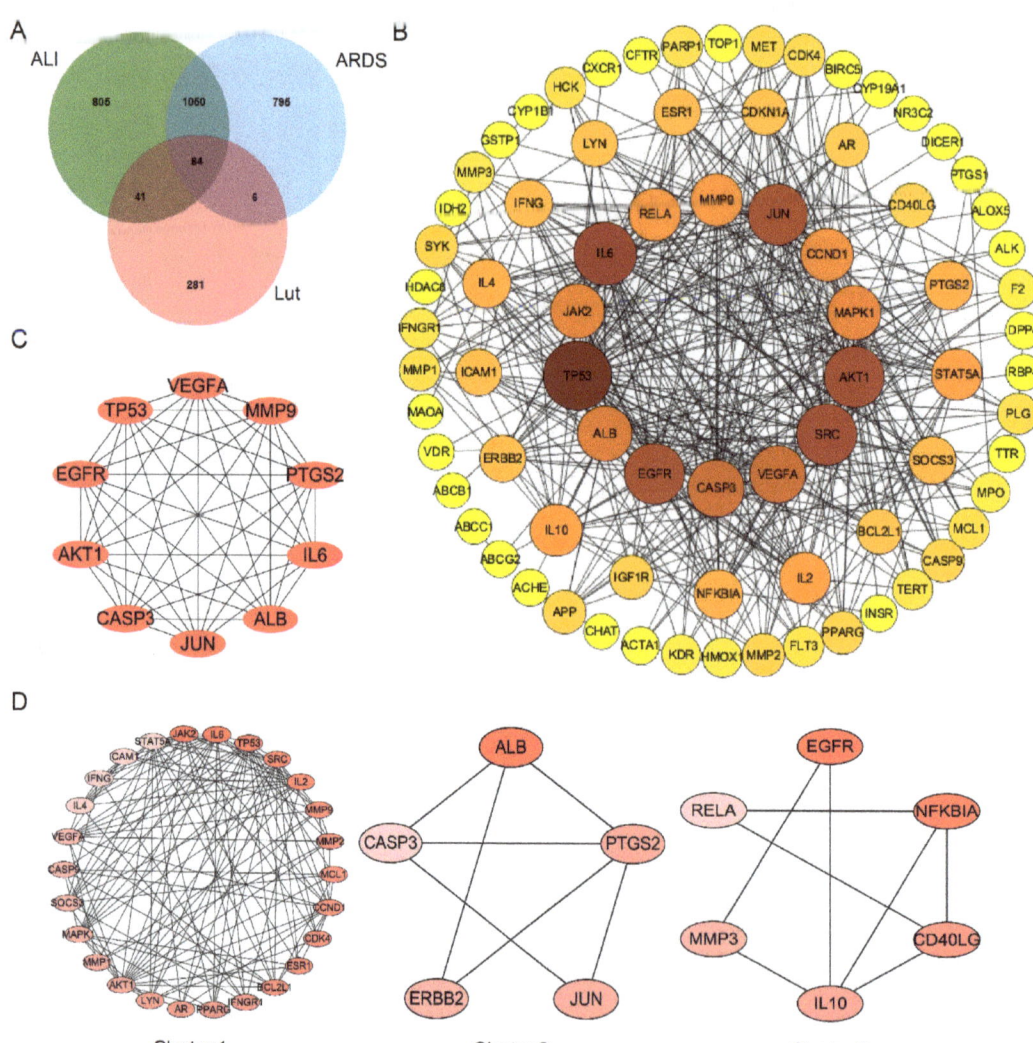

Figure 6. Bioinformatics analysis of overlapping genes. (**A**) Venn diagram of 84 overlapping genes between the predicted targets of Lut and the targets associated with ALI/ARDS. (**B**) PPI network of the 84 overlapping genes. The importance of each gene was analyzed by STRING. The higher the degree, the more crucial the gene. The degree of the outermost circle is 0–10, the middle circle is 11–20, and the smallest circle is >20. The colors of nodes from reddish to yellowish are arranged in descending order on the basis of their degree values. (**C**) Cytohubba, the plug-in of Cytoscape, was used to analyze the top 10 hub gene network of target proteins by MCC algorithm. (**D**) Cluster of the 84 overlapping gene-containing PPI network. Three clusters were identified. Cluster 1 had the highest score of 10.08, and JAK2 was identified as the seed gene. Cluster 2 had a score of 3.5, and ALB was the seed gene. Cluster 3 had a score of 3.2, and EGFR was the seed gene.

The protein–protein interaction (PPI) network was established using the String database to construct a drug–disease target interaction network. After removing free proteins that did not interact, there were 77 nodes (targets) and 430 edges (interactions) in the PPI network. The node size and color were positively correlated with degree, suggesting that darker and larger nodes played an important effect in the fight against ALI/ARDS (Figure 6B).

2.6. Screening of the Hub Genes and Clusters in the PPI Network

We used the MCC algorithm based on Cytoscape plug-in Cytohubba to screen out the top 10 Hub genes of target proteins and constructed the map of Hub gene network. TP53, VEGFA, MMP9, PTGS3, IL6, ALB, JUN, CASP3, AKT1, and EGFR were predicted to be the important targets for Lut intervention of ALI/ARDS (Figure 6C). We obtained three clusters using MCODE, among which Cluster 1 had the highest score of 10.080, and JAK2 was the seed gene (Figure 6D).

2.7. Prediction of the Potential Signaling Pathways of Lut for ALI Treatment

To explore the biological functions of Lut against ALI/ARDS, 84 genes were analyzed by GO analysis. The top 20 significantly enriched terms in GO and KEGG were selected, according to the analysis of GO term (MF) and KEGG pathway with pv < 0.05 and qv < 0.05. MF enrichment analysis was involved mainly with protein kinase and receptor ligand binding activity, which may be closely related to the pathological process of ALI/ARDS (Figure 7A).

The results of the KEGG pathways were related mainly to "PI3K/Akt", "multiplevirus infections", "JAK/STAT", and "HIF-1" (Figure 7B). The critical pathway target visualization network is shown in Figure 7C; the corresponding targets of Lut for treatment of ALI were closely related to the inflammatory reaction, in which the targets were focused mainly on the JAK/STAT pathway.

2.8. Binding Activities of Lut to the JAK/STAT Pathway

Lut was selected as a molecular ligand to dock with the JAK2, STAT3, and SOCS3 (component in the JAK/STAT pathway), respectively. As shown in Figure 8A–C, the affinities between the molecular ligand compound and the receptor proteins were all less than -5.0 kcal/mol, indicating that Lut possessed good binding activity with JAK2, STAT3, and SOCS3 proteins.

2.9. Validation of the Pathways and Targets

In order to verify the dependability of pathways and protein targets predicted by the network pharmacology and molecular docking simulations, we selected the key targets involved in the JAK/STAT pathway, including JAK2, STAT3, and SOCS3, for verification using Western blot assay. We knocked down STAT3 first in the primary AT2 cells, and the efficiency is shown in Figure 8D ($p < 0.05$ vs. Control group). LPS increased phospho-specific forms of JAK2 and STAT3 (Figure 8E, $p < 0.001\sim0.01$ vs. Control group), which were decreased after the Lut treatment ($p < 0.001\sim0.01$ vs. LPS + NC group), and the former was not affected by the knockdown of STAT3. Meanwhile, the LPS-reduced SOCS3 expression ($p < 0.001$ vs. Control group), a negative feedback regulator of JAK/STAT pathway, was inhibited by Lut with or without STAT3 knockdown ($p < 0.001$ vs. LPS + NC group or LPS + siSTAT3 group). As shown in Figure 8E, compared with that in Control, the α/γ-ENaC expression level in the LPS-treated AT2 cells was dramatically suppressed ($p < 0.01\sim0.001$ vs. Control group) and remarkably elevated by either the treatment of Lut or the lack of STAT3 ($p < 0.001\sim0.05$ vs. LPS + NC group). Intriguingly, the Lut-enhanced α/γ-ENaC expression was abolished after the co-administration of the STAT3 knockdown.

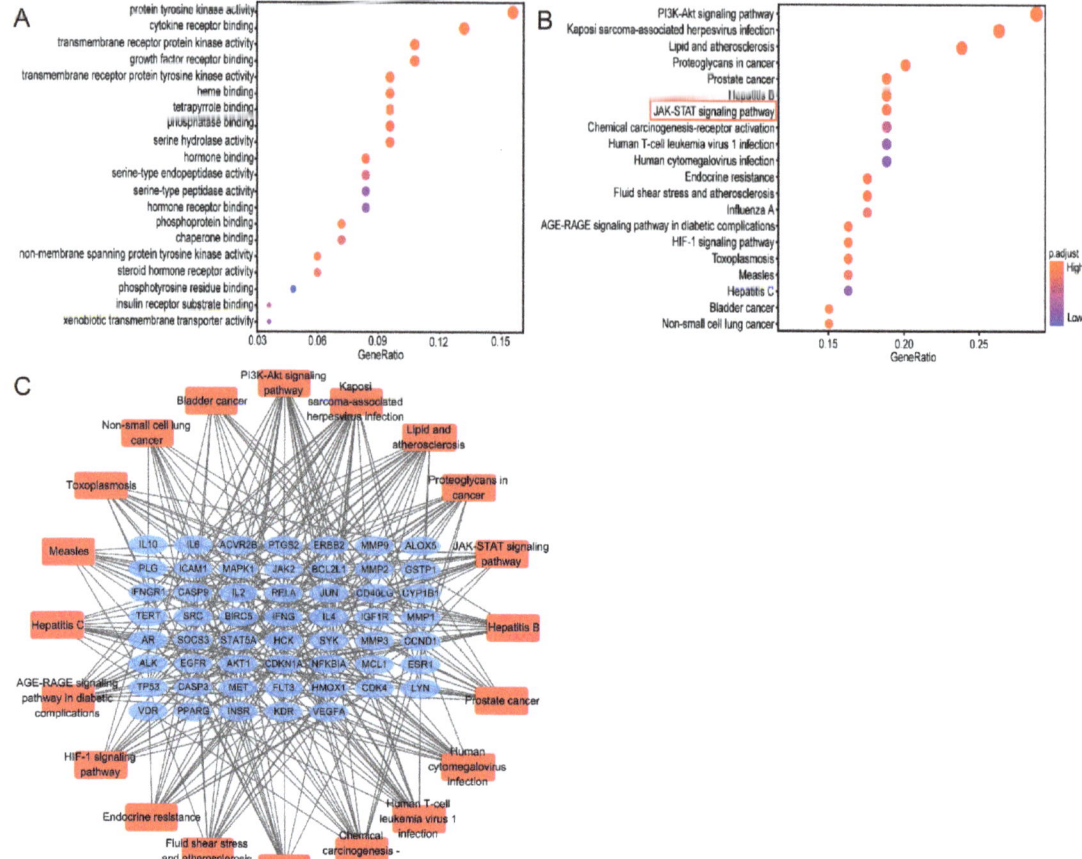

Figure 7. GO and KEGG analysis of 80 common genes. (**A**) A bubble chart of top 20 enriched GO items of potential targets in the molecular function. (**B**) Bubble chart of top 20 KEGG signaling pathways related to the effect of Lut against ALI. The redder the bubble, the smaller the P-value; the larger the bubble, the greater the number of genes that participated in this pathway. (**C**) The critical signaling pathway target visualization network. PPI network of the top 20 KEGG signaling pathways and associated target genes. Red nodes represent top 20 KEGG pathways, and blue nodes indicate the genes that participated.

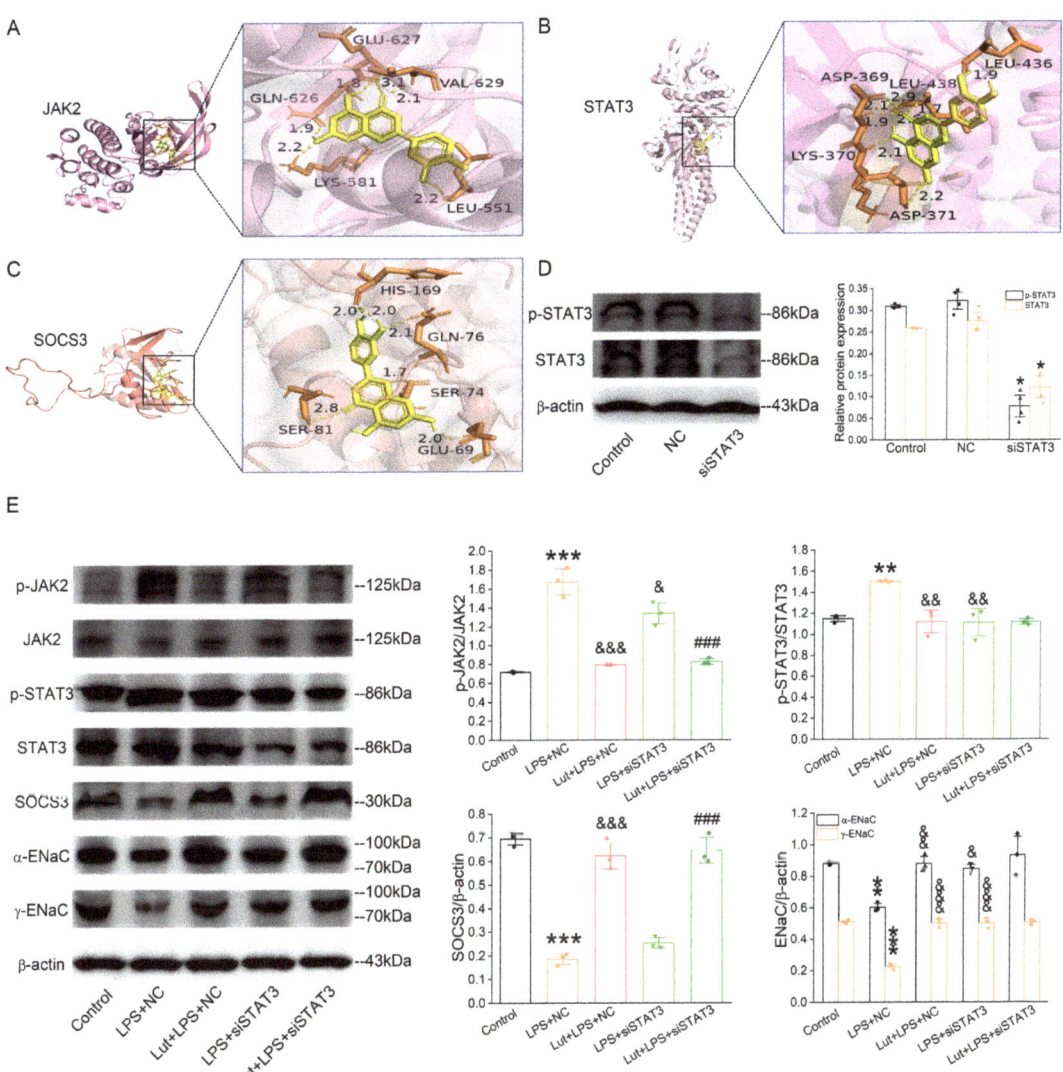

Figure 8. Lut suppressed the activation of JAK/STAT signaling pathway in 3D organoid culture. (**A–C**) Docking diagram of Lut with genes (JAK2, STAT3, and SOCS3) related to core pathway in KEGG of ALI. (**D**) Representative Western blot and corresponding graphical representation for p-STAT3/STAT3 of Control, NC (negative control), and siSTAT3 group in primary AT2 cells. * $p < 0.05$, compared with Control group, $n = 4$. Mann–Whitney U test was used to analyze the difference of the means for significance. (**E**) Representative Western blot and corresponding graphical representation for p-JAK2/JAK2, p-STAT3/STAT3, α/γ-EnaC, and SOCS3 in primary AT2 cells. ** $p < 0.01$, *** $p < 0.001$, compared with Control group. & $p < 0.01$, && $p < 0.01$, &&& $p < 0.001$, compared with LPS + NC group, ### $p < 0.001$, compared with LPS + siSTAT3 group, $n = 3$–4. One-way ANOVA followed by Bonferroni's test was used to analyze the difference of the means for significance.

3. Discussion

Numerous lines of evidence indicate that exposure to LPS stimulation can elicit an inflammatory response and other pulmonary lesions, ultimately leading to the development of respiratory disorders. Serious pulmonary infection involved with LPS is a high risk factor for ALI/ARDS, which can cause inflammatory cells to recruit into the lung, an increase in capillary permeability, and alveolar edema [24–26]. The morphological changes caused by LPS were significant inflammatory cell infiltration, alleviation by hemorrhage, and thickness of the alveolar wall after the Lut treatment. In addition, the pulmonary W/D ratio, which illustrates the amount of exudate in the lungs, was significantly reduced, proving that Lut had a significant anti-edema effect on ALI. Our results also showed that Lut reduced the protein content and inflammatory cytokines in BALF after lung injury, suggesting that Lut alleviated the occurrence of LPS-induced protein-rich alveolar edema and protected the alveolar–capillary barrier.

Na^+ enters AT2 cells mainly through apical ENaC, which is then pumped out by basolateral Na^+ and K^+-ATPase, accompanied by reabsorption of osmotic fluid [27–29]. The main determinant of alveolar fluid clearance is ENaC expressed on the apical side of AT2 cells [30,31]. In this study, primary AT2 cells of mice were isolated, and the results showed that Lut could reverse the LPS-induced decrease in ENaC expression at both the protein and transcription levels, suggesting that Lut could improve transepithelial sodium transport by upregulating ENaC expression.

However, the inability to maintain biological characteristics of primary AT2 cells during culture has been an important obstacle in the research of pulmonary biology. Primary AT2 cells can hardly be passaged by traditional culture methods, and they lose their characteristic cuboid-like appearance with the culture time. Meanwhile, the production of surface active substances decreases, and lamellar bodies are lost [32]. Compared with traditional 2D cell culture, the 3D alveolar epithelial organoids contain a variety of cell types and exhibit closer cellular interactions with the stroma, resulting in functional micro-organs that better simulate the physiological and pathological processes of organ tissues. We, thus, selected AT2 cells and MLg cells of mice to co-culture in matrix glue to construct the lung alveolar model using 3D alveolar epithelial organoids [11]. During the culture, we added a TGF-β inhibitor to prevent excessive proliferation of MLg cells, and we promoted the AT2 cell differentiation by inhibiting the TGF-β receptor signaling. The 3D alveolar epithelial organoids were certified through confocal images by co-expression of AT1 and AT2 cell markers (PDPN/SP-C), as well as alveolar epithelial structure by H&E staining. In addition, immunofluorescence and real-time PCR assay were performed on this model, which showed that Lut could reverse LPS-reduced ENaC expression at both the protein and transcription levels.

LPS can activate the natural immune response and secrete a large number of inflammatory cytokines, such as TNF-α, IL-6, and IL-1β, the contents of which in BALF directly reflect the degree of inflammatory response in the alveolar cavity [33,34]. In addition, current research has suggested that epithelial cells are also involved in regulating inflammation and lung defense, in which AT2 cells serve as one of the main sources of neutrophil chemokines [35]. Our results showed that Lut had a significant anti-inflammatory effect on the LPS-induced mouse ALI model. Meanwhile, Lut reversed the LPS-reduced mRNA expression of IL-1β, IL-6, and TNF-α in primary mouse AT2 cells. The data proved that Lut could alleviate ALI through enhancing ENaC expression in both the primary AT2 cells and 3D alveolar epithelial organoid model, which lays a foundation for the mechanism of Lut relieving inflammation-related pulmonary edema and provides a potential therapeutic strategy for treating ALI (Figure 9).

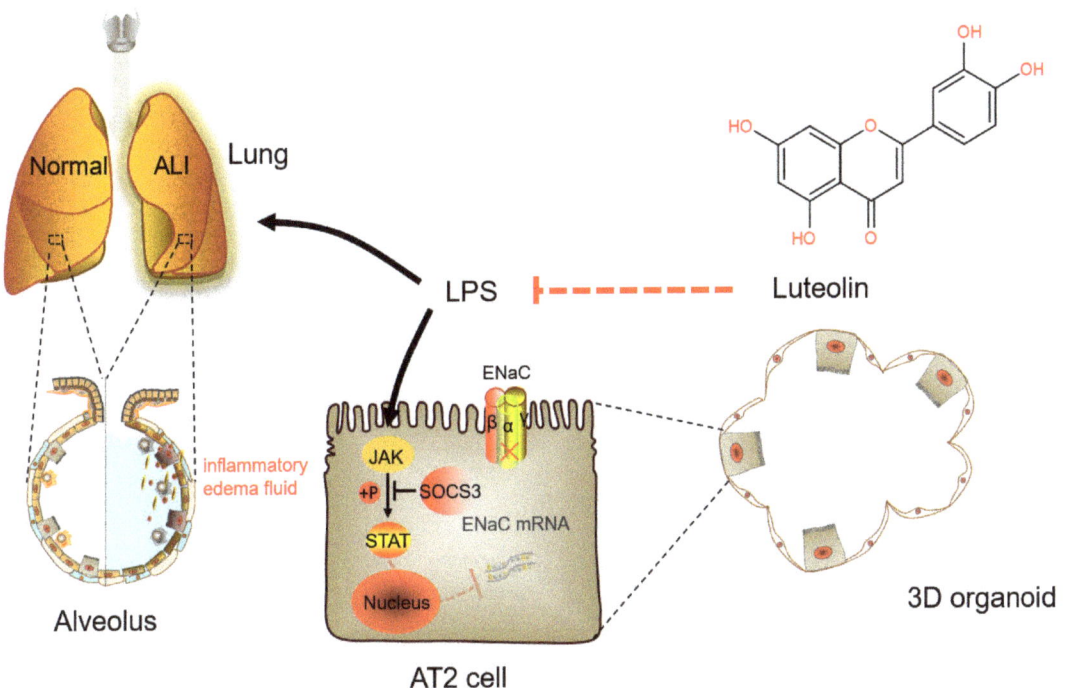

Figure 9. A schematic diagram for Lut to enhance the expression of ENaC in LPS-induced ALI. Lut can interdict the effect of LPS by increasing the expression of ENaC mRNA and protein via JAK/STAT pathway, as well as inhibiting the secretion of inflammatory cytokines in LPS-induced ALI. ALI, acute lung injury; AT2, alveolar epithelial type 2; ENaC, epithelial sodium channel; LPS, lipopolysaccharide.

The network pharmacology was applied to explore the inter-relationship between pharmaceuticals and diseases for various purposes, such as finding new drugs, elucidating pathogenesis, and discovering new targets [36–38]. We used the drug–disease network for topological analysis and applied the corresponding molecular docking method to improve the dependability of the target prediction results. Interactions between Lut and possible protein targets were predicted by combining messages from free databases relating ALI/ARDS, together with revealing the signaling networks in which the Lut targets participated. Hydrogen bonding seemed to be the main interaction form, according to the molecular docking analysis. Pathway relationship uncovered that the Lut-regulated signaling pathways contained mainly PI3K/Akt, multiple virus infections and JAK/STAT in ALI/ARDS. TP53, IL6, AKT1, SRC, JUN, EGFR, VEGFA, CASP3, ALB, JAK2, MAPK1, CCND1, RELA, and MMP9 were key genes with high degree values > 20. Through analyzing the Hub genes and the predominant KEGG pathways, the possible mechanisms of Lut in handling ALI/ARDS might be due to the JAK/STAT signaling pathway, which could modulate oxidative stress, cell apoptosis, and inflammation in an ALI model [39]. In our study, the treatment of Lut enhanced the SOCS3 expression and inhibited the phosphorylation level of JAK2 and STAT3 induced by LPS in the primary mouse AT2 cells. The knockdown of STAT3 did not affect the above effects of Lut on JAK2 phosphorylation or SOCS3 expression, indicating that they were upstream molecules for STAT3. Furthermore, siSTAT3 could abrogate the Lut enhancement of ENaC protein expression, implying a downstream mechanism involved with the STAT3 signal. Overall, Lut could attenuate inflammation-related ALI by enhancing transepithelial sodium transport, at least partially, via the JAK/STAT pathway.

4. Materials and Methods

4.1. Reagents

Lut (CAS: 491-70-3, purity 98%), LPS (purity 98%), and 4′, 6-diamidino-2-phenylindole (DAPI) were purchased from Solarbio Science & Technology Co., Ltd. (Beijing, China). BCA protein detection and H&E kits were purchased from Beyotime Biological Co. (Shanghai, China). Dispase II, DNase I, and Matrigel were provided by Sigma-Aldrich (St. Louis, MO, USA). Low-melting-point agarose and primers were obtained from Sangon Biotech Co., Ltd. (Shanghai, China). Biotinylated antibodies CD16/32 and CD45 were provided by Miltenyi Biotec (Shanghai, China), and the information about specific antibodies are listed in Table 1. ELISA and CCK-8 kits were purchased from Neobioscience Technology Company (Shenzhen, China) and Biosharp Biological Technology Co., Ltd. (Guangzhou, China), respectively.

Table 1. The information about the antibodies.

Antibody	Manufacture	WB	IF	FCM
SP-C	Bioss (Beijing, China)		1:100	1:100
PDPN	Santa Cruz (Dallas, TX, USA)		1:100	
p-STAT3	Affinity (Cincinnati, OH, USA)	1:1000		
p-JAK2	Affinity (Cincinnati, OH, USA)	1:1000		
STAT3	Affinity (Cincinnati, OH, USA)	1:1000		
JAK2	Affinity (Cincinnati, OH, USA)	1:1000		
SOCS3	Affinity (Cincinnati, OH, USA)	1:1000		
α-ENaC	Santa Cruz (Dallas, TX, USA)	1:2000	1:200	
γ-ENaC	Santa Cruz (Dallas, TX, USA)	1:2000	1:200	
β-actin	Santa Cruz (Dallas, TX, USA)	1:1000		
goat anti-mouse	ZSGB-BIO (Beijing, China)	1:5000		
goat anti-rabbit	ZSGB-BIO (Beijing, China)	1:5000		
FITC goat anti-rabbit	ZSGB-BIO (Beijing, China)		1:100	1:200
TRITC goat anti-mouse	ZSGB-BIO (Beijing, China)		1:100	

WB: Western blot, IF: immunofluorescence, FCM: flow cytometry.

4.2. Animals

The Laboratory Animal Center of China Medical University provided the mice, with the certificate number: SYXK (Liao) 2018-0008. Animal experiments were conducted under the guidelines and regulations of Animal Care and Use Ethics Committee. Animals were anesthetized with diazepam (17.5 mg/kg), followed by ketamine (450 mg/kg).

4.3. Primary Mouse AT2 Cell Culture and Cell Viability Analysis

The primary AT2 cells were isolated from mice and cultured as described earlier [40]. Then, the separated primary cells were modulated to 2.5×10^6 cells/mL in DMEM/F12 medium with FBS (10%, Gibco, New York, NY, USA), penicillin (100 IU), and streptomycin (100 µg/mL). The medium was replaced first after 72 h and then every other day thereafter.

The optimal concentration of Lut was detected by CCK8 assay [41]. The primary AT2 cells were incubated with Lut (0, 2.5, 5, 10, 20, and 40 µM) with or without LPS (10 µg/mL) for 24 h. After treatment, the viability of cells was measured by a CCK-8 kit (Biosharp, Guangzhou, China) according to the manufacturer's protocol. In the following cellular experiments, the primary AT2 cells were treated with Lut (10 µM, 24 h) and/or LPS (10 µg/mL, 12 h), respectively.

4.4. Establishment of the ALI Mouse Model

The healthy BALB/c male mice with body weight of 20–25 g were randomly divided into the following 4 groups: Control, LPS, Lut, and Lut + LPS. ALI animal model was established by intraperitoneal injection of LPS (5 mg/kg, Solarbio, Beijing, China) [21]. The mice in Lut and Lut + LPS groups were intraperitoneally injected with Lut (70 μmol/kg, Solarbio, Beijing, China) twice, 12 h before and after LPS injection [42].

4.5. Preparation for 3D Organoid Culture

Adult mouse lungs were used for the isolation of AT2 cells [11]. In brief, the lung was perfused with 4 °C PBS. After trachea intubation, dispase II (3 mg/mL, Corning, New York, NY, USA) was injected into the lung, followed by 1% low-melting-point agarose (42–45 °C, Sangon Biotech, Shanghai, China). Then, the lung was incubated in dispase II for 45 min at 37 °C and gently torn in DMEM/F12 + DNase I (0.01%, Sigma, St. Louis, MO, USA). The cell suspension was passed through serial filters (Solarbio, Beijing, China) and incubated with biotinylated antibodies: CD16/32 and CD45 (Miltenyi Biotec, Shanghai, China) for 10 min. After being incubated with 10 μL Streptavidin MicroBeads (4 °C, Miltenyi Biotec, Shanghai, China) for 15 min in dark, the cells were transferred onto plates pre-coated with 1 mg/mL IgG for 2 h, and the unattached cells were collected. The cell purity was detected by flow cytometry with corresponding antibodies.

4.6. Identification of 3D Alveolar Epithelial Organoid

Mouse AT2 cells (6×10^3) and MLg2908 cells (2×10^5, American Type Culture Collection) were suspended in a 1:1 mixture of growth-factor-reduced Matrigel (Corning, New York, NY, USA) on polyester membrane cell culture transwells (0.4 μm pore size, 0.33 cm^2 area, Corning, New York, NY, USA) and incubated for 30 min to allow the matrix to solidify.

After fixation, permeabilization, and blocking, the 3D organic cultures were incubated with SP-C and PDPN antibody overnight at 4 °C, respectively. The information about the antibodies are listed in Table 1. The nucleus was stained by DAPI. Finally, the sections were imaged by confocal microscopy.

4.7. Determination of Lung Wet/Dry Weight Ratio

The degree of pneumonedema was analyzed by lung W/D ratio to assess the severity of ALI. The lung W/D ratio was acquired by dividing the wet weight by the lung weight after 48 h of oven drying at 60 °C.

4.8. Bronchoalveolar Lavage Fluid Analysis

We collected the BALF to evaluate the extent of lung inflammation [43–45]. Alteration of the barrier between alveolar and capillary was evaluated depending on the BALF protein content via BCA kit (Beyotime Biotechnology, Shanghai, China), and the inflammatory cytokines were tested by ELISA assay (Neobioscience, Shenzhen, China).

4.9. Histological Studies

Freshly harvested lung tissues and 3D organoid cultures were fixed, dehydrated, and embedded in 4% paraformaldehyde, 30% sucrose, and OCT, respectively. To semi-quantify the histopathologic changes in H&E (Beyotime Biotechnology, Shanghai, China) staining, the Szapiel score was used to quantify alveolitis and determine the severity of lung injury through the score of 0 (no injury) to 3 (maximum injury) [46].

4.10. Real-Time PCR

The total RNA (1 μg) in samples was extracted and acquired by TRIzol (Invitrogen, Carlsbad, CA, USA) and used as the template for reverse transcription in triplicate. Real-time PCR was processed with the primers shown in Table 2. Reaction was processed with 95 °C (30 s), followed by 50 cycles of 95 °C (5 s), 52 °C (30 s), and 72 °C (60 s). The relative expression level of mRNA was obtained by $2^{-\Delta(\Delta CT)}$ comparative method.

Table 2. The information about the primers.

Primer Name	Forward (5′–3′)	Reverse (5′–3′)
α-ENaC	AAC AAA TCG GACTGC TTC TAC	AGC CAC CAT CAT CCA TAA A
β-ENaC	GGG ACC AAA GCA CCA AT	CAG ACG CAG GGA GTC ATAG
γ-ENaC	GCACCG TTC GCC ACC TTC TA	AGG TCA CCA GCA GCT CCT CA
IL-1β	AGA AGC TGT GGC AGC TAC CTG	GGA AAA GAA GGT GCT CAT GTC C
IL-6	GCT ACC AAA CTG GAT ATA ATC AGG A	CCA GGT AGC TAT GGT ACT CCA GAA
TNF-α	TCT TCT CAT TCC TGC TTG TGG	GGT CTG GGG CCA TAG AAC TGA
GAPDH	AGA AGG CTG GGG CTC ATT TG	AGG GGC CAT CCA CAG TCT TC

4.11. Immunofluorescence Assay

The AT2 cells were incubated with primary α-ENaC and γ-ENaC antibodies, respectively, and then with secondary antibody (Table 1). After the nuclei were stained by DAPI, the sections were observed by a fluorescence microscope, and target proteins were quantified through Image J software.

4.12. Target Prediction

The potential targets of Lut were acquired from Traditional Chinese Medicine Systems Pharmacology (TCMSP, https://tcmsp-e.com/tcmsp.php), SwissTargetPredictive (http://www.swisstargetprediction.ch), and PharmMapper (http://www.lilab-ecust.cn/pharmmapper). By converting protein targets into gene targets by the database of UniProt (http://www.uniprot.org) and removing duplicate genes, we obtained 412 related genes.

The disease targets of ALI/ARDS were obtained from databases including DrugBank (https://go.drugbank.com), GeneCards (https://www.genecards.org, accessed on 3 November 2022), PharmGKb (https://www.pharmgkb.org), and Online Mendelian Inheritance in Man (OMIM, https://omim.org). The 1980/1935 related genes in ALI/ARDS were obtained by merging the 4 disease database targets and deleting the duplicates.

4.13. Constructing Protein–Protein Interaction Networks

The intersection between disease and drug targets was captured by Venny 2.1 (https://bioinfogp.cnb.csic.es/tools/venny), and the Venn diagram was drawn. There were 84 common targets between Lut and ALI/ARDS.

By using the limitation to "Homo sapiens" and confidence score ≥ 0.7, the 84 overlapped target PPI networks were obtained by the database of String (https://string-db.org). The PPI network containing the degree values of nodes was generated by Cytoscape v3.7.2. In Cytohubba plugin of CytoScape, PPI network Hub genes for Lut against ALI/ARDS were calculated by MCC algorithm, and 10 core targets were acquired to construct the related protein target networks. The major dense regions were selected from the network of 84 overlapped genes using Cytoscape plugin Molecular Complex Detection, in which seed genes were present in clusters with the largest MCODE Score. The following settings were used: Degree Cut-off = 2, Node Score Cut-off = 0.2, K-Core = 2, and Max Depth = 100.

4.14. Pathway Enrichment Analysis

Annotation, Visualization, Integrated Discovery (https://david.ncifcrf.gov), and Kyoto Encyclopedia of Genes and Genomes (KEGG, www.kegg.jp/kegg) were used for pathway enrichment analysis. $p < 0.05$ in KEGG enrichments was considered significant.

4.15. Molecular Docking Analysis

The docking ligand of Lut 3D structure in PDBQT format was obtained from the PubChem database and Chem3D software. PyMol (https://pymol.org/2) was used to delete water molecules and add hydrogen bonds of protein conformation, which was acquired from the PDB (https://www.rcsb.org). AutoDock Tools V1.5.6 (http://autodock.scripps.edu) software was used to detect the roots, set the rotatable key, calculate the Gasteiger charge, and identify the binding pockets. Then, AutoDockVinaV1.1.2 was used for molecular docking, and the results were visualized using PyMol software.

4.16. Western Blot Assay

Proteins were separated and transferred to PVDF membranes (Invitrogen, Waltham, MA, USA), which were then incubated with primary and secondary antibodies, respectively. The information about the antibodies is also listed in Table 1. Finally, the protein bands were visualized by ECL kit and quantitatively analyzed by the Image J.

4.17. Statistical Analysis

We applied Origin 2021 software to process the data as mean ± SE and assessed the power of sample size firstly to meet $p < 0.05$. When the data passed the Levene's test for normality and Shapiro–Wilk's test for heteroscedasticity, one-way analysis of variance (ANOVA) and Bonferroni's test was used for comparison among multiple groups. If the data did not pass the normality and heteroscedasticity tests, the non-parametric t-test (Mann–Whitney U test) was applied.

Author Contributions: Conceptualization, Y.D. and L.C.; methodology, T.Y.; software, Y.D. and T.Y.; validation, Y.D. and X.L.; formal analysis, L.C. and Y.Z.; investigation, X.L.; resources, Y.D.; data curation, L.C.; writing—original draft preparation, L.C.; writing—review and editing, Y.D. and H.N.; visualization, Y.D.; supervision, X.L.; project administration, H.N.; funding acquisition, H.N. All authors have read and agreed to the published version of the manuscript.

Funding: This research was funded by National Natural Science Foundation of China, grant number 82170093.

Institutional Review Board Statement: The animal study protocol was approved by the guidelines and regulations of Animal Care and Use Ethics Committee. The experimental protocols were approved by China Medical University, and the certificate number is SYXK (Liao) 2018-0008.

Informed Consent Statement: Not applicable.

Data Availability Statement: All data/code generated or analyzed during this study are available from the corresponding author on reasonable request.

Acknowledgments: The authors appreciated the support from Aixin Han in manuscript preparation and technical assistance.

Conflicts of Interest: The authors declare no conflict of interest.

References

1. Xie, X.; Yu, T.; Hou, Y.; Han, A.; Ding, Y.; Nie, H.; Cui, Y. Ferulic acid ameliorates lipopolysaccharide-induced tracheal injury via cGMP/PKGII signaling pathway. *Respir. Res.* **2021**, *22*, 308. [CrossRef] [PubMed]
2. Jiang, Y.; Xia, M.; Xu, J.; Huang, Q.; Dai, Z.; Zhang, X. Dexmedetomidine alleviates pulmonary edema through the epithelial sodium channel (ENaC) via the PI3K/Akt/Nedd4-2 pathway in LPS-induced acute lung injury. *Immunol. Res.* **2021**, *69*, 162–175. [CrossRef] [PubMed]
3. Guillot, L.; Nathan, N.; Tabary, O.; Thouvenin, G.; Le Rouzic, P.; Corvol, H.; Amselem, S.; Clement, A. Alveolar epithelial cells: Master regulators of lung homeostasis. *Int. J. Biochem. Cell Biol.* **2013**, *45*, 2568–2573. [CrossRef] [PubMed]
4. Ruaro, B.; Salton, F. The history and mystery of alveolar epithelial type II cells: Focus on their physiologic and pathologic role in lung. *Int. J. Mol. Sci.* **2021**, *22*, 2566–2582. [CrossRef] [PubMed]
5. Wu, A.; Song, H. Regulation of alveolar type 2 stem/progenitor cells in lung injury and regeneration. *Acta Biochim. Biophys. Sin.* **2020**, *52*, 716–722. [CrossRef] [PubMed]
6. Zhou, W.; Yu, T.; Hua, Y.; Hou, Y.; Ding, Y.; Nie, H. Effects of hypoxia on respiratory diseases: Perspective view of epithelial ion transport. *Am. J. Physiol. Lung Cell. Mol. Physiol.* **2022**, *323*, L240–L250. [CrossRef] [PubMed]
7. Wu, W.; Zhong, W.; Lin, Z.; Yan, J. Blockade of Indoleamine 2,3-Dioxygenase attenuates lipopolysaccharide-induced kidney injury by inhibiting TLR4/NF-κB signaling. *Clin. Exp. Nephrol.* **2023**, *27*, 495–505. [CrossRef] [PubMed]
8. Peng, K.; Yang, F.; Qiu, C.; Yang, Y.; Lan, C. Rosmarinic acid protects against lipopolysaccharide-induced cardiac dysfunction via activating Sirt1/PGC-1α pathway to alleviate mitochondrial impairment. *Clin. Exp. Pharmacol. Physiol.* **2023**, *50*, 218–227. [CrossRef]

9. Yang, T.; Zhao, S.; Sun, N.; Zhao, Y.; Wang, H.; Zhang, Y.; Hou, X.; Tang, Y.; Gao, X.; Fan, H. Network pharmacology and in vivo studies reveal the pharmacological effects and molecular mechanisms of Celastrol against acute hepatic injury induced by LPS. *Int. Immunopharmacol.* **2023**, *117*, 109898. [CrossRef]
10. Zhang, H.; Cui, Y.; Zhou, Z.; Ding, Y.; Nie, H. Alveolar type 2 epithelial cells as potential therapeutics for acute lung injury/acute respiratory distress syndrome. *Curr. Pharm. Des.* **2019**, *25*, 4077–4082. [CrossRef]
11. Zhang, M.; Ali, G.; Komatsu, S.; Zhao, R.; Ji, H.L. Prkg2 regulates alveolar type 2-mediated re-alveolarization. *Stem Cell Res. Ther.* **2022**, *13*, 111. [CrossRef] [PubMed]
12. Li, Y.; Wu, Q.; Sun, X.; Shen, J.; Chen, H.Y. Organoids as a powerful model for respiratory diseases. *Stem Cells Int.* **2020**, *2020*, 5847876. [CrossRef] [PubMed]
13. Ahmed, H.M. Ethnomedicinal, phytochemical and pharmacological investigations of *Perilla frutescens* (L.) britt. *Molecules* **2018**, *24*, 102. [CrossRef] [PubMed]
14. Yu, H.; Qiu, J.F.; Ma, L.J.; Hu, Y.J.; Li, P.; Wan, J.B. Phytochemical and phytopharmacological review of *Perilla frutescens* L. (Labiatae), a traditional edible-medicinal herb in China. *Food Chem. Toxicol.* **2017**, *108*, 375–391. [CrossRef] [PubMed]
15. Chen, X.; Xu, X.; Lv, J.; Huang, J.; Lyu, L.; Liu, L. Potential mechanisms of perillae folium against COVID-19: A network pharmacology approach. *J. Med. Food* **2023**. *ahead of print*. [CrossRef] [PubMed]
16. Zhang, M.; He, L.; Liu, J.; Zhou, L. Luteolin attenuates diabetic nephropathy through suppressing inflammatory response and oxidative stress by inhibiting STAT3 pathway. *Exp. Clin. Endocrinol. Diabetes* **2021**, *129*, 729–739. [CrossRef]
17. Imran, M.; Rauf, A.; Abu-Izneid, T.; Nadeem, M.; Shariati, M.A.; Khan, I.A.; Imran, A.; Orhan, I.E.; Rizwan, M.; Atif, M.; et al. Luteolin, a flavonoid, as an anticancer agent: A review. *Biomed. Pharmacother.* **2019**, *112*, 108612–108621. [CrossRef]
18. Ganai, S.A.; Sheikh, F.A.; Baba, Z.A.; Mir, M.A.; Mantoo, M.A.; Yatoo, M.A. Anticancer activity of the plant flavonoid luteolin against preclinical models of various cancers and insights on different signalling mechanisms modulated. *Phytother. Res.* **2021**, *35*, 3509–3532. [CrossRef]
19. Park, E.J.; Kim, Y.M.; Kim, H.J.; Chang, K.C. Luteolin activates ERK1/2− and Ca^{2+}-dependent HO$_{-1}$ induction that reduces LPS-induced HMGB1, iNOS/NO, and COX$_{-2}$ expression in RAW264.7 cells and mitigates acute lung injury of endotoxin mice. *Inflamm. Res.* **2018**, *67*, 445–453. [CrossRef]
20. Xie, K.; Chai, Y.S.; Lin, S.H. Luteolin regulates the differentiation of regulatory T cells and activates IL-10 dependent macrophage polarization against acute lung injury. *J. Immunol. Res.* **2021**, *2021*, 8883962. [CrossRef]
21. Hou, Y.; Li, J.; Ding, Y.; Cui, Y.; Nie, H. Luteolin attenuates lipopolysaccharide-induced acute lung injury/acute respiratory distress syndrome by activating alveolar epithelial sodium channels via cGMP/PI3K pathway. *J. Ethnopharmacol.* **2022**, *282*, 114654. [CrossRef] [PubMed]
22. Yang, R.; Yang, H.; Wei, J.; Li, W.; Yue, F.; Song, Y.; He, X.; Hu, K. Mechanisms underlying the effects of Lianhua Qingwen on sepsis-induced acute lung injury: A network pharmacology approach. *Front. Pharmacol.* **2021**, *12*, 717652. [CrossRef] [PubMed]
23. Djeujo, F.M.; Stablum, V.; Pangrazzi, E.; Ragazzi, E. Luteolin and vernodalol as bioactive compounds of leaf and root vernonia amygdalina extracts: Effects on α-glucosidase, glycation, ROS, cell Viability, and in silico ADMET parameters. *Pharmaceutics* **2023**, *15*, 1541. [CrossRef] [PubMed]
24. Mu, M.; Gao, P.; Yang, Q.; He, J.; Wu, F.; Han, X.; Guo, S.; Qian, Z.; Song, C. Alveolar epithelial cells promote IGF-1 production by alveolar macrophages through TGF-β to suppress endogenous inflammatory signals. *Front. Immunol.* **2020**, *11*, 1585–1598. [CrossRef]
25. Gong, T.; Zhang, X.; Peng, Z.; Ye, Y.; Liu, R. Macrophage-derived exosomal aminopeptidase N aggravates sepsis-induced acute lung injury by regulating necroptosis of lung epithelial cell. *Commun. Biol.* **2022**, *5*, 543. [CrossRef]
26. Li, J.; Bai, Y.; Tang, Y.; Wang, X.; Cavagnaro, M.J.; Li, L.; Li, Z.; Zhang, Y.; Shi, J. A 4-benzene-Indol derivative alleviates LPS-induced acute lung injury through inhibiting the NLRP3 inflammasome. *Front. Immunol.* **2022**, *13*, 812164. [CrossRef]
27. Moore, P.J.; Tarran, R. The epithelial sodium channel as a therapeutic target for cystic fibrosis lung disease. *Expert. Opin. Ther. Targets* **2018**, *22*, 687–701. [CrossRef]
28. Yang, Q.; Xu, H.R.; Xiang, S.Y.; Zhang, C.; Ye, Y.; Shen, C.X.; Mei, H.X.; Zhang, P.H.; Ma, H.Y.; Zheng, S.X.; et al. Resolvin conjugates in tissue regeneration 1 promote alveolar fluid clearance by activating alveolar epithelial sodium channels and Na, K-ATPase in lipopolysaccharide-induced acute lung injury. *J. Pharmacol. Exp. Ther.* **2021**, *379*, 156–165. [CrossRef]
29. Han, J.; Li, H.; Bhandari, S.; Cao, F.; Wang, X.Y.; Tian, C.; Li, X.Y.; Zhang, P.H.; Liu, Y.J.; Wu, C.H.; et al. Maresin conjugates in tissue regeneration 1 improves alveolar fluid clearance by up-regulating alveolar ENaC, Na, K-ATPase in lipopolysaccharide-induced acute lung injury. *J. Cell. Mol. Med.* **2020**, *24*, 4736–4747. [CrossRef]
30. Deng, W.; Qi, D.; Tang, X.M.; Deng, X.Y.; He, J.; Wang, D.X. The WNK4/SPAK pathway stimulates alveolar fluid clearance by up-regulation of epithelial sodium channel in mice with lipopolysaccharide-induced acute respiratory distress syndrome. *Shock* **2022**, *58*, 68–77. [CrossRef]
31. Hua, Y.; Han, A.; Yu, T.; Hou, Y.; Ding, Y.; Nie, H. Small extracellular vesicles containing miR-34c derived from bone marrow mesenchymal stem cells regulates epithelial sodium channel via targeting MARCKS. *Int. J. Mol. Sci.* **2022**, *23*, 5196. [CrossRef] [PubMed]
32. Lamers, M.M.; van der Vaart, J. An organoid-derived bronchioalveolar model for SARS-CoV-2 infection of human alveolar type II-like cells. *EMBO J.* **2021**, *40*, e105912. [CrossRef] [PubMed]

33. Wang, Y.M.; Ji, R.; Chen, W.W.; Huang, S.W.; Zheng, Y.J.; Yang, Z.T. Paclitaxel alleviated sepsis-induced acute lung injury by activating MUC1 and suppressing TLR-4/NF-κB pathway. *Drug. Des. Devel Ther.* **2019**, *13*, 3391–3404. [CrossRef] [PubMed]
34. Li, Y.; Li, G.; Zhang, L.; Li, Y.; Zhao, Z. G9a promotes inflammation in Streptococcus pneumoniae induced pneumonia mice by stimulating M1 macrophage polarization and H3K9me2 methylation in FOXP1 promoter region. *Ann. Transl. Med.* **2022**, *10*, 583. [CrossRef] [PubMed]
35. Wichmann, L.; Althaus, M. Evolution of epithelial sodium channels: Current concepts and hypotheses. *Am. J. Physiol. Regul. Integr. Comp. Physiol.* **2020**, *319*, R387–R400. [CrossRef] [PubMed]
36. Zhou, W.; Wang, Y.; Lu, A.; Zhang, G. Systems pharmacology in small molecular drug discovery. *Int. J. Mol. Sci.* **2016**, *17*, 246. [CrossRef]
37. Wang, Z.Y.; Li, M.Z.; Li, W.J.; Ouyang, J.F.; Gou, X.J.; Huang, Y. Mechanism of action of Daqinjiao decoction in treating cerebral small vessel disease explored using network pharmacology and molecular docking technology. *Phytomedicine* **2023**, *108*, 154538. [CrossRef]
38. Zhu, W.; Li, Y.; Zhao, J.; Wang, Y.; Li, Y.; Wang, Y. The mechanism of triptolide in the treatment of connective tissue disease-related interstitial lung disease based on network pharmacology and molecular docking. *Ann. Med.* **2022**, *54*, 541–552. [CrossRef]
39. Zhao, X.; Zhao, B.; Zhao, Y.; Zhang, Y.; Qian, M. Protective effect of anisodamine on bleomycin-induced acute lung injury in immature rats via modulating oxidative stress, inflammation, and cell apoptosis by inhibiting the JAK2/STAT3 pathway. *Ann. Transl. Med.* **2021**, *9*, 859. [CrossRef]
40. Zhang, H.; Ding, Y.; Hou, Y.; Liu, Y.; Zhou, Z.; Nie, H. Bone marrow mesenchymal stem cells derived miRNA-130b enhances epithelial sodium channel by targeting PTEN. *Respir. Res.* **2020**, *21*, 329–343. [CrossRef]
41. Liu, H.; Hou, Y.; Jin, R.; Zhou, Z.; Zhang, H.; Wang, L.; Ding, Y.; Nie, H. Luteolin affects lung epithelial ion transport by regulating epithelial sodium channels. *Tradit. Chin. Drug Res. Clin. Pharmacol.* **2020**, *31*, 402–408. [CrossRef]
42. Kuo, M.Y.; Liao, M.F.; Chen, F.L.; Li, Y.C.; Yang, M.L.; Lin, R.H.; Kuan, Y.H. Luteolin attenuates the pulmonary inflammatory response involves abilities of antioxidation and inhibition of MAPK and NFκB pathways in mice with endotoxin-induced acute lung injury. *Food Chem. Toxicol.* **2011**, *49*, 2660–2666. [CrossRef] [PubMed]
43. Ding, Y.; Hou, Y.; Liu, Y.; Yu, T.; Cui, Y.; Nie, H. MiR-130a-3p alleviates inflammatory and fibrotic phases of pulmonary fibrosis through proinflammatory factor TNF-α and profibrogenic receptor TGF-βRII. *Front. Pharmacol.* **2022**, *13*, 863646. [CrossRef]
44. Hu, A.; Chen, W.; Wu, S.; Pan, B.; Zhu, A.; Yu, X.; Huang, Y. An animal model of transfusion-related acute lung injury and the role of soluble CD40 ligand. *Vox Sang.* **2020**, *115*, 303–313. [CrossRef] [PubMed]
45. Zhou, Y.; Liu, T.; Duan, J.X.; Li, P.; Sun, G.Y.; Liu, Y.P.; Zhang, J.; Dong, L.; Lee, K.S.S.; Hammock, B.D.; et al. Soluble epoxide hydrolase inhibitor attenuates lipopolysaccharide-induced acute lung injury and improves survival in mice. *Shock* **2017**, *47*, 638–645. [CrossRef] [PubMed]
46. Wang, J.; Wang, H.; Fang, F.; Fang, C. Danggui buxue tang ameliorates bleomycin-induced pulmonary fibrosis by suppressing the TLR4/NLRP3 signaling pathway in rats. *Evid. Based Complement. Altern. Med.* **2021**, *2021*, 8030143. [CrossRef] [PubMed]

Disclaimer/Publisher's Note: The statements, opinions and data contained in all publications are solely those of the individual author(s) and contributor(s) and not of MDPI and/or the editor(s). MDPI and/or the editor(s) disclaim responsibility for any injury to people or property resulting from any ideas, methods, instructions or products referred to in the content.

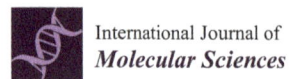

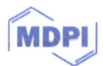

Article

Naringin's Alleviation of the Inflammatory Response Caused by *Actinobacillus pleuropneumoniae* by Downregulating the NF-κB/NLRP3 Signalling Pathway

Qilin Huang [1,2,3], Wei Li [4], Xiaohan Jing [1,2,3], Chen Liu [1,2,3], Saad Ahmad [1,2,3], Lina Huang [5], Guanyu Zhao [1,2,3], Zhaorong Li [1,2,3], Zhengying Qiu [1,2,3,*] and Ruihua Xin [1,2,3,*]

1. Lanzhou Institute of Husbandry and Pharmaceutical Sciences of Chinese Academy of Agricultural Sciences (CAAS), Lanzhou 730050, China; 82101215691@caas.cn (Q.H.); xhanjing306@gmail.com (X.J.); 82101225773@caas.cn (C.L.); saadahmad.uaf@gmail.com (S.A.); zhaogy517@gmail.com (G.Z.); lizr@st.gsau.edu.cn (Z.L.)
2. Engineering and Technology Research Center of Traditional Chinese Veterinary Medicine of Gansu Province, Lanzhou 730050, China
3. Key Laboratory of Veterinary Pharmaceutical Development of Ministry of Agriculture and Rural Affairs of China, Lanzhou 730050, China
4. Lanzhou Center for Disease Control and Prevention, Lanzhou 730050, China; liwei@lzcdc.cn
5. State Key Laboratory of Applied Organic Chemistry, School of Pharmacy, Lanzhou University, Lanzhou 730013, China; 220220943870@lzu.edu.cn
* Correspondence: qiuzhengying@caas.cn (Z.Q.); xinruihua@caas.cn (R.X.)

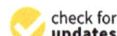

Citation: Huang, Q.; Li, W.; Jing, X.; Liu, C.; Ahmad, S.; Huang, L.; Zhao, G.; Li, Z.; Qiu, Z.; Xin, R. Naringin's Alleviation of the Inflammatory Response Caused by *Actinobacillus pleuropneumoniae* by Downregulating the NF-κB/NLRP3 Signalling Pathway. *Int. J. Mol. Sci.* **2024**, *25*, 1027. https://doi.org/10.3390/ijms25021027

Academic Editors: Marilena Gilca and Adelina Vlad

Received: 11 December 2023
Revised: 4 January 2024
Accepted: 7 January 2024
Published: 14 January 2024

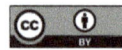

Copyright: © 2024 by the authors. Licensee MDPI, Basel, Switzerland. This article is an open access article distributed under the terms and conditions of the Creative Commons Attribution (CC BY) license (https://creativecommons.org/licenses/by/4.0/).

Abstract: *Actinobacillus pleuropneumoniae* (APP) is responsible for causing Porcine pleuropneumonia (PCP) in pigs. However, using vaccines and antibiotics to prevent and control this disease has become more difficult due to increased bacterial resistance and weak cross-immunity between different APP types. Naringin (NAR), a dihydroflavonoid found in citrus fruit peels, has been recognized as having significant therapeutic effects on inflammatory diseases of the respiratory system. In this study, we investigated the effects of NAR on the inflammatory response caused by APP through both in vivo and in vitro models. The results showed that NAR reduced the number of neutrophils (NEs) in the bronchoalveolar lavage fluid (BALF), and decreased lung injury and the expression of proteins related to the NLRP3 inflammasome after exposure to APP. In addition, NAR inhibited the nuclear translocation of nuclear factor kappa-B (NF-κB) P65 in porcine alveolar macrophage (PAMs), reduced protein expression of NLRP3 and Caspase-1, and reduced the secretion of pro-inflammatory cytokines induced by APP. Furthermore, NAR prevented the assembly of the NLRP3 inflammasome complex by reducing protein interaction between NLRP3, Caspase-1, and ASC. NAR also inhibited the potassium (K$^+$) efflux induced by APP. Overall, these findings suggest that NAR can effectively reduce the lung inflammation caused by APP by inhibiting the over-activated NF-κB/NLRP3 signalling pathway, providing a basis for further exploration of NAR as a potential natural product for preventing and treating APP.

Keywords: *Actinobacillus pleuropneumoniae* (APP); inflammatory injury; NLRP3 inflammasome; protein interactions; naringin (NAR); anti-inflammatory mechanism

1. Introduction

Actinobacillus pleuropneumoniae (APP) is responsible for causing porcine pleuropneumonia (PCP), which is characterized by acute haemorrhagic necrotizing pneumonia, as well as chronic fibrinous pleuropneumonia [1]. The spread of APP between pig herds occurs mainly through direct contact, aerosols, and manure [2]. The various virulence factors of APP trigger cascade reactions after infection, leading to an "inflammatory storm" characterized by lung haemorrhage, necrosis, and fibrinous exudate [1], resulting in a mortality rate of up to 80–100%. Commonly used antibiotics like florfenicol, tetracycline, and enrofloxacin are usually employed for treating PCP. However, the effectiveness of antibiotics in preventing and controlling the disease is being diminished by growing bacterial resistance [3]. Additionally, the frequent international trade of newly developed species has led to the emergence of more complex APP serotypes, resulting in poor cross-immunity between different serotypes, which has created a bottleneck in vaccine prevention and control [4,5]. As a result, the development of natural drugs for preventing and controlling APP has become a topic of increasing interest among researchers.

Naringin (NAR) is a dihydroflavonoid compound abundantly found in the dried unripe peel of the citrus "Tomentosa" or "*mandarin* (L.)" [6,7], which has traditional pharmacological traceability and is known for its antitussive and expectorant effects [8]. Recent studies have revealed that NAR has beneficial consequences including anti-inflammatory, antioxidant, and anti-apoptotic responses [9–11]. After NAR enters the body, its active metabolite naringenin protects endothelial cells from apoptosis and inflammation by regulating the Hippo-YAP pathway [12]. Most notably, NAR has shown effectiveness in repairing inflammatory damage in the respiratory tract, and reducing sputum secretion and inflammatory infiltration in lungs [13]. NAR can improve lung inflammation by inhibiting the release of interleukin (IL)-8, leukotriene B4, tumour necrosis factor (TNF)-α, and persistent neutrophilic infiltration due to infection [14]. Furthermore, NAR can prevent ovalbumin-induced airway inflammation by regulating the T1/T2 cell ratio [15]. However, it has not been confirmed whether NAR has the ability to repair the inflammatory damage caused by APP.

Porcine alveolar macrophages (PAM) are widely distributed on the alveolar and bronchial surfaces, forming a vital defence barrier for innate lung immunity [16]. When APP invades, pathogen-associated molecular patterns (PAMP) and damage-associated molecular patterns (DAMP) in PAM are activated, causing it to release an excess of inflammatory cytokines [13,16]. When lung tissue is overloaded with inflammatory factors, it activates the NLRP3 inflammatory vesicle classical/non-classical pathway in turn, which mediates apoptosis as well as cellular pyroptosis via the caspase-1, caspase-8, and caspase-9 pathways, further exacerbating inflammation [17,18]. A large number of studies have demonstrated that NLRP3 inflammasomes are associated with the pathogenesis of a variety of respiratory diseases [19], such as rhinitis [20], asthma [21], and chronic obstructive pulmonary disease (COPD) [22]. It has been found that the virulence factors Lipopolysaccharide (LPS) [23] and *Actinobacillus pleuropneumoniae* toxin (Apx) [17] of APP could initiate activation of the NLRP3 inflammasome signalling pathway, which is closely associated with the lung inflammatory injury of PCP. Therefore, in the present study, we investigated the role of NAR in repairing inflammatory lung injury through an APP-induced mice pneumonia model and a PAM inflammatory cell model, and elucidated the mechanism by which NAR exerts anti-inflammatory effects by inhibiting the NF-κB/NLRP3 inflammasome signalling pathway.

2. Results

2.1. Effects of NAR on Body Weight, Food Intake, and Macroscopic Lesions of Lung Tissue after APP Infection

In the study, we observed weight changes and symptoms in mice after APP infection. Before infection, all groups of mice showed continuous weight gain from day 1 to day 7; after APP infection on the 7th day, mice in the model group experienced significant weight loss, decreased appetite, depression, and loose stool. The results showed that the intervention of NAR was able to reverse the weight loss (Figure 1A). Before APP infection, there were no differences in the food intake among the groups of mice. However, the model group showed a decreasing trend in food intake compared to the control group after infection, and NAR administration reversed the feed intake decline to some extent (Figure 1B). The lung tissue was congested, haemorrhagic, purplish-red, and hardened in texture after APP infection and the lesions were alleviated after NAR intervention, with the highest concentration of NAR showing the most pronounced effect (Figure 1C). We further analysed total cell counts, as well as the percentage of neutrophils (NEs) and CRP in the bronchoalveolar lavage fluid (BALF). The results showed that both entire cells and NEs were significantly increased by the induced APP infection. However, after NAR intervention, both the total cell count and the percentage of NEs decreased considerably, which positively correlated with the NAR dosage (Figure 1D–F). Similarly, the levels of C-reactive protein (CRP) were significantly increased by the APP infection, and NAR intervention reduced the secretion of CRP in a dose-dependent manner (Figure 1G).

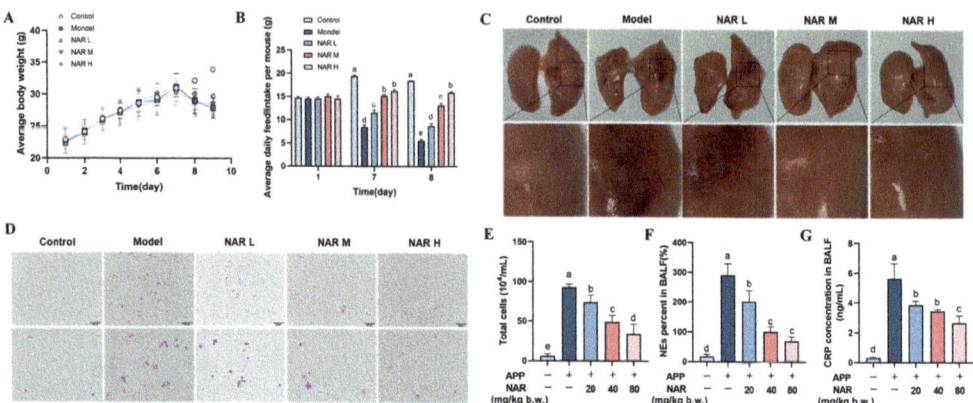

Figure 1. Effects of NAR on APP-induced lesions in mice. (**A**) Effect of NAR on weight loss in APP-induced mice. (**B**) Effect of NAR on food intake of mice. (**C**) Effect of NAR observed during lung dissection after APP infection. (**D**) Observation of Swiss-Giemsa staining after BALF smears of mice (100 μm). (**E**) Effect of NAR on the total number of cells in APP-induced BALF in mice. (**F**) Effect of NAR on the percentage of NEs in APP-induced BALF in mice. (**G**) Effect of NAR on CRP in BALF of APP-induced mice. (Different lowercase letters indicate statistically significant differences between groups $p < 0.05$, while the same lowercase letters indicate no significant differences between groups $p > 0.05$).

2.2. Effect of NAR on Histopathological Damage in the Lungs of Mice after APP Infection

After performing H&E staining on the lung tissues, we observed that the bronchial mucosa in the control group remained intact, the lung lobules had a clear structure, and the alveolar lumen was also unharmed. However, in the model group infected with APP, the lung tissues showed degeneration and necrotic shedding of alveolar epithelial cells, interstitial oedema, and haemorrhage. We also observed inflammatory cell infiltration, alveolar dilation, and interstitial widening, with a predominant infiltration of NEs. After administering NAR in different doses, we observed a reduction of tissue lesions in different treated groups. Particularly in the high-dose group (Figure 2A), the infiltration of NEs decreased, the degree of alveolar haemorrhage lessened, and the structure of the alveolar wall was restored with the increased number of inflated alveolar lumens. To judge more objectively, we used ImageJ software (Image Pro Plus version 6.0) to analyse the degree of inflammatory cell infiltration, lung parenchyma, and alveolar wall thickness in the mice's lung tissue. The results showed that the model group had significantly higher levels of inflammatory cell infiltration, parenchymatous lung tissue, and alveolar thickening compared to the control group. However, after the intervention of NAR, these judging indicators were significantly reduced to a certain extent (Figure 2B). Since myeloperoxidase (MPO) is mainly found in myeloid cells—such as NEs and monocytes—and closely associated with inflammation, the results showed that MPO content was elevated in the model group and significantly reduced after treatment of NAR in a dose-dependent manner, which was consistent with the results for NEs in BALF (Figure 2C).

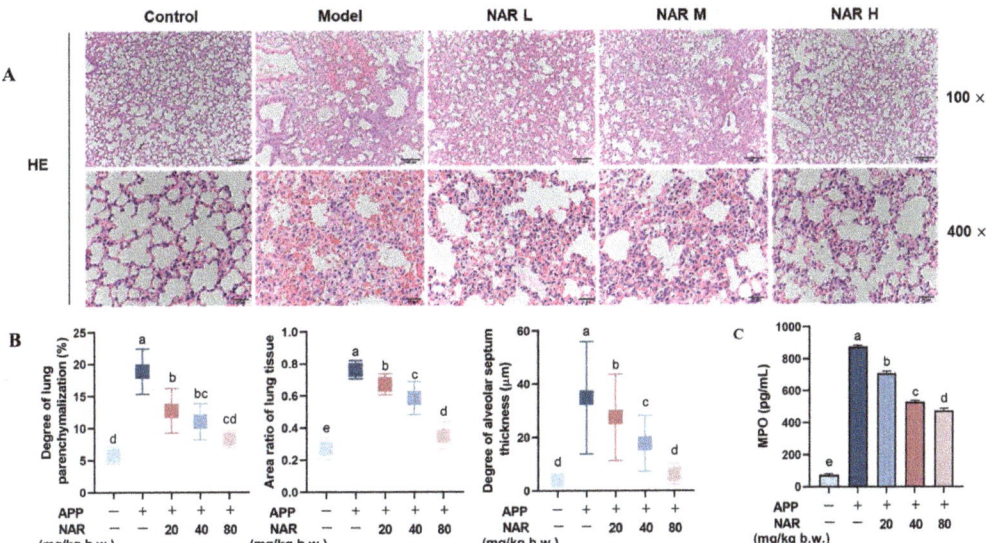

Figure 2. Effect of NAR on APP-induced histopathological damage of lung tissue. (**A**) Pathological tissue observation of mouse lung tissue under H&E staining. (**B**) Effect of NAR on the degree of inflammatory cell infiltration, lung parenchyma, and alveolar wall thickness of mouse lung tissue. (**C**) Effect of NAR on the content of MPO in lung tissue detected by ELISA. Scale bar: 100 μm (100×), 20 μm (400×). (Different lowercase letters indicate statistically significant differences between groups $p < 0.05$, while the same lowercase letters indicate no significant differences between groups $p > 0.05$).

2.3. NAR Exerts Anti-Inflammatory Effects by Inhibiting the NLRP3 Inflammasome Signalling Pathway in the Lungs

NLRP3 inflammasomes are considered to be closely associated with lung inflammation. After an NLRP3 inflammasome is activated, the matured Caspase-1 lead cleaves Gasder-minD (GSDMD), leading to cellular pyroptosis. We examined the expression of essential proteins involved in the NLRP3 inflammasome signalling pathway using Western blotting. The results showed that the phosphorylation level of the P65 protein increased after APP infection, and the expression of NLRP3, Caspase-1, GSDMD, and IL-18 proteins was also significantly elevated ($p < 0.05$). However, administration of NAR effectively inhibited the expression of p-P65, NLRP3, Caspase-1, GSDMD, and IL-18 proteins (Figure 3A). Gene expression analysis also confirmed that NAR could reduce the gene expression of NLRP3, Caspase-1, and GSDMD (Figure 3B). Furthermore, ELISA assay results demonstrated that the protein expression of IL-1β and IL-18 significantly increased after APP stimulation, but decreased after NAR administration (Figure 3C). These findings suggest that NAR provides anti-inflammatory effects by preventing the overactivation of crucial proteins in the NLRP3 inflammasome signalling pathway induced by APP in vivo.

2.4. NAR Inhibits the First Signalling of NLRP3 Inflammasome Activation in PAMs

It is reported that activating the NF-κB signalling pathway is necessary to activate the NLRP3 inflammasome. Specifically, the nuclear translocation of NF-κBP65 plays a crucial role in regulating gene transcription and promoting the release of inflammatory factors such as TNF-α and IL-6 (Figure 4A). In this study, we observed that the expression levels of these inflammatory factors (TNF-α and IL-6) were significantly ($p < 0.05$) higher in PAMs caused by APP, but decreased after NAR intervention. The results were consistent at both the genetic and protein levels (Figure 4A,B). Furthermore, we analysed the protein levels of P65 in the nucleus and cytoplasm, respectively, and found that the levels of P65 in the nucleus were significantly increased after APP infection, but decreased after NAR intervention.

Meanwhile, the protein levels of P65 in the cytoplasm were significantly decreased after APP infection and rebounded after NAR intervention. This result suggests that NAR could inhibit the entry of P65 into the nucleus and maintain normal levels of P65 in the cytoplasm (Figure 4C). Immunofluorescence results also supported that the expression of P65 decreased in the cytoplasm and increased in the nucleus after APP infection, which suggests that the NF-κB signalling pathway is over-activated. After NAR treatment, the amount of P65 in the nucleus was significantly reduced ($p < 0.05$) (Figure 4D). Overall, our results indicate that NAR exhibits anti-inflammatory effects by inhibiting the entry of P65 into the nucleus, reducing the activation of the first signal of NLRP3 inflammasomes.

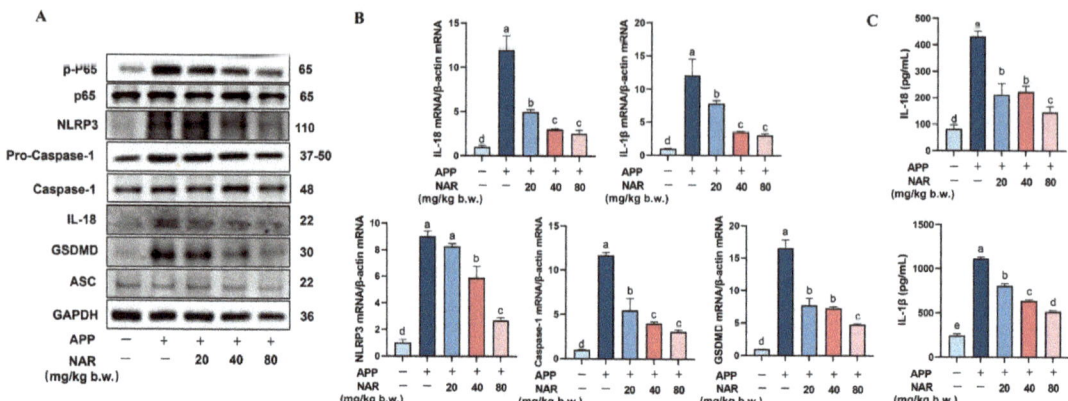

Figure 3. Effect of NAR on APP-induced NLRP3 inflammasome activation in mice lung tissue. (**A**) Effect of NAR on the expression of essential proteins in the NLRP3 inflammasome signalling pathway in lung tissue after APP infection. (**B**) Effect of NAR on the expression of critical genes in the NLRP3 inflammasome signalling pathway in lungs after APP infection. (**C**) Effect of NAR on the expression of IL-18 and IL-1β proteins in lung tissues, shown by ELISA assay. (Different lowercase letters indicate statistically significant differences between groups $p < 0.05$, while the same lowercase letters indicate no significant differences between groups $p > 0.05$).

2.5. NAR Exerts Anti-Inflammatory Effects by Inhibiting the NLRP3 Inflammasome Signalling Pathway in PAMs

We observed a significant increase in the expression of NLRP3 and Caspase-1 in PAMs after APP infection. However, after NAR introduction, a notable reduction in the expression of NLRP3 and Caspase-1 was observed (Figure 5A,B). Meanwhile, NAR was also found to significantly reduce the gene expression of inflammatory cytokines IL-1β and IL-18, which are closely related to the NLRP3 inflammasome. We also examined the key factor GSDMD, which is closely related to cellular pyroptosis, and whose cleavage at the Asp-275 site triggers cellular pyroptosis. The results indicate that the protein and gene expression levels of GSDMD were higher after APP stimulation compared to the control group, and the protein expression of FL-GSDMD (275) also significantly increased ($p < 0.05$). However, the expression of these factors was inhibited considerably after NAR treatment (Figure 5B). Additionally, the protein expression levels of IL-18 and IL-1β in the cell supernatant increased significantly during infection, but decreased after NAR intervention in a dose-dependent manner (Figure 5A–C). These results indicate that NAR effectively inhibits the expression of essential proteins and genes in the NLRP3 signalling pathway induced by APP infection, reduces the cleavage of GSDMD by Caspase-1, decreases cellular pyroptosis, and exerts anti-inflammatory effects.

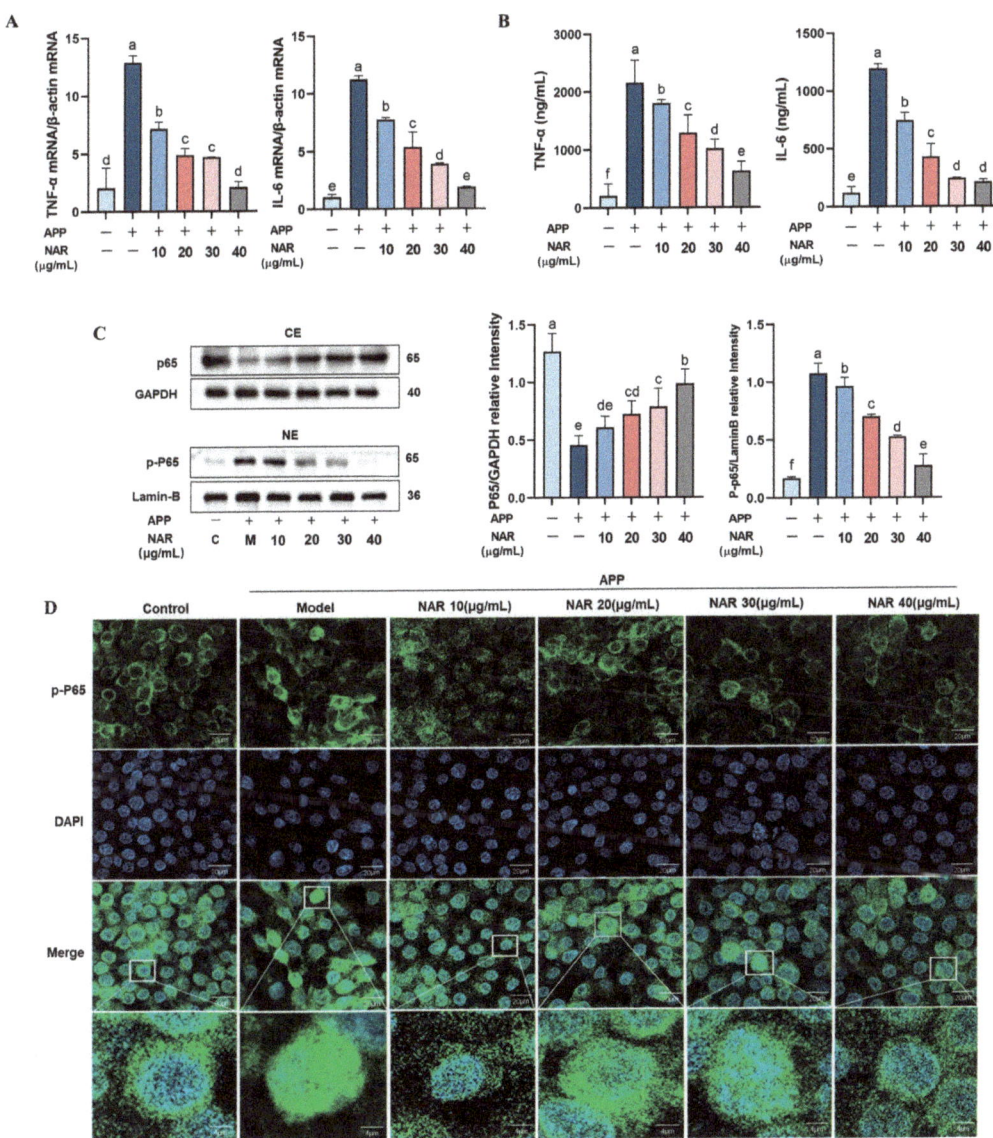

Figure 4. Effect of NAR on APP-induced nuclear translocation of P65 protein in PAMs. (**A**) Effect of NAR on relative mRNA expression of TNF-α and IL-6 in APP infection-induced PAM cells. (**B**) ELISA detection of TNF-α and IL-6 in PAM cells. (**C**) Effect of NAR intervention on APP-induced P65 protein nuclear translocation. (**D**) Confocal microscopy shows that NAR can reduce the nuclear load of P65 in APP-induced PAM cells. Note: Green fluorescence represents P65, blue fluorescence represents DAPI. Scale bar indicates 4 and 20 μm. (Different lowercase letters indicate statistically significant differences between groups $p < 0.05$, while the same lowercase letters indicate no significant differences between groups $p > 0.05$).

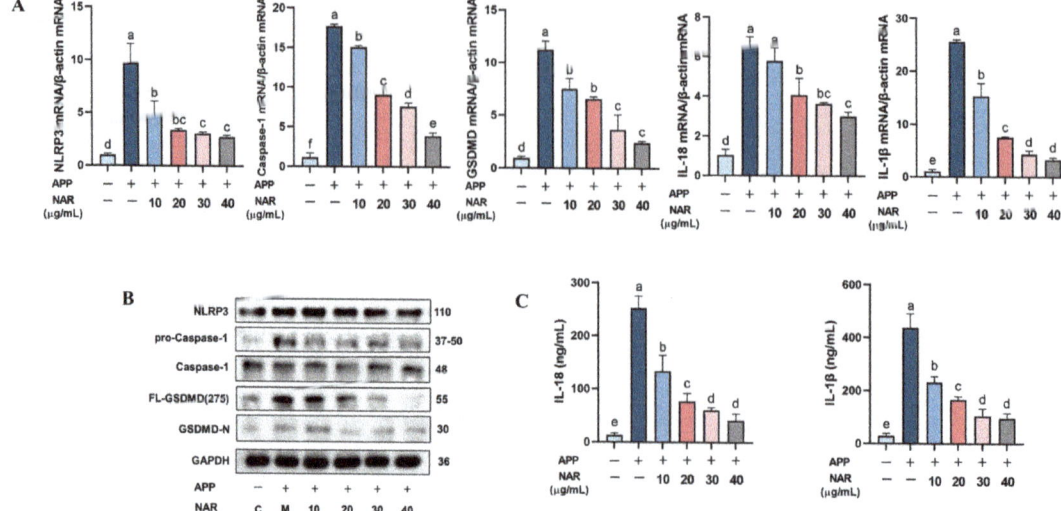

Figure 5. Effect of NAR on the APP-induced NLRP3 inflammasome signalling pathway in PAMs. (**A**) Effect of NAR on the expression of critical genes of the NLRP3 inflammatory vesicle signalling pathway in PAMs. (**B**) Effect of NAR on the expression of essential proteins of the NLRP3 inflammasome in PAMs. (**C**) Effect of NAR on the expression of IL-18 and IL-1β proteins in PAMs. (Different lowercase letters indicate statistically significant differences between groups $p < 0.05$, while the same lowercase letters indicate no significant differences between groups $p > 0.05$).

2.6. NAR Exerts Anti-Inflammatory Effects by Interfering with the Assembly of NLRP3 Inflammasome Complex Proteins

In this study, we investigated the impact of NAR on the activation of the NLRP3 inflammasome's initiating factors. Since ASC plays a crucial role in activating NLRP3 inflammasome complex proteins, we probed the level of oligomerization of the ASC protein. Our findings revealed that after APP stimulation, the level of ASC aggregation increased in PAMs compared to the control group, and the oligomerization level of ASC was significantly reduced ($p < 0.05$) to some extent after NAR intervention (Figure 6A). To further understand the assembly of NLRP3 inflammasome complex proteins, we used the immunoprecipitation technique (Co-IP) to explore the interactions between receptor protein NLRP3, effector protein Caspase-1, and junction protein ASC. The results showed that APP stimulation increased the amount that NLRP3 and Caspase-1 proteins interacted with ASC, indicating an improved assembly of NLRP3 inflammasome complex proteins. However, NAR intervention downregulated the protein expression of NLRP3, as well as Caspase-1's interaction with ASC, suggesting that NAR inhibited the assembly of NLRP3 inflammasome complex proteins (Figure 6B). Additionally, intracellular potassium (K^+) efflux also triggers the activation of the NLRP3 inflammasome's second signalling pathway. Through turbidimetric assay, we measured the intracellular K^+ content, and the results showed that the model group had significantly reduced K^+ content compared to the control group ($p < 0.05$). However, the cells treated with NAR showed a dose-dependent increase in intracellular K^+ content, indicating that NAR could significantly inhibit APP-induced intracellular K^+ efflux and subsequently inhibit the activation of the NLRP3 inflammasome (Figure 6C).

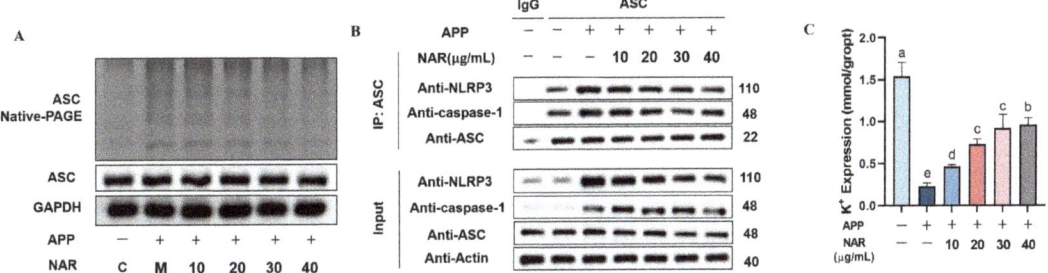

Figure 6. Effect of NAR on assembly of NLRP3 inflammasome complex proteins in PAMs induced by APP. (**A**) Effect of NAR on the level of ASC oligomerization in APP-induced PAMs. (**B**) Effect of NAR on the assembly of complex proteins of the NLRP3 inflammasome in APP-induced PAM cells. (**C**) Effect of NAR on intracellular K$^+$ efflux. (Different lowercase letters indicate statistically significant differences between groups $p < 0.05$, while the same lowercase letters indicate no significant differences between groups $p > 0.05$).

3. Discussion

Frequent international trade introductions have resulted in the continued spread of APP worldwide and the severe blow it has inflicted on the pig economy. The effectiveness of antibiotic and vaccine prophylaxis is greatly hampered by antibiotic resistance and poor cross-immunity between serotypes [23]. In recent years, many natural drugs have been found to possess anti-inflammatory properties. Therefore, we hope that the addition of natural plant drugs to diets will reduce the inflammatory damage caused by pathogens to the tissues of the organism, thus reducing the use of antibiotics and indirectly lowering the risk of bacterial resistance, which is ultimately conducive to healthy farming and food safety. NAR is an active flavonoid that is not only found in the peel of citrus fruits, but also widely found in grapefruit, tomatoes, cherries, and other plants. It has the advantages of being easy to extract, widely available, inexpensive, and safe to use [23]. Studies have proved that NAR has a good repairing effect on respiratory inflammatory injury, which can significantly reduce sputum secretion and inflammatory infiltration in the lungs, and also decrease goblet cell proliferation and mucus secretion [24]. Therefore, we investigated the protective effect of NAR on APP-induced lung inflammatory injury, which provides a theoretical basis for developing natural drugs for treating PCP. The results of this study showed that NAR was able to improve APP-induced symptoms such as loss of weight and appetite, alleviate lung tissue lesions in mice, and significantly reduce inflammatory cell infiltration, lung parenchymatous, and alveolar thickening in lung tissues. Through further analysis, we discovered that the mechanisms of these actions may inhibit the overactivation of the NF-κB/NLRP3 inflammasome signalling pathway, thereby exerting its effect on alleviating the inflammatory injury of the lungs.

The pathogenesis of APP is mainly through the secretion of multiple virulence factors that enter the lungs from the respiratory tract [20,25], adhere to and deposit in the alveolar epithelium, and persistently stimulate PAMs, which form an essential immune barrier in the lungs' cell surface. Intracellular pattern recognition receptors (PRRs) activate pathogen-associated molecular patterns (PAMPs) by recognizing virulence factors, or activate damage-associated molecular patterns (DAMPs), and phosphorylate Toll-like receptors (TLRs) through the TLR4 signalling pathway; this subsequently activates the NF-κB/MAKE/AP-1 pathway, promotes the transcription of NLRP3, proIL-1β, and proIL-18, and regulates the intensity of the natural immune response [26]. When intense stimuli and inflammatory responses persist, the dynamic immune balance is disrupted. The early production of pro-inflammatory factors further promotes the release of cytokines, such as macrophage inflammatory protein 1α (MIP-1α), macrophage inflammatory protein 1β (MIP-1β), IL-6, IL-8, IL-12, etc., leading to a series of cytokine cascade responses that promote NEs to accumulate in large numbers in the alveoli, causing an inflammatory storm [18], and at the same time inducing platelets to agglutinate in the lung tissues, causing capillary rupture, leading to cell necrosis [27] and tissue damage [28]. We found that NAR significantly reduced the number of NEs in BALF of APP mice, inhibited the secretion of pro-inflammatory factors TNF-α and IL-6, reduced APP-induced lung congestion and necrosis, and reduced inflammatory cell infiltration, lung parenchyma, and alveolar thickening, which significantly ameliorated the inflammatory injury of the lungs induced by APP.

The activation of the classical NLRP3 inflammasome requires two crucial signals: signal 1 is the transcription of inflammatory cytokines, which involves the activation of the NF-κB signalling pathway, thus activating the transcription of inflammatory cytokines such as NLRP3, pro-Caspase-1, and pro-IL 1β [29], while signal 2 is the binding of NLRP3 and Caspase-1 to ASC to form NLRP3 inflammasome [30]. The LRR structural domain of NLRP3 is usually in a state of autoinhibition; its protein spatial structure will change after stimulation, and the NACHT structural domain of NLRP3 will mediate its own oligomerization, recruiting ASC through the PYD structural domain and then recruiting pro-Caspase-1 to form an inflammasome through the CARD structural domain of ASC proteins, and the activated Caspase-1 not only cleaves and activates pro-IL-1β and pro-IL-18 precursor proteins into mature forms of IL-1β and IL-18, but also cleaves Gasdermin D, which plays a vital role in cellular pyroptosis [19] in our study. We found that NAR reduced the nuclear translocation of NF-κB P65 and IL-6, as well as the TNF-α expression induced by APP, thereby inhibiting NLRP3 inflammasome's first signalling activation. Immediately after that, we explored the effect of NAR on the second signalling of NLRP3. As oligomerization of ASC is a critical step in the activation of the second signalling of NLRP3 inflammasome, the assay results revealed that NAR was able to reduce the level of ASC oligomerization dose-dependently, and also inhibit the protein interactions between NLRP3, Caspase-1, and ASC, thus inhibiting the NLRP3 inflammasome complex protein assembly. Meanwhile, NAR reduced the expression of IL-18, IL-1β, NLRP3, Caspase-1, and GSDMD at the gene level, as well as NLRP3, Caspase-1, IL-18, GSDMD, and FL-GSDMD (275) at the protein level, suggesting that NAR could play an essential role in inhibiting the NF-κB/NLRP3 signalling pathway's activation and also inhibit the NLRP3 inflammasome complex protein, thus exerting an inhibitory effect on the inflammatory response. Since intracellular K^+ efflux could enhance the assembly of NLRP3 proteins and activate the NLRP3 inflammasome, the results suggest that NAR could reduce APP-induced K^+ efflux and avoid exacerbating inflammatory responses.

In summary, NAR was able to alleviate pathological damage in mouse lung tissue due to APP-induced injury; reduce the content of NEs in BALF; and decrease the expression of crucial proteins and genes in the NLRP3 inflammasome signalling pathway in lung tissue. Meanwhile, in the APP-induced PAMs inflammatory cell model, NAR was able to not only reduce the nuclear translocation of the NF-κB P65 protein and thereby inhibit the NLRP3 first signal activation, but also inhibit the oligomerization of ASC protein, as well as reduce the protein interactions between NLRP3, Caspase-1, and ASC, thereby interfering with the assembly of the NLRP3 inflammasome complex protein. Further, NAR treatment could lessen the intracellular K^+ efflux from the PAMs, thus exerting anti-inflammatory effects. It was shown that NAR ameliorates inflammatory injury in the lungs caused by APP induction by inhibiting the NF-κB/NLRP3 signalling pathway (Figure 7).

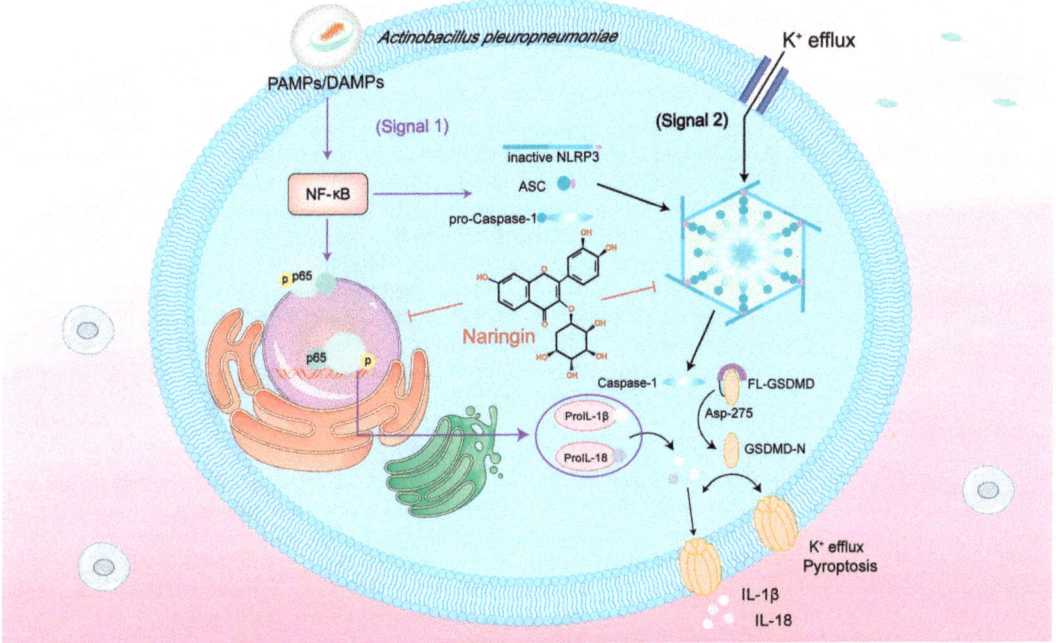

Figure 7. Effect of NAR on APP-induced activation of the NLRP3 inflammasome signalling pathway. The activation of the NLRP3 inflammasome is a dual-signalling activation mechanism. Firstly, APP enters the organism and activates NF-κB via pathogen-associated molecular patterns (PAMPs) or damage-associated molecular patterns (DAMPs). This prompts the entry of the P65 subunit into the nucleus for transcription, thereby promoting the transcription and release of inflammatory factors such as NLRP3, pro-Caspase-1, pro-IL-1β, and other inflammatory cytokines. Transcription and release is the preparatory stage of NLRP3 inflammatory vesicle activation. The second signal is stimulated by APP, K$^+$ efflux, or other factors, which activates the assembly of the NLRP3 inflammasome and, in turn, elicits pro-Caspase-1 to form activated Caspase-1. The activated Caspase-1 can cause cellular death by cleaving Gasdermin D and can activate the NLRP3–ASC–Caspase-1 pathway to increase the maturation and release of IL-1β and IL-18. It was found that NAR could alleviate the APP-induced inflammatory response by inhibiting the dual signalling activation mechanism of the NLRP3 inflammasome.

4. Materials and Methods

4.1. Chemicals and Reagents

NAR was purchased from Sigma Aldrich Chemical (St. Louis, MO, USA. HPLC ≥ 98%, chemical formula $C_{27}H_{32}O_{14}$, molecular weight 580.54, CAS No. 10236-47-2); 1640 medium (Gibco, Grand Island, NY, USA) and trypsin were purchased from JS Biosciences Co., Ltd. (Lanzhou, Gansu Province, China); foetal bovine serum (FBS) and penicillin–streptomycin antibiotics were purchased from Thermo Fisher Scientific (Waltham, MA, USA); nuclear protein extraction kit was purchased from Solarbio Science & Technology Co., Ltd. (Beijing, China); ELISA kits for IL-6, TNF-α, IL-1β, and IL-18 were purchased from Jianglai Industry Co., Ltd. (Beijing, China); RNA extraction kit, TRIzol® Reagent RT-PCR kit, and SYBR® green PCR master mix were purchased from TaKaRa (Tokyo, Japan); NLRP3, Caspase-1, pro-Caspase-1, ASC, NF-κB P65, p-P65, IL-18, GAPDH, Lamin B, HRP-conjugated goat anti-rabbit IgG, HRP-conjugated goat anti-mouse primary IgG, and Alexa Flour 488-labelled anti-mouse IgG were purchased from Cell Signaling Technology, Inc. (Beverly, MA, USA); bovine serum albumin (BSA) and ECL assay kits were obtained from Thermo Fisher

Scientific (Waltham, MA, USA); bovine serum albumin (BSA) and ECL assay kits were provided by Thermo Fisher Scientific (Waltham, MA, USA); and McConkay's medium was purchased from Sigma–Aldrich (Merk, Darmstadt, Germany)

4.2. Bacteria, Cellular Inflammation Models, and NAR Treatment

Actinobacillus pleuropneumoniae (APP) isolated from swine farms and verified through Blast sequencing was conserved in our laboratory and resuscitated in TSA medium (additionally supplemented with 5% foetal bovine serum and 1% NAD) at 37 °C. PAMs were purchased from Procell Life Science & Technology Co., Ltd. (Wuhan, China), then cultured in 1640 medium, containing 1% penicillin–streptomycin and 10% FBS, at 37 °C in a humidified atmosphere containing 5% CO_2. After the cell fusion reached about 70–80%, they were digested with trypsin and passaged for culture. The cells were pretreated with NAR (10 µg/mL, 20 µg/mL, 30 µg/mL, and 40 µg/mL) for 12 h, then stimulated with APP bacterial solution (1×10^7 CFU/mL) for 1 h. After removing the bacterial solution, the cells were cultured as usual for 12 h and collected for Western blotting and RT-PCR assays, and the supernatant was collected for ELISA tests.

4.3. Establishment of Animal Model and Treatment with NAR

Sixty Kunming mice (18–22 g) were provided by the Lanzhou Veterinary Institute of CAAS (License No. SCXK Gansu 2023–016). Animal welfare statement: institutional ethical and animal care guidelines were observed, and all experimental processes were conducted according to the China Guide for the Care and Use of Laboratory Animals (protocol number: IACUC-157031). The mice were randomly divided into five groups, namely the control group (gavage with water), the model group (gavage with water + 10^8 CFU/mL APP infection), the naringin low-dose group (gavage with 20 mg/kg NAR + 10^8 CFU/mL APP infection), the naringin medium-dose group (gavage with 40 mg/kg + 10^8 CFU/mL APP infection), and the naringin high-dose group (gavage with 80 mg/kg + 10^8 CFU/mL APP infection) (n = 12). The drugs were administered by gavage continuously for eight d. Saline was given to the control and model groups. On day 7, the mice were anaesthetized through intraperitoneal injection of sodium pentobarbital (50 mg/kg b.w.) and infected through tracheal intubation with mice from the model group and the administered group (100 µL/each mouse, APP bacterial concentration of 1×10^8 CFU/mL), while the control group was injected with an equal volume of sterile saline. The daily number of deaths, body weight, and feed intake of the animals were recorded. The mice in each group were anesthetized and executed 48 h after successful modelling, and different samples were taken using the following steps.

4.4. Bronchoalveolar Lavage Fluid (BALF) Preparation and Analysis

Three mice were randomly picked from each group and fixed on the dissection table in the supine position. The skin, subcutaneous tissue, and muscular layer were cleaned and sequentially incised about 5 mm above the sternal pedicle, the lungs were exposed, and the right lobe of the lung was ligated. The trachea was carefully cut into with an oblique incision. The tracheal tube was introduced and placed 10–15 mm above the tracheal eminence and then tied with a fine thread. The lungs were rinsed with pre-cooled PBS (refrigerated at 4 °C in advance) and rinsed three times, 0.5 mL each time, for about 1.2 mL of irrigating fluid (80% recovery rate). The BALF was then stained with Swiss-Giemsa reagent solution, and the total cell and neutrophil counts were calculated using a blood cell counter. Then, the BALF was centrifuged at 4 °C, $5000 \times g$ for 10 min, and the supernatant was taken to detect the concentration of C-reactive protein (CRP).

4.5. Histopathologic Examination

Fresh mouse lung tissues were fixed in 4% paraformaldehyde for 3 d, dehydrated, and embedded in paraffin wax. The wax blocks were cut into 5 µm thick sections with a microtome, stained with haematoxylin–eosin (H&E), and finally sealed with neutral gum.

The sections were placed under a microscope (DM 4000B, Leica, Wetzlar, Germany) to observe the mouse lung tissue. The extent of lung injury and inflammatory cell infiltration was analysed using ImageJ software.

4.6. Quantitative Real-Time PCR Analysis

Total RNA was isolated from cells or lung tissues using TRIzol reagent (15596026, Invitrogen Life Technologies, Carlsbad, CA, USA), RNA was reverse transcribed into cDNA according to the PrimeScript RT Reverse Transcription Kit (RR047Q, Takara, Dalian, China), and mRNA expression was quantified using the Applied Biosystems Real-Time Fluorescence Quantitative PCR System and the SYBR premix Ex Taq II (R075A, Takara, Dalian, China). Quantification results were calculated using the $2^{®-\Delta\Delta Ct}$ method compared to β-actin as the reference mRNA (Table 1).

Table 1. Primer sequences of the target genes.

Target	Sequence (5'-3')	Gene Bank Accession No.
IL-1β	5'-GCAGGCAGTATCACTCATTGT-3' 5'-GGCTTTTTTGTTGTTCATCTC-3'	LT727274.1
IL-6	5'-CTGCAGTCACAGAACGAGTG-3' 5'-GACGGCATCAATCTCAGGTG-3'	XM_047753916.1
TNF-α	5'-AAGGGAGAGTGGTCAGGTTGC-3' 5'-CAGAGGTTCAGTGATGTAGCG-3'	NM_001278601.1
IL-10	5'-GCTCCTAGAGCTGCGGACTGC-3' 5'-TGCTTCTCTGCCTGGGGCATCA-3'	XM_021175612.1
IL-18	5'-GCTTGAATCTAAATTATCAGT-3' 5'-GAAGATTCAAATTGCATCTTAT-3'	EF444989.1
NLRP3	5'-AGACCTCCAAGACCACTAC-3' 5'-ACATAGCAGCGAAGAACTC-3'	XR_004607107.1
Caspase-1	5'-TGCCCAGAGCACAAGACTTC-3' 5'-TCCTTGTTTCTCTCCACGGC-3'	XM_032910338.1
β-actin	5'-GGTCACCAGGGCTGCTTT-3' 5'-ACTGTGCCGTTGACCTTGC-3'	OY781925.1

4.7. Western Blotting Analysis

Collected lung tissues or cells were lysed with lysate supplemented with PMSF, and then centrifuged at 4 °C for 10 min at 15,000× g. The supernatant was collected as protein extracts, and the concentration of protein samples was measured according to the bicinchoninic acid assay (BCA). Equal protein samples were separated using 8–12% SDS-PAGE and then electrotransferred into a nitrocellulose membrane (Millipore, Billerica, MA, USA). The membranes were immersed in 5% skimmed milk powder and enclosed at room temperature for 1 h. The membranes were incubated with NLRP3 (1:1000), Caspase-1 (1:1000), pro-Caspase-1 (1:1000), ASC (1:1000), NF-κB P65 (1:1000), NF-κB p-P65 (1:1000), FL- GSDMD (275) (1:1000), GSDMD (1:1000), and IL-18 (1:1000). Then HRP-coupled goat anti-mouse IgG secondary antibody (1:5000) or HRP-coupled goat anti-rabbit IgG secondary antibody (1:5000) was added and incubated at 37 °C for 1 h. The luminescent solution was configured by mixing WesternBright Sirius HRP substrate's solution A and solution B in a ratio of 1:1. The moisture on the surface of the membrane was sucked off with filter paper, and the luminescent solution was added dropwise. Ultimately, the membranes were visualized with the chemiluminescence detection kit and examined with a Biosciences Imager. GAPDH or Lamin-B served as the internal control normalized against the overall proteins. Further, the phosphorylated proteins were normalized against their respective total proteins.

4.8. ELISA Test

(1) The collected lung tissues from different groups of mice were removed, about 1 g was placed in 800 μL of pre-cooled TRIzol reagent, and an appropriate amount of

zirconium oxide beads were added to homogenize the tissue in a tissue homogenizer. After centrifugation for 10 min at 4 °C, 3000 r/min, the supernatant was collected. The levels of TNF-α, IL-1β, IL-18, IL-6, and MPO were determined by referring to the instructions of the mouse ELISA kit.

(2) Cytokine assay: The collected cell supernatant was kept on ice and immediately added to the enzyme wells according to the instructions, and the absorbance value was read at 450 nm on the enzyme labeller (Hong Kong Genetics Limited, Hong Kong, China). The detailed steps were the same as above.

4.9. Immunofluorescence Staining

PAMs were placed on coverslips in 24-well plates and left to fuse to 70% for subsequent experiments. After treatment, the cells were treated with NAR for 1 h before APP infection and collected 30 min after APP infection for subsequent experiments. To the cell culture plate, 1 mL of 4% paraformaldehyde was added for fixation, 0.03% Triton X-100 was permeabilised for 20 min at room temperature, and 5% BSA was bound for 30 min at room temperature, after which the binding solution was discarded. The cells were then incubated overnight with P65 primary antibody (1:100) at 4 °C. After washing three times with PBS, the cells were incubated with Alexa Fluor 488 coupled to goat anti-mouse secondary antibody (1:1000) at room temperature for 1 h. Before the end of the incubation, 1 μg/mL of blue fluorescent DAPI dye was added to the plate and incubated for 10 min to stain the nuclear DNA of the cells. Using an IF laser scanning confocal microscope (German Zeiss Z800), the cells were observed at 488 nm (green) and 405 nm (blue) excitation wavelengths for cell fluorescence images.

4.10. Co-Immunoprecipitation

Cells were lysed with RIPA lysis buffer, and 50% proteinA/G-agarose working solution was prepared using PBS; 50% proteinA/G-agarose working solution was added to the samples at the rate of 100 μL proteinA agarose beads per 1 mL, and the samples were shaken for 10 min at 4 °C on a horizontal shaker to remove the non-specifically bound proteins. Specifically bound proteins were centrifuged at 4 °C, 14,000× g for 15 min, and the supernatant was transferred to a new centrifuge tube to remove proteinA/G-agarose microspheres; after measuring the concentration of the protein samples using a BCA, a particular volume of primary antibody was added. The antigen–antibody mixture was shaken slowly with a shaker, and the model was incubated at 4 °C overnight; the precipitate was collected through centrifugation at 14,000× g rpm and washed three times with pre-cooled PBS; the supernatant was collected, and protein denaturation was carried out by adding PAS and Protein Sample Loading Buffer (Denaturing, Reducing, 5×) in a metal bath at 100 °C for 10 min. The supernatant was collected and subjected to SDS-PAGE.

4.11. Statistical Analysis

The results were analysed using various statistical tests in GraphPad Prism version 9 (GraphPad Software, San Diego, CA, USA). All the data were statistically analysed through one-way ANOVA using IBM SPSS 27 (SPSS Inc., Chicago, IL, USA). Values were expressed as mean ± SEM. Differences between groups in body-related parameters were analysed using a one-way analysis of variance (ANOVA) and Tukey's post hoc test. For all tests, a probability value (p) of less than 0.05 ($p < 0.05$) was considered statistically significant. Different lowercase letters on the error bars indicate statistically significant differences ($p < 0.05$).

5. Conclusions

In short, this study has revealed that NAR has the potential to alleviate the inflammatory response caused by APP by inhibiting the activation mechanism of the NLRP3 inflammasome. It also provides a theoretical basis for the use of NAR as an animal feed additive in the future. Thus, we can fully use the "vaccine-antibiotic-natural drug" triangular defence system to prevent and control lung bacterial infections in pig farms and promote healthy breeding and a safe food supply.

Author Contributions: Conceptualization, R.X. and Q.H.; methodology, Q.H. and X.J.; software, W.L. and Q.H.; validation, G.Z., W.L. and X.J.; formal analysis, Q.H. and C.L.; investigation, L.H., Z.L. and W.L.; data curation, Q.H.; writing—original draft preparation, Q.H., S.A. and Z.Q.; writing—review and editing, R.X., W.L. and Z.Q.; project administration, R.X.; funding acquisition, W.L., R.X. and Z.Q. All authors have read and agreed to the published version of the manuscript.

Funding: This work was supported by the National Key Research and Development Program of China (2022YFD180110304), the National Natural Science Foundation of China (32002328), the Natural Science Foundation of Gansu Province (22JR5RA038), and the Key Research and Development fund of Gansu Province, China (21YF5FA166, 23YFNA0010, 23YFFA0014). The central government guides local science and technology development fund projects in Gansu province (22ZY1QA012). Lanzhou Science and Technology Project, China (2021-1-159, 2022-RC-21).

Institutional Review Board Statement: All mice were provided by the Lanzhou Veterinary Institute of CAAS (license no. SCXK Gansu 2023–016). Animal welfare statement: institutional ethical and animal care guidelines were observed, and all procedures were conducted according to the China Guide for the Care and Use of Laboratory Animals (protocol number: IACUC-157031).

Informed Consent Statement: Not applicable.

Data Availability Statement: The data presented in this study are available upon request from the corresponding authors.

Acknowledgments: We are very grateful that X.P. (Xiangyi Pan) was involved in organizing the data for this paper.

Conflicts of Interest: The authors declare that they have no known competing financial interest or personal relationship that could have appeared to influence the work reported in this paper.

References

1. Nahar, N.; Turni, C.; Tram, G.; Blackall, P.J.; Atack, J.M. Actinobacillus pleuropneumoniae: The molecular determinants of virulence and pathogenesis. *Adv. Microb. Physiol.* **2021**, *78*, 179–216. [PubMed]
2. Cohen, L.M.; Grøntvedt, C.A.; Klem, T.B.; Gulliksen, S.M.; Ranheim, B.; Nielsen, J.P.; Valheim, M.; Kielland, C. A descriptive study of acute outbreaks of respiratory disease in Norwegian fattening pig herds. *Acta Vet. Scand.* **2020**, *62*, 35. [CrossRef]
3. Tobias, T.J.; Bouma, A.; Daemen, A.J.; Wagenaar, J.A.; Stegeman, A.; Klinkenberg, D. Association between transmission rate and disease severity for *Actinobacillus pleuropneumoniae* infection in pigs. *Vet. Res.* **2013**, *44*, 2. [CrossRef] [PubMed]
4. Hathroubi, S.; Loera-Muro, A.; Guerrero-Barrera, A.L.; Tremblay, Y.D.N.; Jacques, M. *Actinobacillus pleuropneumoniae* biofilms: Role in pathogenicity and potential impact for vaccination development. *Anim. Health Res. Rev.* **2018**, *19*, 17–30. [CrossRef] [PubMed]
5. Donà, V.; Ramette, A.; Perreten, V. Comparative genomics of 26 complete circular genomes of 18 different serotypes of Actinobacillus pleuropneumoniae. *Microb. Genom.* **2022**, *8*, 000776. [CrossRef]
6. Ma, X.; Zheng, B.; Wang, J.; Li, G.; Cao, S.; Wen, Y.; Huang, X.; Zuo, Z.; Zhong, Z.; Gu, Y. Quinolone Resistance of *Actinobacillus pleuropneumoniae* Revealed through Genome and Transcriptome Analyses. *Int. J. Mol. Sci.* **2021**, *22*, 10036. [CrossRef] [PubMed]
7. Guo, F.; Guo, J.; Cui, Y.; Cao, X.; Zhou, H.; Su, X.; Yang, B.; Blackall, P.J.; Xu, F. Exposure to Sublethal Ciprofloxacin Induces Resistance to Ciprofloxacin and Cross-Antibiotics, and Reduction of Fitness, Biofilm Formation, and Apx Toxin Secretion in Actinobacillus pleuropneumoniae. *Microb. Drug Resist.* **2021**, *27*, 1290–1300. [CrossRef] [PubMed]
8. Pereira, M.F.; Rossi, C.C.; Seide, L.E.; Martins Filho, S.; Dolinski, C.M.; Bazzolli, D.M.S. Antimicrobial resistance, biofilm formation and virulence reveal *Actinobacillus pleuropneumoniae* strains' pathogenicity complexity. *Res. Vet. Sci.* **2018**, *118*, 498–501. [CrossRef]
9. Yang, C.P.; Liu, M.H.; Zou, W.; Guan, X.L.; Lai, L.; Su, W.W. Toxicokinetics of naringin and its metabolite naringenin after 180-day repeated oral administration in beagle dogs assayed by a rapid resolution liquid chromatography/tandem mass spectrometric method. *J. Asian Nat. Prod. Res.* **2012**, *14*, 68–75. [CrossRef]
10. Mohamed, E.E.; Ahmed, O.M.; Zoheir, K.M.A.; El-Shahawy, A.A.G.; Tamur, S.; Shams, A.; Burcher, J.T.; Bishayee, A.; Abdel-Moneim, A. Naringin-Dextrin Nanocomposite Abates Diethylnitrosamine/Acetylaminofluorene-Induced Lung Carcinogenesis by Modulating Oxidative Stress, Inflammation, Apoptosis, and Cell Proliferation. *Cancers* **2023**, *15*, 5102. [CrossRef]
11. Zhao, G.; Huang, Q.; Jing, X.; Huang, L.; Liu, C.; Pan, X.; Li, Z.; Li, S.; Qiu, Z.; Xin, R. Therapeutic Effect and Safety Evaluation of Naringin on Klebsiella pneumoniae in Mice. *Int. J. Mol. Sci.* **2023**, *24*, 15940. [CrossRef] [PubMed]

12. Zhang, H.H.; Zhou, X.J.; Zhong, Y.S.; Ji, L.T.; Yu, W.Y.; Fang, J.; Ying, H.Z.; Li, C.Y. Naringin suppressed airway inflammation and ameliorated pulmonary endothelial hyperpermeability by upregulating Aquaporin1 in lipopolysaccharide/cigarette smoke-induced mice. *Biomed. Pharmacother.* **2022**, *150*, 113035. [CrossRef] [PubMed]
13. AmeliMojarad, M.; AmeliMojarad, M. Interleukin-6 inhibitory effect of natural product naringenin compared to a synthesised monoclonal antibody against life-threatening COVID-19. *Rev. Med. Virol.* **2023**, *33*, e2445. [CrossRef]
14. Liu, Y.; Wu, H.; Nie, Y.C.; Chen, J.L.; Su, W.W.; Li, P.B. Naringin attenuates acute lung injury in LPS-treated mice by inhibiting NF-κB pathway. *Int. Immunopharmacol.* **2011**, *11*, 1606–1612. [CrossRef] [PubMed]
15. Bissonnette, E.Y.; Lauzon-Joset, J.F.; Debley, J.S.; Ziegler, S.F. Cross-Talk Between Alveolar Macrophages and Lung Epithelial Cells is Essential to Maintain Lung Homeostasis. *Front. Immunol.* **2020**, *11*, 583042. [CrossRef] [PubMed]
16. Shilpa, V.S.; Shams, R.; Dash, K.K.; Pandey, V.K.; Dar, A.H.; Ayaz Mukarram, S.; Harsányi, E.; Kovács, B. Phytochemical Properties, Extraction, and Pharmacological Benefits of Naringin: A Review. *Molecules* **2023**, *28*, 5623. [CrossRef]
17. Li, S.C.; Cheng, Y.T.; Wang, C.Y.; Wu, J.Y.; Chen, Z.W.; Wang, J.P.; Lin, J.H.; Hsuan, S.L. *Actinobacillus pleuropneumoniae* exotoxin ApxI induces cell death via attenuation of FAK through LFA-1. *Sci. Rep.* **2021**, *11*, 1753. [CrossRef] [PubMed]
18. Wang, L.; Qin, W.; Zhang, J.; Bao, C.; Zhang, H.; Che, Y.; Sun, C.; Gu, J.; Feng, X.; Du, C.; et al. Adh enhances *Actinobacillus pleuropneumoniae* pathogenicity by binding to OR5M11 and activating p38 which induces apoptosis of PAMs and IL-8 release. *Sci. Rep.* **2016**, *6*, 24058. [CrossRef]
19. Tang, H.; Zhang, Q.; Han, W.; Wang, Z.; Pang, S.; Zhu, H.; Tan, K.; Liu, X.; Langford, P.R.; Huang, Q.; et al. Identification of FtpA, a Dps-Like Protein Involved in Anti-Oxidative Stress and Virulence in Actinobacillus pleuropneumoniae. *J. Bacteriol.* **2022**, *204*, e0032621. [CrossRef]
20. Bao, C.; Jiang, H.; Zhu, R.; Liu, B.; Xiao, J.; Li, Z.; Chen, P.; Langford, P.R.; Zhang, F.; Lei, L. Differences in pig respiratory tract and peripheral blood immune responses to Actinobacillus pleuropneumoniae. *Vet. Microbiol.* **2020**, *247*, 108755. [CrossRef]
21. Xi, Y.; Chi, Z.; Tao, X.; Zhai, X.; Zhao, Z.; Ren, J.; Yang, S.; Dong, D. Naringin against doxorubicin-induced hepatotoxicity in mice through reducing oxidative stress, inflammation, and apoptosis via the up-regulation of SIRT1. *Environ. Toxicol.* **2023**, *38*, 1153–1161. [CrossRef] [PubMed]
22. Zhai, X.; Dai, T.; Chi, Z.; Zhao, Z.; Wu, G.; Yang, S.; Dong, D. Naringin alleviates acetaminophen-induced acute liver injury by activating Nrf2 via CHAC2 upregulation. *Environ. Toxicol.* **2022**, *37*, 1332–1342. [CrossRef] [PubMed]
23. Syed, A.A.; Reza, M.I.; Shafiq, M.; Kumariya, S.; Singh, P.; Husain, A.; Hanif, K.; Gayen, J.R. Naringin ameliorates type 2 diabetes mellitus-induced steatohepatitis by inhibiting RAGE/NF-κB mediated mitochondrial apoptosis. *Life Sci.* **2020**, *257*, 118118. [CrossRef] [PubMed]
24. Zeng, X.; Su, W.; Liu, B.; Chai, L.; Shi, R.; Yao, H. A Review on the Pharmacokinetic Properties of Naringin and Its Therapeutic Efficacies in Respiratory Diseases. *Mini Rev. Med. Chem.* **2020**, *20*, 286–293. [CrossRef] [PubMed]
25. Guihua, X.; Shuyin, L.; Jinliang, G.; Wang, S. Naringin Protects Ovalbumin-Induced Airway Inflammation in a Mouse Model of Asthma. *Inflammation* **2016**, *39*, 891–899. [CrossRef] [PubMed]
26. Martin, F.P.; Jacqueline, C.; Poschmann, J.; Roquilly, A. Alveolar Macrophages: Adaptation to Their Anatomic Niche during and after Inflammation. *Cells* **2021**, *10*, 2720. [CrossRef] [PubMed]
27. Sassu, E.L.; Bossé, J.T.; Tobias, T.J.; Gottschalk, M.; Langford, P.R.; Hennig-Pauka, I. Update on Actinobacillus pleuropneumoniae-knowledge, gaps and challenges. *Transbound. Emerg. Dis.* **2018**, *65*, 72–90. [CrossRef]
28. Zhang, F.; Zhao, Q.; Tian, J.; Chang, Y.F.; Wen, X.; Huang, X.; Wu, R.; Wen, Y.; Yan, Q.; Huang, Y.; et al. Effective Pro-Inflammatory Induced Activity of GALT, a Conserved Antigen in A. Pleuropneumoniae, Improves the Cytokines Secretion of Macrophage via p38, ERK1/2 and JNK MAPKs Signal Pathway. *Front. Cell Infect. Microbiol.* **2018**, *8*, 337. [CrossRef]
29. Sipos, W.; Cvjetković, V.; Dobrokes, B.; Sipos, S. Evaluation of the Efficacy of a Vaccination Program against *Actinobacillus pleuropneumoniae* Based on Lung-Scoring at Slaughter. *Animals* **2021**, *11*, 2778. [CrossRef]
30. Wu, C.M.; Chen, Z.W.; Chen, T.H.; Liao, J.W.; Lin, C.C.; Chien, M.S.; Lee, W.C.; Hsuan, S.L. Mitogen-activated protein kinases p38 and JNK mediate *Actinobacillus pleuropneumoniae* exotoxin ApxI-induced apoptosis in porcine alveolar macrophages. *Vet. Microbiol.* **2011**, *151*, 372–378. [CrossRef]

Disclaimer/Publisher's Note: The statements, opinions and data contained in all publications are solely those of the individual author(s) and contributor(s) and not of MDPI and/or the editor(s). MDPI and/or the editor(s) disclaim responsibility for any injury to people or property resulting from any ideas, methods, instructions or products referred to in the content.

Article

In Vivo Biocompatibility Study on Functional Nanostructures Containing Bioactive Glass and Plant Extracts for Implantology

Laura Floroian [1,*] and Mihaela Badea [2]

1. Faculty of Electrical Engineering and Computer Science, Transilvania University of Brasov, Romania, No. 1, Politehnicii St., 500031 Brașov, Romania
2. Faculty of Medicine, Transilvania University of Brasov, Romania, No. 56, Nicolae Bălcescu St., 500019 Brașov, Romania; mihaela.badea@unitbv.ro
* Correspondence: lauraf@unitbv.ro

Abstract: In this paper, the in vivo behavior of orthopedic implants covered with thin films obtained by matrix-assisted pulsed laser evaporation and containing bioactive glass, a polymer, and natural plant extract was evaluated. In vivo testing was performed by carrying out a study on guinea pigs who had coated metallic screws inserted in them and also controls, following the regulations of European laws regarding the use of animals in scientific studies. After 26 weeks from implantation, the guinea pigs were subjected to X-ray analyses to observe the evolution of osteointegration over time; the guinea pigs' blood was collected for the detection of enzymatic activity and to measure values for urea, creatinine, blood glucose, alkaline phosphatase, pancreatic amylase, total protein, and glutamate pyruvate transaminase to see the extent to which the body was affected by the introduction of the implant. Moreover, a histopathological assessment of the following vital organs was carried out: heart, brain, liver, and spleen. We also assessed implanted bone with adjacent tissue. Our studies did not find significant variations in biochemical and histological results compared to the control group or significant adverse effects caused by the implant coating in terms of tissue compatibility, inflammatory reactions, and systemic effects.

Keywords: in vivo study; plant extract; orthopedic implant

1. Introduction

Orthopedic implants play a crucial role in the field of medical science by providing support and restoring functionality to damaged or diseased bones and joints. To improve the success and longevity of these implants, researchers have been exploring the use of thin films from various materials or combinations of materials as coatings on implant surfaces [1–6]. Thin films offer a range of benefits, including enhanced biocompatibility [7], improved osseointegration [8], reduced infection rates [9], and controlled drug release [10]. Most modern approaches in this field involve the use of films containing plant extracts for implant covering; this is an area of research that explores the potential benefits of incorporating natural compounds into thin-film coatings [11–14]. Plant extracts contain a wide range of bioactive compounds, such as polyphenols, flavonoids, terpenoids, and alkaloids, which have shown various beneficial properties, including antioxidant, antimicrobial, anti-inflammatory, and osteogenic activities. These compounds have the potential to enhance the performance of orthopedic implants when incorporated into thin-film coatings.

Researchers have been exploring various plant extracts and their incorporation into thin-film coatings for orthopedic implants. Commonly used plant extracts include green tea extract [15], curcumin (from turmeric) [16], aloe vera [17], chamomile, and ginkgo biloba, among others. These extracts have shown promising results in enhancing biocompatibility, antimicrobial activity, and tissue regeneration in preclinical studies.

The fabrication techniques for incorporating plant extracts into thin films can vary, including methods such as electrospinning, layer-by-layer assembly, and physical vapor deposition. The choice of technique depends on the specific properties of the plant extract, the desired film characteristics, and the intended application.

While the use of plant extract-containing films for implant covering is still an active area of research, it shows potential for improving the performance of orthopedic implants by harnessing the natural properties of these plant-derived compounds.

Our team has proposed and implemented a thin double-layered structure fabricated by matrix-assisted pulsed laser evaporation (MAPLE) to cover a metallic implant [18]. The synthesized nanostructure consists of two overlapping layers: the lower layer comprises a biocompatible polymer for anticorrosive protection, and the upper one consists of bioactive glass incorporating antimicrobial plant extract, acting as a drug delivery system. Morphology, composition, adherence, ability for drug delivery, and biological properties (cytotoxicity and antimicrobial effect) were studied and validated by in vitro tests. The structures proved compact and stable, conserving a remarkable drug delivery ability for more than 21 days, i.e., enough to ensure long-term microbe eradication.

The bioactive compounds from plant extracts promote cell adhesion, proliferation, and differentiation, thereby enhancing tissue integration and reducing the risk of implant rejection. Plant extracts possess natural antimicrobial properties, making them effective in preventing bacterial colonization and reducing the risk of implant-associated infections. By incorporating plant extracts with antimicrobial activity into thin-film coatings, the films can create a protective barrier against bacteria, enhancing the long-term success of orthopedic implants.

Inflammation is a common response after implantation, which can hinder proper healing and the integration of the implant. Certain plant extracts have demonstrated anti-inflammatory properties by modulating inflammatory pathways and reducing inflammatory markers [19,20]. Thin-film coatings containing these extracts can help minimize inflammation at the implant site and promote better healing. Also, plant extracts have been found to stimulate bone formation and enhance osteogenic activity. When incorporated into thin-film coatings, these extracts can promote osseointegration, leading to improvements in the stability and longevity of orthopedic implants [21–23]. This work describes the final validation of a structure deposited over implants by in vivo tests, which are crucial. The study was conducted according to the international standards [24].

These types of tests involve the evaluation of implant performance and biocompatibility in living organisms, typically animal models. First, in vivo tests provide valuable information about the biocompatibility of thin-film coatings. They help determine the tissue response, inflammatory reactions, and the body's acceptance of the implant with the coating. These tests are essential to ensure that the coating does not cause adverse reactions such as inflammation, infection, or immune responses. At the same time, in vivo studies assess the integration of the implant with the surrounding tissues [25]. They help to determine the degree of osseointegration, which is the direct structural and functional connection between the implant and the bone. In vivo tests provide insights into the strength and stability of the implant-coating system and its long-term performance. Moreover, in vivo testing allows for the evaluation of the functional performance of the implant with thin-film coating. This can include assessing the range of motion, load-bearing capacity, and biomechanical properties. Such evaluations provide valuable data on the ability of the coating to support normal physiological function.

In our work, some blood was used immediately after harvesting to quantify urea, creatinine, glycemia, alkaline phosphatase, pancreatic amylase, total serum protein, and glutamate pyruvate transaminase (TGP) to analyze how the body was affected by implant insertion. Also, enzyme activity was evaluated by measuring superoxide dismutase, catalase, and glutathione peroxidase.

Urea is the main nitrogenous final product of the metabolism of amino acids [26], originating from the splitting of proteins in the stomach and intestine under the action of proteolytic enzymes and their absorption through the intestinal wall [27]. The main seat of urea formation is the liver, but growing tissue (for example, embryonic or tumor tissue) also has the ability to form urea from arginine. Most of the urea is eliminated by glomerular filtration; 40–60% is redistributed in the blood depending on the tubular flow and the antidiuretic hormone.

Urea in blood and urine varies in direct proportion to the protein diet and is inversely proportional to cellular anabolism during growth, pregnancy, and convalescence [28]. Serum urea is primarily used as a measure of renal or metabolic dysfunction, but it also provides important information about liver function and dietary protein intake [29].

Creatinine is creatine anhydride (methylguanidylacetic acid) and represents its elimination form; it is formed in the muscle tissue. Creatine is synthesized in the liver, and after its release, it is taken up by the muscles in a percentage of 98.6%, where phosphorylation takes place, with this form having an important role in storing muscle energy [30]. When this muscle energy is required for the needs of metabolic processes, phosphocreatine is split to creatinine. The amount of creatine converted into creatinine is maintained at a constant level, which is directly related to the body's muscle tissue mass.

The main utility of serum creatinine determination is the diagnosis of renal failure [31]. The disturbance of renal function reduces creatinine excretion, causing an increase in serum creatinine. Thus, creatinine concentrations provide an approximation of the glomerular filtration rate.

Amylase is an enzyme produced in the pancreas and salivary glands that hydrolyzes starch, glycogen, and related polysaccharides to simple sugars. Amylase is also secreted by the lining of the small intestine, ovaries, placenta, and fallopian tubes [32]. Pancreatic amylase is more thermally labile than salivary amylase, has tissue specificity, and is secreted by acinar cells. The dosage of pancreatic amylase gives indications about how the pancreas works, with the values obtained being important for establishing a diagnosis. Pancreatic amylase is generally the screening test for the diagnosis of acute pancreatitis, with its values increasing 4–6 times above the reference limit [33].

Proteins have a vital role in the normal functioning of the body; therefore, a test that determines total serum proteins is usually included in the list of investigations carried out periodically as a screening method. More than 300 proteins are found in plasma. The test that analyzes the level of total proteins does not count them but determines whether we have enough for our body to function normally. A protein level that is too high or too low can lead to weight loss, fatigue, and inflammatory diseases [34]. The determination of total serum proteins can help diagnose liver and kidney diseases, among others. Proteins are found as a component in enzymes, enzyme inhibitors, clotting factors, antibodies, and transporter proteins. Proteins play the most important role in maintaining osmotic pressure.

Establishing the level of total serum proteins [35] helps in the investigation of edematous syndromes, the diagnosis of conditions accompanied by hypercatabolism such as hyperthyroidism, inflammations, neoplasias, chronic diseases, screening for the detection of gammopathy.

Alkaline phosphatase is an enzyme that belongs to the class of hydrolases and is found in the liver, digestive system, kidneys, and bones. Bone alkaline phosphatase is produced in osteoblasts and plays a role in the formation of bone tissue [36]. The laboratory test measures the activity of enzymes in the body and helps detect liver or bone disorders.

Increased values for alkaline phosphatase indicate the presence of a condition but cannot show whether the liver or bile ducts are functioning problematically. For this reason, in most cases, alkaline phosphatase is determined together with other specific analyses. It can also be used in oncological diagnosis [37], especially for bone tumors, Paget's disease, and liver cancers [38].

Low alkaline phosphatase, that is a value below the reference range for the patient's age and sex, can be seen in those with familial bone disease (hypophosphatasia), achondroplasia, cretinism, malnutrition, vitamin C deficiency, zinc deficiency, and magnesium deficiency, as well as in women with osteoporosis who have entered menopause [39].

Glutamate pyruvate transaminase is an enzyme found mostly in the liver and, to a lesser extent, in the kidneys, myocardium, skeletal muscles, and pancreas, with a role in enzymatic reactions that use proteins as an energy source [40]. The absolute values of the enzyme do not correlate directly with the severity of the organ's suffering, as serial, periodic determinations of the compound are necessary to monitor the evolution of the disease and establish a prognosis in patients with this condition. The administration of medication (acetaminophen) or substances with a liver-toxic effect (e.g., alcohol consumption) represent other situations in which an increase in TGP values is recorded.

Increases of up to 20–100 times compared to the normal value are specific to acute viral and toxic drug hepatitis, while multiplication by 2 or 3 of the physiological values occurs in hepatic steatosis (fatty liver). Liver metastases are accompanied by moderate increases in TGP, and in the case of a diagnosis of primary hepatoma, the changes are minimal [41].

Decreases in TGP values are found in urinary infections, neoplasia (hepatocellular carcinoma), and pyridoxal phosphate deficiency (found in malnutrition and alcoholic hepatitis [42].

Superoxide dismutase (SOD) is an enzyme that catalyzes the dismutation of superoxide ($O_2\bullet$) into hydrogen peroxide (H_2O_2) and molecular oxygen (O_2). Superoxide is a reactive oxygen species that can be produced in excess in inflammatory and oxidative processes [43]. SOD helps to eliminate superoxide and prevent the formation of other more harmful reactive oxygen species. This can protect tissues against implant-induced oxidative stress and promote healing and regeneration processes. SOD is widely distributed in humans, in all other mammals, and in most chordates. It occurs in high concentrations in the liver, heart, brain, kidney, and erythrocytes. Some enzymes (such as NADPH oxidase) are used by human white blood cells to generate superoxide and other reactive oxygen species to kill bacteria. The amount of SOD present in cellular and extracellular environments is crucial for the prevention of diseases linked to oxidative stress [44].

Catalase (oxidoreductase, CAT) is an omnipresent antioxidant enzyme that exists in most aerobic cells. Catalase is involved in the detoxification of hydrogen peroxide (H_2O_2), a reactive oxygen species, which is a toxic product of both pathogenic reactive oxygen species production and normal aerobic metabolism. In human beings, the highest levels of CAT are in the kidney, liver, and erythrocytes, where it is believed to account for the majority of H_2O_2 decomposition [45]. The measurement of catalase activity can provide information about the ability of the antioxidant system to cope with the stress induced by orthopedic implants.

Glutathione peroxidase (GPx) is an intracellular antioxidant enzyme that reduces hydrogen peroxide to water and limits its harmful effects [46]. By limiting hydrogen peroxide accumulation, GPx also modulates processes that involve it, like mitochondrial function, growth factor-mediated signal transduction, and the maintenance of normal thiol redox balance. The regulation and removal of hydrogen peroxide prevents the formation of the highly reactive and damaging hydroxyl radical, which can be formed by the reaction of hydrogen peroxide with Fe^{2+} (Fenton reaction) and may protect against oxidative stress [47]. GPx-1 is an isoform of GPx, one of several cellular enzymes that may modulate overall redox stress. Decreased GPx-1 activity can promote susceptibility to oxidative stress by allowing for the accumulation of harmful oxidants, whereas excess GPx-1 may promote reductive stress, characterized by a lack of essential ROS needed for cellular signaling processes. Excess oxidants or the loss of essential ROS can lead to diminished cell growth and promote apoptotic pathways [48].

2. Results and Discussion

Because the processes in the guinea pig body are carried out much faster than in humans [49], to obtain information on the behavior of the implant and the human body for a long time after implantation, we analyzed the implant and the body of each guinea pig at just 26 weeks after implantation. At that moment, the guinea pigs were subjected to another surgical procedure to remove the implant from the body, and at the same time, blood and organ harvests were collected from all the animals studied.

2.1. X-ray Imaging

At 26 weeks after implantation, the guinea pigs were again subjected to X-ray analyses to observe the evolution of osteointegration over time. Shown below are some radiographs and the significant details of them (Figure 1). There is good bone implant stability and good fixation (Figure 1a,b). In the case of a single guinea pig, the implant moves out of the bone and becomes parallel to the bone, as shown in Figure 1c. This could be due not necesarily an incorrect implantation but also to the fact that the animal feels a foreign body under the skin and does its best to remove it. For this reason, the implantations were performed carefully in areas where guinea pigs cannot reach with their teeth or claws.

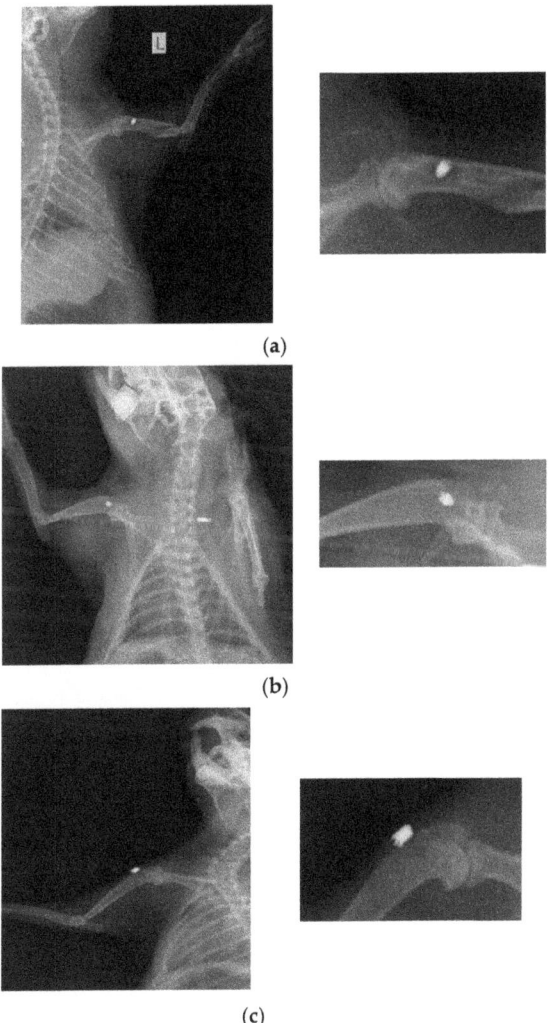

Figure 1. RX images of implants inserted in the humerus of guinea pigs: (**a**) lot I, (**b**) lot II, and (**c**) lot III.

2.2. EDS Analyses on Implants Removed from the Body

The results of the quantitative compositional analysis of stainless steel (OL) implant coated with BG + neem/PMMA layer (referred to as BGN) are presented in Table 1. In addition to the components of hydroxyapatite (HA) (i.e., Ca, P, and O), EDS analyses revealed the presence of some trace elements (Na, Mg, F) characteristic of the bone mineral phase. In addition to the above-mentioned elements, which are naturally found in the chemical composition of healthy bone tissue, other species characteristic of the steel substrate could also be detected

Table 1. Chemical compositions in wt% of the coatings obtained by MAPLE.

Sample	Element									
	Ca	P	Na	Mg	C	O	Al	Cr	Fe	Ni
	Concentration (wt. %)									
BGN	8.56	6.58	1.9	2.82	16.83	41.7	0.28	3.37	11.59	1.01

The Ca/P molar ratio of the material was ~1.30, indicating, according to FTIR results, the presence of carbonate apatite [50], which means that consistent osteointegration has taken place.

2.3. Blood Analyses

The harvested blood was used immediately after collection to measure values for urea, creatinine, blood glucose, alkaline phosphatase, pancreatic amylase, total protein, and TGP to see the extent to which the body was affected by the introduction of the implant of titanium (Ti), stainless steel, or stainless steel coated. The obtained values are presented in Table 2, also for guinea pigs without implant (WI). That table also contains normal blood analysis values for guinea pigs from the literature [51].

Table 2. Blood analysis results for study groups.

Analysis	Normal Values	Lot I Ti	Lot II OL	Lot III BGN	Lot IV WI
Urea (mmol/L)	2.04–11.28	3.21	3.07	3.13	3.13
Creatinine (µmol/L)	23.90–73.45	59.4	58.67	52.8	61.6
Blood glucose (mmol/L)	4.62–19.55	15.44	12.90	14.74	10.22
Pancreatic amylase (U/L)	726.93–1831.55	1421	1420.33	1479	1707.25
Total protein (g/dL)	5.00–7.09	4.85	4.27	4.25	4.88
Alkaline phosphatase (U/L)	50.80–328.10	42	28	27	41
TGP (U/L)	41.45–165.35	23	22.33	21	22.25

The graphs in Figures 2–6 compare all the values with those measured for the titanium implant because the process for the validation of the in vivo tests requires reporting related to an implant made from a commonly used and accepted material, with established characteristics, which, in bone implantology, is titanium.

Figure 2a shows that the process of urea formation and elimination worked properly. Lower urea values compared to Ti values can suggest a more rapid formation of new bone tissue, as in vitro tests have demonstrated [18].

Figure 2b does not show an increase in serum creatinine in the case of implantation, instead showing a slight decrease, which proves the good functioning of the kidneys is not affected by the introduction or presence of the implant.

From the point of view of blood glucose determination, Figure 3a contains values obtained for all four groups of study, and we observed a slight increase in all cases with implants (Ti, OL, or BGN) compared to the cases without implants (WI), a normal reaction for a stressed body in which a foreign body is introduced.

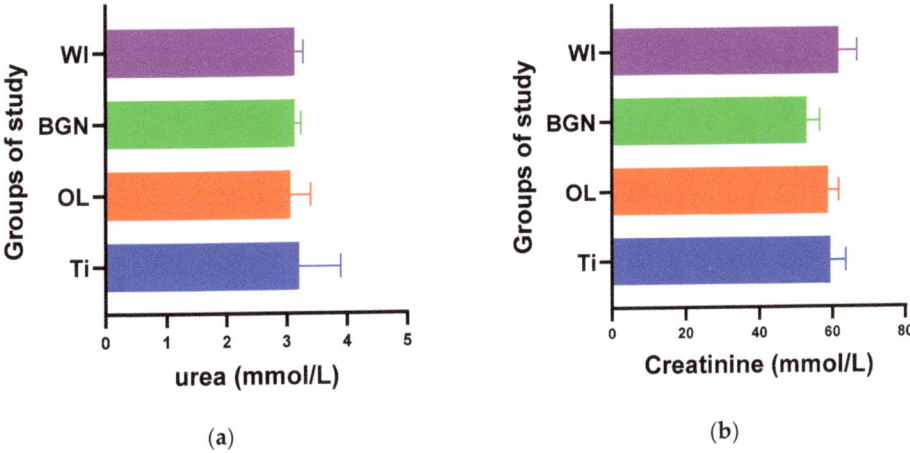

Figure 2. Urea (**a**) and creatinine (**b**) values of guinea pig groups.

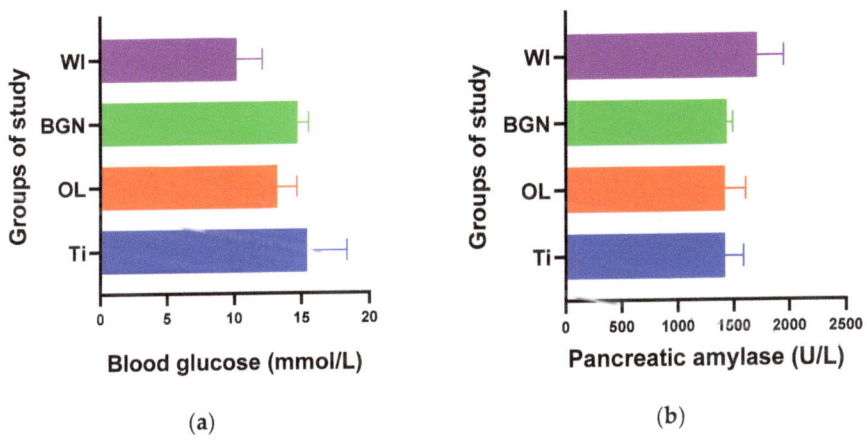

Figure 3. Blood glucose (**a**) and pancreatic amylase (**b**) values of guinea pig groups.

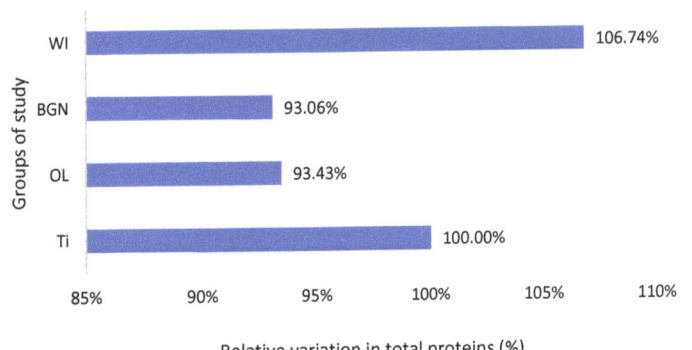

Figure 4. Relative variation in total proteins of guinea pig groups versus the group with the Ti implant.

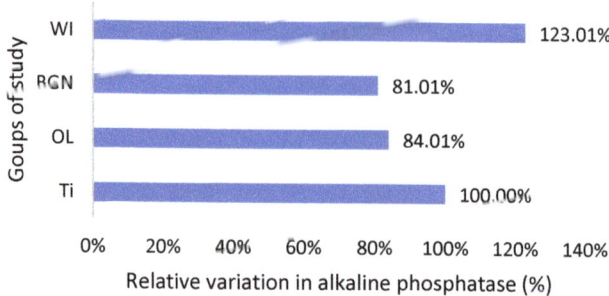

Figure 5. Relative variation in alkaline phosphatase of guinea pig groups versus the group with the Ti implant.

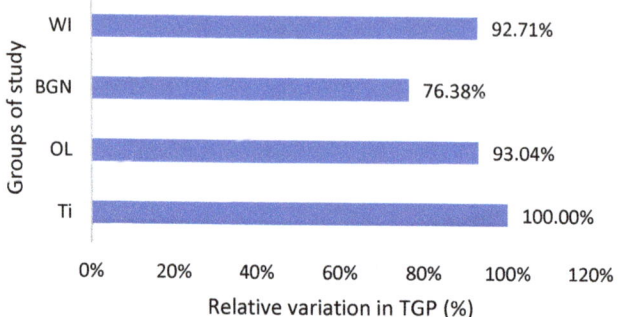

Figure 6. Relative variation in TGP of guinea pig groups versus the group with the Ti implant.

Comparing the Ti and BGN groups, we observed smaller blood glucose values in the animals with implants coated with BGN because of its plant component, neem, which is recognized for such an effect [52].

In our experiment, measured values of pancreatic amylase were in the normal range in both the implanted and not-implanted guinea pigs, which underlined that the pancreas is not affected by the presence of the implant in the body.

Also, the measured values of total protein are slightly lower than the normal ones, including those of animals without implants, but very close to each other (Figure 4). This fact, along with the results of the analyses described below, leads to the hypothesis of the existence of a lower-protein diet of the animals during the study. Proteins can adsorb on metal surfaces, and such protein adsorption layers can induce corrosion protection by blocking the active sites of the surface [53].

Regarding the alkaline phosphatase values obtained for the guinea pigs implanted with all types of implants, they are smaller than those for the pigs without implants (Figure 5). This could be related to the fact that bone tissue reconstruction is magnesium-consuming. Those with the BGN implant demonstrated a bigger rate of bone growth [18], as determined by in vitro testing, and the relative variation in alkaline phosphatase was bigger, which shows a good correlation.

Magnesium is a very important component of bone structure, an indispensable component for the absorption of calcium from food and its fixation at the bone level [54]. Magnesium stored in bones is not passive but contributes to bone stabilization, growth, and mineralization. During the bone synthesis process, intensified by the coating of the implant, the need for magnesium increases, and its consumption leads to increased absorption from the blood, hence the existing magnesium deficit.

As can be seen in Table 2, the TGP values are not in the normal range; instead, they are almost half of the minimum normal value for all study groups, which is bad news. Also, there are lower alkaline phosphatase and total protein values, all of which suggest that the nutrition of the guinea pigs was insufficient. In the studies that will follow, it will be necessary to change guinea pigs' diet with a much more protein-rich one. The good news is that the TGP values measured for the guinea pigs with BGN or OL implants do not show an increase, but they are smaller than for the animals with the Ti implants (Figure 6). Low levels are generally considered good and are usually not a cause for concern. However, in some cases, a low TGP can be a result of an underlying medical condition, such as vitamin B6 deficiency.

2.4. Detection of Other Enzymatic Activity

The introduction of an implant into the body naturally produces oxidative stress [55], a fact highlighted by the significant changes in enzyme activity for all three monitored enzymes.

Analyzing the obtained results, we noticed that the presence of the BGN implant in the body causes it to release the largest amounts of SOD (see Figure 7), which can help to quickly eliminate superoxide and prevent the formation of other more harmful reactive oxygen species. This protects the tissues against the oxidative stress induced by the implant and promotes the healing and regeneration processes.

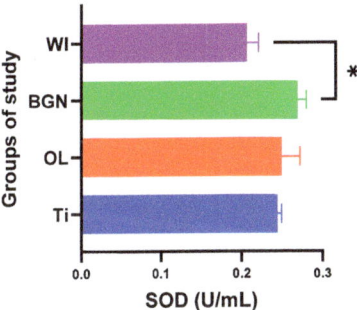

Figure 7. Superoxide dismutase values of guinea pig groups (* level of significance $p < 0.5$).

Analyzing the values obtained for CAT, we noticed that the introduction of the titanium implant in the body leads to a slight decrease in catalase activity, and it seems that the antioxidant system has a weak capacity to deal with the oxidative stress induced by the implant. Things are completely different in the cases of the OL and BGN implants, where catalase has a pronounced activity, especially in the BGN group, the calculations for which generated statistically significant results (see Figure 8).

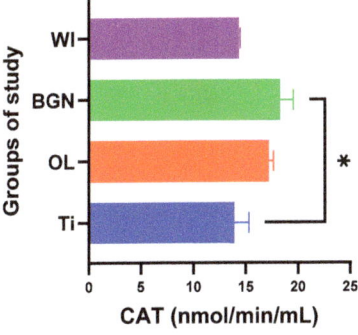

Figure 8. Catalase values of guinea pig groups (* level of significance $p < 0.5$).

Regarding GPx, the body reaction closest to the case of the guinea pigs with a titanium implant was obtained in the BGN group (Figure 9).

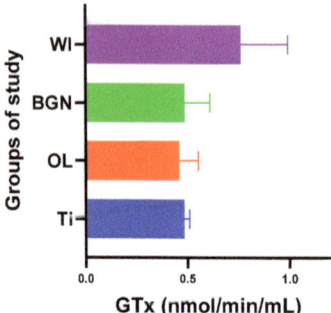

Figure 9. Glutathione peroxidase values of guinea pig groups.

All this shows that the best response to the oxidative stress generated by the introduction of the implant into the body was recorded in guinea pigs with thin film-coated implants rather than those with Ti or stainless-steel implants.

The results obtained for the SOD, CAT, and GPx activities are summarized in Table 3.

Table 3. Calculated values for enzymatic activity.

Lot	SOD (U/mL)	CAT (nmol/min/mL)	GPx (nmol/min/mL)
I Ti	0.244	13.98	0.480
II OL	0.250	17.26	0.462
III BGN	0.270	18.39	0.486
IV WI	0.206	14.43	0.739

Oxidative stress is a factor of the initiation of inflammation, fibrosis in various organs, genotoxicity, the inhibition of cell multiplication, and, finally, cell death, and obtaining lower values for oxidative stress in our work means there is a lower risk of these effects occurring when implanting screws coated with such nanocomposite thin films into the human body.

2.5. Histopathology Studies

Figure 10 shows histopathological images for guinea pigs' organs after 26 weeks from implantation: liver (a, b), spleen (c, d), brain (e, f), heart (g, h), bone, (i) and muscle (j).

A liver sample of approximately 7 × 5 × 2.4 cm was sectioned through the left and right lateral lobes, processed, and embedded in paraffin. Figure 10a,b are diffuse; the hepatocytes show predominantly optically empty cytoplasm, rarely (periportal) with granular appearance, eosinophilic, central nucleus, rarely binucleated. The blood vessels and bile ducts do not show changes. Panlobular hepatic glycogenosis can be interpreted. Glycogenosis can be caused by increased glycogen synthesis (diets rich in carbohydrates, the administration of corticosteroids, etc.) or in glycogen storage diseases with systemic manifestation.

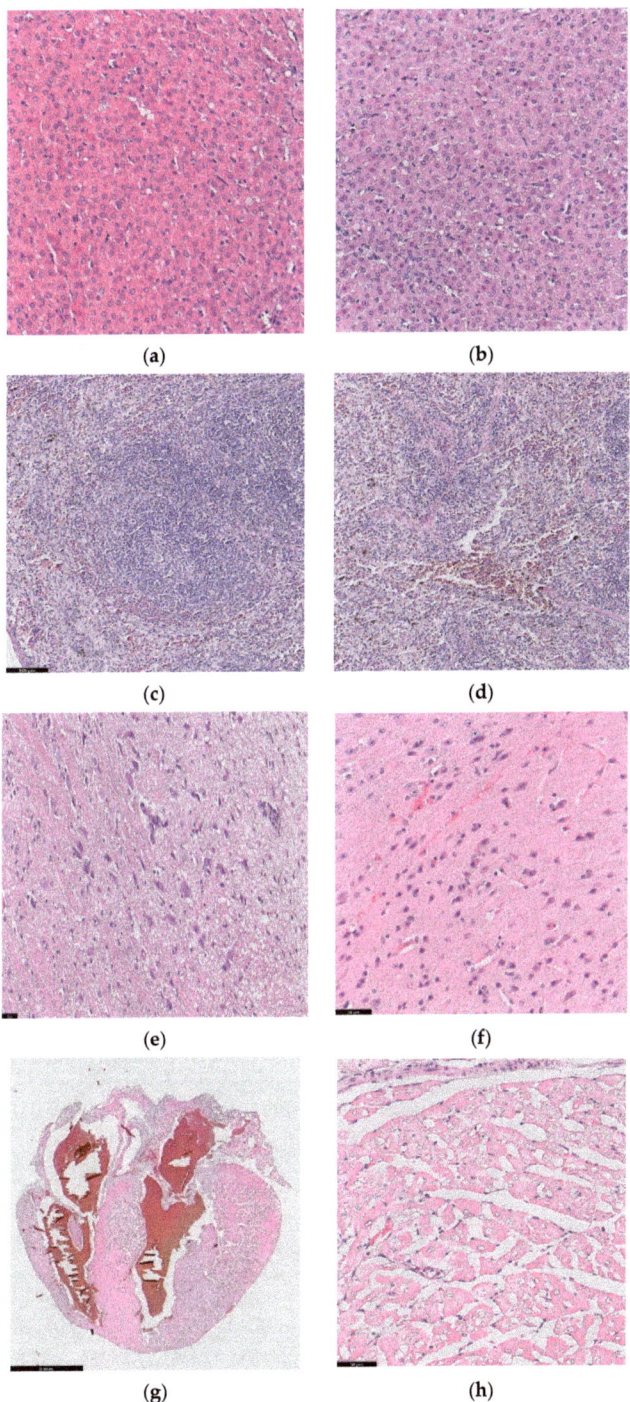

Figure 10. *Cont.*

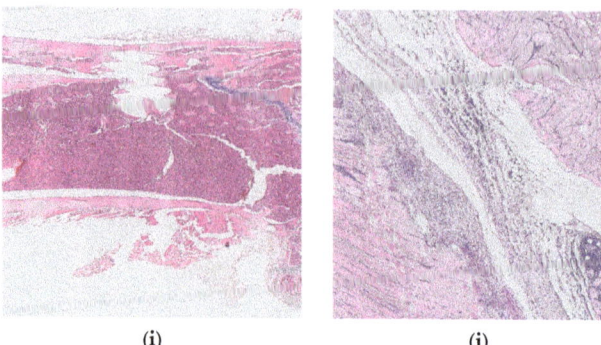

(i)   (j)

Figure 10. Histopathological images for liver (**a**,**b**), spleen (**c**,**d**), brain (**e**,**f**), heart (**g**,**h**), bone (i), and muscle (j).

Spleen samples (2.9 × 1.6 × 0.5 cm) were sectioned in four slices parallel to the longitudinal axis, and two of which were processed and embedded in paraffin. Red pulp is well represented, with areas of extramedullary hematopoiesis and the accumulation of hemosiderin, and white pulp is represented by splenic follicles, occasionally with hyperplasia of the germinal centers. No pathological changes in the spleen were detected in the examined sections.

Two longitudinal sections, one paramedian and one sagittal through half of the hemisphere of brain, were processed and embedded in paraffin. In the examined sections, the nervous tissue did not show any pathological changes.

Cord of 2.5 × 2 × 1.6 cm with hemopericardium was examined. Parasagittal sectioning through the heart, including the four chambers and, partially, the great vessels, was performed, and we also analyzed ectized blood and lymphatic vessels. Muscle fibers have optically empty intracytoplasmic vacuoles (glycogen accumulations) of variable sizes. No pathological changes were detected.

We should mention that the existence of glycogenosis in the liver and heart was also observed in the control groups that did not receive implants, so it is not related to the implant materials.

Histopathological examinations about bone and muscle are presented in Figure 10i,j, which show antero-lateral musculature sectioned longitudinally parallel to the axis of the humerus. After the decalcification of the bone (24 h), three slices parallel to the longitudinal axis were made, of which the one that included the trajectory of the implant was included.

Focal periosteal reaction with proliferation of fibroblasts and osteogenic layer, abundant adjacent fibrous tissue with reduced cellularity and a reduced number of capillaries of uniform diameter, perpendicular or oblique to the surface of the periosteum (scar tissue). The bone compact in the vicinity of the implant shows an irregular subperiosteal surface, well-represented osteoid tissue, with rare, reduced foci of chondrocytes. Growth cartilage, scapulohumeral articular surface and bone marrow do not show changes.

The muscles show discrete lipid infiltration and numerous eosinophilic cells focally and peripherally aggregated among the connective tissue fibers, around a group of foamy macrophages. Eosinophils are also present perivascularly, in variable numbers, and multifocal.

Interpretation: Periosteal hyperplasia. Callus in resolution. Discreet eosinophilic myositis. Osseointegration is good, without inflammatory reactions or other adverse effects. The presence of eosinophils in the tissue may indicate a parasitic infection or a hypersensitivity response.

3. Materials and Methods

3.1. Fabrication of the Structure for Implantation

Were made two lots of metallic screws—one lot of stainless-steel screws and one lot of titanium grade 4 screws—with the proper dimensions for implantation: 3 mm long and 2 mm diameter, with M2 thread and a rounded tip achieved with 2 drilling channels (Figure 11). The implants were screwed with a cross key specially made for this experiment. The stainless-steel screws composition is as follows: 64.26% Fe, 18.51% Cr, 13% Ni, 2.13% Mo, 1.44% Mn, 0.48% Cu, 0.56% Si, 0.0265% C, 0.0036% S, and a smaller concentration of other elements, in accordance with the ISO 5832-1:2016(E) International Standard [56].

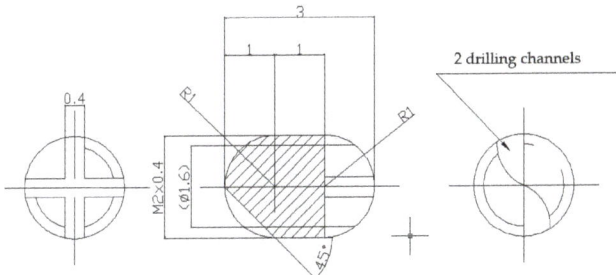

Figure 11. Metallic screws for implantation.

Some of the implants were covered with nanometric films containing bioactive glass (BG) from SiO_2-Na_2O-K_2O-CaO-MgO-P_2O_5 system, plant extract of Azadirachta indica (neem), an Indian medicinal plant used in traditional Ayurveda treatment of various infections, and Poly(methyl methacrylate) (PMMA) in two layered structures- BG + neem/PMMA/OL- using an advanced laser-based technique (matrix assisted pulsed laser evaporation), like in [18].

3.2. Surgery and Implantation Procedure

For our in vivo studies, the chosen subjects for implant surgery (Figure 12) were guinea pigs (*Cavia porcellus*), which have similar developmental and physiological characteristics to humans and, in some ways, are better models than mice because of their relatively larger body size and higher stress resistance to experimental manipulation [57]. The studies were carried out at the Department of Sanitary, Veterinary and Public Health of Brasov County (DSVSA).

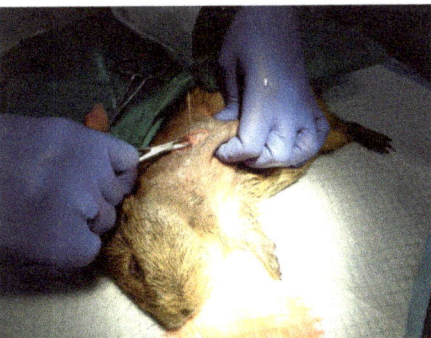

Figure 12. Implant surgery.

From the existing biobase, healthy animals (males) of the same age (one year) and approximately the same weight (650–700 g) were selected and grown in optimal conditions, as required by Law 149/2019 on the protection of animals used for scientific purposes, published in Official Monitor, MO, Part I nr. 619 of 25 June 2019, and also EU regulations on animal research [24,57,58]. Ten guinea pigs for each material and ten control guinea pigs were used.

Special cages with a minimum enclosure area of 2500 cm^2, a minimum enclosure height of 23 cm, and a floor area of 900 cm^2 per animal were constructed. The heating, ventilation, and lighting systems were inspected to ensure that the inside of the cages had a constant temperature of 22 °C, constant humidity, and 12 h light/12 h darkness cycles.

Important notes:
- The persons conducting or participating in the experiments, as well as the persons who cared for the animals, including those that supervised them, had received specialized training and had experience with such studies.
- A minimum number of animals of low neurophysiological sensitivity (guinea pigs) was used.
- All experiments were set up to prevent the experimental animals from suffering and experiencing undue pain; hence, general anesthesia was used, and if the animals suffered pain after the effect of anesthesia had passed, they were treated early with analgesics applied for 5 days post-operation.

3.3. In Vivo Study

Screws consisting of the tested materials (steel, titanium, and steel coated with special thin films) were implanted into the humerus bones of guinea pigs from three groups, and the fourth group contained animals without implants, as shown in Table 4.

Table 4. The study groups.

Group	Substrate	Coating	Name
I	Ti	without coating	Ti
II	OL	without coating	OL
III	OL	BG + neem/PMMA	BGN
IV	unimplanted guineea pigs		WI

In the beginning, the pigs were weighed before being placed into a tucked position to enable one to chip into the implantation area. Kanamycin sulfate ophthalmic ointment (Antibiotice a+, Iasi, Romania) was applied to prevent corneal dryness during the surgery. Implantation was performed under general anesthesia by the neuroleptic analgesic method using a combination of ketamine (80 mg/kg body weight) and xylazine (10 mg/kg body weight), following ISO 10993-6:2016 [24].

Before the effect of anesthesia had finished and for 5 days after the surgery, analgesic injections (meloxicam) were applied for pain relief, and local treatment with both povidone iodine and spray containing zinc was applied to avoid infections.

At the end of the intervention, each guinea pig was microcipated for full control and handling without the risk of mistaking their belonging to one of the lots. X-ray post-implantation radiographs were made to visualize the correct insertion of the implant into the body.

For 26 weeks, the animals were kept, cared for, and supervised in accordance with the Care and Housing Standards set out in ANNEX NO. 3, Law 149/2019 [57].

Remarks:
- The wounds of guinea pigs from Lot III healed after 7 days;
- After 7 days, 2 guinea pigs from Lot I required sewing to close their wounds and anti-inflammatory treatment because they had a 1–2 cm long sore wound;
- One guinea pig from Lot II showed a 2 cm wound with a slight amount of blood-swelling exudate and needed 2-wire emergency stitching, as well as an anti-inflammatory injection;

- The occurrence of wounds may have been due to the stitching initially carried out on the inside, which proved to be too weak. It may be useful in subsequent studies to apply a "stitch in points" approach, which can lead to greater resistance.

To draw conclusions related to the influence of the implant on the guinea pigs' body, X-ray and energy-dispersive spectroscopy (EDS) analyses were performed, as well as blood analyses, five months after implantation.

EDS was performed on all samples removed from the body after 26 weeks using a SiLi detector (EDAX Inc., Philips, Edinburgh, The Netherlands) that has eZAF Smart Quant Results software and operates at 15 kV.

Some blood was used immediately after harvesting to quantify urea, creatinine, glycemia, alkaline phosphatase, pancreatic amylase, total serum protein, and glutamate pyruvate transaminase to analyze how the body was affected by implant insertion.

3.4. Detection of Enzymatic Activity

Moreover, another part of the collected blood was harvested in EDTA anticoagulant containers and centrifuged at $1000 \times g$ for 10 min to obtain plasma, which was then stored at -20 °C. Using special kits (Cayman Chemical, Ann Arbor, Mi, USA), enzyme activity was evaluated by measuring superoxide dismutase, catalase, and glutathione peroxidase. Changes in the values of these parameters compared to the non-implanted group will indicate the level of oxidative stress in the body and the degree of damage to the body caused by inserting the implant, and comparisons with the group of guinea pigs implanted with SS will show whether there are any advantages of implant coating.

The introduction of an orthopedic implant into the body triggers an inflammatory response as a response of the immune system to the presence of a foreign body. This inflammatory response involves the release of pro-inflammatory cytokines such as interleukin-1 (IL-1), interleukin-6 (IL-6), and tumor necrosis factor-alpha (TNF-α), as well as the formation of reactive oxygen species (ROS). These reactions can impact the performance and durability of orthopedic implants.

Superoxide dismutase (SOD), glutathione peroxidase (GPx), and catalase (CAT) are antioxidant enzymes involved in neutralizing and eliminating reactive oxygen species from the body. These enzymes have an important role in protecting tissues against oxidative stress and may be relevant in the context of coated implants.

Their activity is often measured to assess the level of oxidative stress induced by orthopedic implants. Oxidative stress occurs when there is an imbalance between the production of reactive oxygen species and the ability of the body's antioxidant system to neutralize them. Enzyme activity is therefore considered an important marker of the cellular ability to combat superoxide free radicals and maintain the redox balance around the implants.

3.4.1. Determination of Superoxide Dismutase

In this work, tetrazolium salt was utilized for the detection of superoxide radicals in blood plasma. One unit of SOD is defined as the amount of enzyme needed to exhibit 50% dismutation of the superoxide radical. Triplicate standards and samples were put on a well plate up to a volume of 210 µL in a well-determined order.

Into the SOD standard wells, 10 µL of the standard solution of bovine erythrocyte (Cu/Zn) with 7 different concentrations (and activity) and 200 µL of the diluted Radical Detector (tetrazolium salt solution) were added. The sample wells contained 10 µL of sample and 200 µL of the diluted Radical Detector. A reaction was initiated by adding 20 µL of diluted xanthine oxidase to all the wells; the well plates were shaken for a few seconds and incubated on a shaker at room temperature for 30 min. Then, the absorbance was read at 440–460 nm using a plate reader.

The average absorbance of each standard and sample was calculated, and sample background absorbance was subtracted from the sample. The activity of superoxide dismutase was determined (Table 3) using the formula below (where the necessary corrections are made) using the slope of the calibration curve (Figure 13) and the linearized SOD standard rate (LR) as a function of final SOD Activity (U/mL):

$$\text{SOD}\left(\frac{U}{mL}\right) = \left[\left(\frac{\text{sample LR} - \text{y intercept}}{\text{slope}}\right) \times \frac{0.23\ mL}{0.01\ mL}\right] \times \text{sample dilution}$$

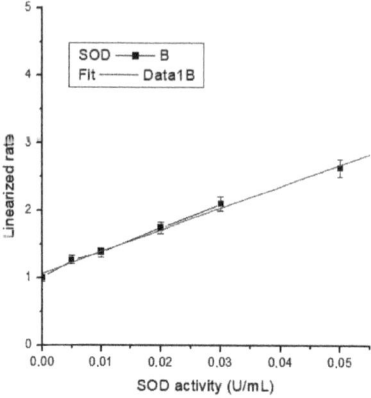

Figure 13. Calibration curve of SOD activity.

The equation of the calibration line is y = 1.06582 + 32.38154x, with a very good correlation coefficient (R^2 = 0.997), almost unitary.

3.4.2. Determination of Catalase

We used the peroxidatic function of CAT for the determination of enzyme activity. This method is based on the reaction between the enzyme and methanol in the presence of an optimal H_2O_2 concentration. The formaldehyde produced is measured using 4-amino-3-hydrazino-5-mercapto-1,2,4-triazole (Purpald) as the chromogen.

The preparation of the formaldehyde standards was carried out by diluting catalase formaldehyde standard with diluted sample buffer to obtain formaldehyde stock solution with different concentrations: 0, 5, 15, 30, 45, 60, and 75 µM formaldehyde.

The standards, positive control (lyophilized powder of bovine liver CAT), and samples were put in triplicate on a well plate up to a volume of 240 µL in a very well-established order, following the assay protocol. The reactions were initiated by adding 20 µL of diluted hydrogen peroxide to all the wells, and after 20 min of incubation at room temperature, 30 µL potassium hydroxide was added to each well to end the reactions. We put 30 µL of catalase Purpald (chromogen) in each well, followed by incubation on a shaker for 10 min at room temperature.

Absorbance was read at 540 nm, and the calibration curve was built. Using the curve slope and the formula below, with necessary corrections, formaldehyde was determined.

$$\text{Formaldechyde}(\mu M) = \left[\frac{\text{sample absorbance} - \text{y intercept}}{\text{slope}}\right] \times \frac{0.17\ mL}{0.02\ mL}$$

The CAT activity of the sample was calculated (Table 3) using the following equation and considering that one unit is the amount of enzyme that will cause the formation of 1.0 nmol of formaldehyde per minute at 25 °C.

$$\text{CAT activity} = \frac{\mu m\ \text{of Formaldehide sample}}{20\ min} \times \text{sample dilution} = \frac{nmoL}{min}/mL$$

3.4.3. Determination of Glutathione Peroxidase

In this work, GPX activity was measured indirectly by the oxidation of NADPH, which was accompanied by a decrease in absorbance at 340 nm.

On a well plate, in triplicate, the background (assay buffer), positive controls (bovine erythrocyte GPX, lyophilized glutathione, and glutathione reductase), and the samples were measured up to a volume of 190 µL in a very well- determined order, and the reaction was initiated by quickly adding 20 µL of cumene hydroperoxide to all the wells.

Absorbance was read at 340 nm once per minute to obtain more than five readings; the mean absorbance was calculated, and the calibration curve for each reading was constructed. Using its slope and the formula below, where the necessary corrections are made, GPX activity was determined (Table 3).

$$\text{GPx activity} = \frac{\text{slope}}{0.00373} \times \frac{0.19 \text{ mL}}{0.02 \text{ mL}} \times \text{sample dilution}$$

3.5. Histopathological Evaluation

The histopathological evaluation of orthopedic medical devices involves the examination of tissue samples collected from around the implant site to assess the local tissue response and potential adverse reactions associated with the device, as well as the examination of vital organs, including the heart, liver, pancreas, spleen, and kidneys. This comprehensive evaluation provides a broader understanding of the systemic effects and potential adverse reactions associated with the medical device [59–61]. It is an important component of preclinical and clinical studies to evaluate the biocompatibility and safety of orthopedic implants.

Our histopathological evaluation of the different types of studied implants had multiple aims, the first of which was to assess tissue response to the implant. This involved examining the cellular and structural changes, inflammation, fibrosis, vascularization, and presence of foreign body reactions in the tissue surrounding the implant. This evaluation provided insights into the biocompatibility and local tissue integration of the device [62].

The second aim was the identification of adverse reactions. Histopathological evaluations help identify any adverse reactions or complications associated with the orthopedic device. This may include the presence of necrosis, granuloma formation, chronic inflammation, excessive fibrosis, or other tissue abnormalities. The detection of adverse reactions is crucial for understanding the potential risks and improving the design and performance of medical devices and is of great importance in determining the possible hospital-associated infections [63].

The third goal was the assessment of the potential systemic effects and toxicity caused in vital organs, which involves any pathological changes, inflammation, or organ-specific reactions that may result from the presence of the implant, as well as organ-specific toxicity such as hepatotoxicity, nephrotoxicity, and cardiotoxicity, which may occur due to the implant or its interaction with the body. Our histopathological evaluation of vital organs also provided information on organ function and viability. It helped to assess the impact of the implant on organ health and functioning, allowing for the detection of any abnormalities or functional impairments.

The procedure used for our histopathological evaluation was the usual one. Tissue samples were collected from the implant site during post-mortem examination. The samples included samples of peri-implant tissue, adjacent bone, surrounding soft tissue, and vital organs. The collected tissue samples were carefully dissected, fixed, processed, and embedded in paraffin wax or frozen for sectioning. Paraffin sections were stained with histological stains like Hematoxylin and Eosin (H&E) for general tissue assessment, while other specialized stains were used to evaluate specific tissue components or reactions. Then, the stained tissue sections were examined under a microscope.

4. Conclusions

Our biochemical blood analysis and histological analysis of the guinea pigs' organs and of the tissues surrounding the implants did not show significant adverse effects caused by the implant coating containing bioactive glass, a polymer, and natural plant extract in terms of tissue compatibility, inflammatory reactions, and systemic effects.

Author Contributions: Conceptualization, L.F.; methodology, L.F. and M.B.; validation, L.F. and M.B.; writing—original draft preparation, L.F.; writing—review and editing, L.F. and M.B.; funding acquisition, L.F. All authors have read and agreed to the published version of the manuscript.

Funding: This research was funded by the European Union, structural funds project PRO-DD (POS-CCE, O.2.2.1., ID 123, SMIS 2637, ctr. No 11/2009), and UEFISCDI Romania, PN-III-P2-2.1-PED-2016-0621 no. 146PED/2017.

Institutional Review Board Statement: All of the experimental procedures involving animals were conducted in accordance with the Law 43/2014 on the Protection of animals used for scientific purposes, published in the Official Monitor, Part I no. 326 of 6 May 2014, and approved by the National Veterinary Sanitary and Food Safety Authority, Veterinary Sanitary and Food Safety Directorate of Brașov County, Romania, endorsement no. 9191/16.06.2016.

Data Availability Statement: The raw data supporting the conclusions of this article will be made available by the authors on request.

Acknowledgments: We are grateful to veterinary doctor Gabriel Stan (NatiVet, Brasov, Romania) for performing implantation surgeries, to Claudiu Gal, Synevovet Laboratory, Bucharest, Romania, for his technical expertise in histopathology, and Laser-Surface-Plasma Interactions Laboratory from INFLPR Magurele, Romania, for thin films deposition on implants.

Conflicts of Interest: The authors have no conflicts of interest to declare.

References

1. Wang, X.; Honda, Y.; Zhao, J.; Morikuni, H.; Nishiura, A.; Hashimoto, Y.; Matsumoto, N. Enhancement of Bone-Forming Ability on Beta-Tricalcium Phosphate by Modulating Cellular Senescence Mechanisms Using Senolytics. *Int. J. Mol. Sci.* **2021**, *22*, 12415. [CrossRef]
2. Vladescu, A.; Badea, M.; Padmanabhan, S.C.; Paraschiv, G.; Floroian, L.; Gaman, L.; Morris, M.A.; Marty, J.L.; Cotrut, C.M. Nanomaterials for medical applications and their antimicrobial advantages. In *Materials for Biomedical Engineering*; Holban, A.-M., Grumezescu, A.M., Eds.; Elsevier Inc.: Amsterdam, The Netherlands, 2019; pp. 409–431.
3. Saruta, J.; Ozawa, R.; Okubo, T.; Taleghani, S.R.; Ishijima, M.; Kitajima, H.; Hirota, M.; Ogawa, T. Biomimetic Zirconia with Cactus-Inspired Meso-Scale Spikes and Nano-Trabeculae for Enhanced Bone Integration. *Int. J. Mol. Sci.* **2021**, *22*, 7969. [CrossRef] [PubMed]
4. Hussain, M.; Askari Rizvi, S.H.; Abbas, N.; Sajjad, U.; Shad, M.R.; Badshah, M.A.; Malik, A.I. Recent Developments in Coatings for Orthopedic Metallic Implants. *Coatings* **2021**, *11*, 791. [CrossRef]
5. Floroian, L.; Ristoscu, C.; Mihailescu, N.; Negut, I.; Badea, M.; Ursutiu, D.; Chifiriuc, M.C.; Urzica, I.; Dyia, H.M.; Bleotu, C.; et al. Functionalized antimicrobial composite thin films printing for stainless steel implant coatings. *Molecules* **2016**, *21*, 740. [CrossRef] [PubMed]
6. Cristea, D.; Cunha, L.; Gabor, C.; Ghiuta, I.; Croitoru, C.; Marin, A.; Velicu, L.; Besleaga, A.; Vasile, B. Tantalum Oxynitride Thin Films: Assessment of the Photocatalytic Efficiency and Antimicrobial Capacity. *Nanomaterials* **2019**, *9*, 476. [CrossRef] [PubMed]
7. Subramanian, B.; Sasikumar, P.; Thanka Rajan, S.; Gopal Shankar, K.; Veerapandian, M. Fabrication of Zr-Ti-Si glassy metallic overlay on 3D printed Ti-6Al4V implant prototypes for enhanced biocompatibility. *J. Alloys Compd.* **2023**, *960*, 170933. [CrossRef]
8. Zhu, G.; Wang, G.; Li, J.J. Advances in implant surface modifications to improve osseointegration. *Mater. Adv.* **2021**, *2*, 6901–6927. [CrossRef]
9. Ul Haq, I.; Krukiewicz, K. Antimicrobial approaches for medical implants coating to prevent implants associated infections: Insights to develop durable antimicrobial implants. *Appl. Surf. Sci. Adv.* **2023**, *18*, 100532–100544. [CrossRef]
10. Chen, X.; Zhou, J.; Qian, Y.; Zhao, L.Z. Antibacterial coatings on orthopedic implants. *Mater. Today Bio* **2023**, *19*, 100586–100592. [CrossRef] [PubMed]
11. Floroian, L.; Ristoscu, C.; Candiani, G.; Pastori, N.; Moscatelli, M.; Mihailescu, N.; Negut, I.; Badea, M.; Gilca, M.; Chiesa, R.; et al. Antimicrobial thin films based on ayurvedic plants extracts embedded in a bioactive glass matrix. *Appl. Surf. Sci.* **2017**, *417*, 224–233. [CrossRef]
12. Jeevanandam, J.; Danquah, M.K.; Pan, S. Plant-derived nanobiomaterials as a potential next generation dental implant surface modifier. *Front. Mater.* **2021**, *8*, 666202. [CrossRef]

13. Hassan, S.; Khan, T.J.; Ali, M.N.; Bilal, N. Development of plant based bioactive, anticoagulant and antioxidant surface coatings for medical implants. *Mater. Today Commun.* **2022**, *33*, 104516. [CrossRef]
14. Ghafoor, B.; Najabat Ali, M. Synthesis and in vitro evaluation of natural drug loaded polymeric films for cardiovascular applications. *J. Bioact. Compat. Polym.* **2022**, *37*, 98–114. [CrossRef]
15. Kharat, Z.; Sadri, M.; Kabiri, M. Herbal Extract Loaded Chitosan/PEO Nanocomposites as Antibacterial Coatings of Orthopaedic Implants. *Fibers Polym.* **2021**, *22*, 989–999. [CrossRef]
16. Virk, R.S.; Rehman, M.A.U.; Munawar, M.A.; Schubert, D.W.; Goldmann, W.H.; Dusza, J.; Boccaccini, A.R. Curcumin-Containing Orthopedic Implant Coatings Deposited on Poly-Ether-Ether-Ketone/Bioactive Glass/Hexagonal Boron Nitride Layers by Electrophoretic Deposition. *Coatings* **2019**, *9*, 572. [CrossRef]
17. Raj, R.; Duraisamy, N.; Raj, V. Drug loaded chitosan/aloe vera nanocomposite on Ti for orthopedic applications. *Mater. Today Proc.* **2022**, *51*, 1714–1719.
18. Negut, I.; Floroian, L.; Ristoscu, C.; Mihailescu, C.N.; Mirza Rosca, J.C.; Tozar, T.; Badea, M.; Grumezescu, V.; Hapenciuc, C.; Mihailescu, I.N. Functional bioglass—Biopolymer double nanostructure for natural antimicrobial drug extracts delivery. *Nanomaterials* **2020**, *10*, 385. [CrossRef] [PubMed]
19. Yontar, A.K.; Çevik, S. Electrospray deposited plant-based polymer nanocomposite coatings with enhanced antibacterial activity for Ti-6Al-4V implants. *Prog. Org. Coat.* **2024**, *186*, 107965. [CrossRef]
20. Park, J.; Chi, L.; Kwon, H.Y.; Lee, J.; Kim, S.; Hong, S. Decaffeinated green tea extract as a nature-derived antibiotic alternative: An application in antibacterial nano-thin coating on medical implants. *Food Chem.* **2022**, *383*, 132399. [CrossRef]
21. Schuhladen, K.; Roether, J.A.; Boccaccini, A.R. Bioactive glasses meet phytotherapeutics: The potential of natural herbal medicines to extend the functionality of bioactive glasses. *Biomaterials* **2019**, *217*, 119288. [CrossRef]
22. Ilyas, K.; Singer, L.; Akhtar, M.; Bourauel, C.P.; Boccaccini, A.R. Boswellia sacra Extract-Loaded Mesoporous Bioactive Glass Nano Particles: Synthesis and Biological Effects. *Pharmaceutics* **2022**, *14*, 126. [CrossRef]
23. Negut, I.; Grumezescu, V.; Ficai, A.; Grumezescu, A.M.; Holban, A.M.; Popescu, R.C.; Savu, D.; Vasile, B.S.; Socol, G. MAPLE deposition of Nigella sativa functionalized Fe3O4 nanoparticles for antimicrobial coatings. *Appl. Surf. Sci.* **2018**, *455*, 513–521. [CrossRef]
24. *ISO 10993-6:2016*; Biological Evaluation of Medical Devices Part 6: Tests for Local Effects after Implantation. Available online: https://www.iso.org/standard/61089.html (accessed on 14 February 2018).
25. Almeida, D.; Sartoretto, S.C.; Calasans-Maia, J.A.; Ghiraldini, B.; Bezerra, F.J.B.; Granjeiro, J.M.; Calasans-Maia, M.D. In vivo osseointegration evaluation of implants coated with nanostructured hydroxyapatite in low density bone. *PLoS ONE* **2023**, *18*, e0282067. [CrossRef]
26. Weiner, I.D.; Mitch, W.E.; Sands, J.M. Urea and Ammonia Metabolism and the Control of Renal Nitrogen Excretion. *Clin. J. Am. Soc. Nephrol.* **2015**, *10*, 1444–1458. [CrossRef] [PubMed]
27. Kurz, A.; Seifert, J. Factors Influencing Proteolysis and Protein Utilization in the Intestine of Pigs: A Review. *Animals* **2021**, *11*, 3551. [CrossRef] [PubMed]
28. Tesfa, E.; Munshea, A.; Nibret, E.; Mekonnen, D.; Sinishaw, M.A.; Gizaw, S.T. Maternal serum uric acid, creatinine and blood urea levels in the prediction of pre-eclampsia among pregnant women attending ANC and delivery services at Bahir Dar city public hospitals, northwest Ethiopia: A case-control study. *Heliyon* **2022**, *8*, e11098. [CrossRef]
29. Kellum, J.A.; Romagnani, P.; Ashuntantang, G.; Ronco, C.; Zarbock, A.; Anders, H.J. Acute kidney injury. *Nat. Rev. Dis. Primers* **2021**, *7*, 52–67. [CrossRef] [PubMed]
30. Buford, T.W.; Kreider, R.B.; Stout, J.R.; Greenwood, M.; Campbell, B.; Spano, M.; Ziegenfuss, T.; Lopez, H.; Landis, J.; Antonio, J. International Society of Sports Nutrition position stand: Creatine supplementation and exercise. *J. Int. Soc. Sports Nutr.* **2007**, *30*, 6–18. [CrossRef]
31. Gounden, V.; Bhatt, H.; Jialal, I. Renal Function Tests. In *StatPearls [Internet]*; StatPearls Publishing: Treasure Island, FL, USA, 2023. Available online: https://www.ncbi.nlm.nih.gov/books/NBK507821/ (accessed on 12 November 2023).
32. Date, K.; Yamazaki, T.; Toyoda, Y.; Hoshi, K.; Ogawa, H. α-Amylase expressed in human small intestinal epithelial cells is essential for cell proliferation and differentiation. *J. Cell. Biochem.* **2020**, *121*, 1238–1249. [CrossRef] [PubMed]
33. Matull, W.R.; Pereira, S.P.; O'Donohue, J.W. Biochemical markers of acute pancreatitis. *J. Clin. Pathol.* **2006**, *59*, 340–344. [CrossRef]
34. Vihinen, M. Types and effects of protein variations. *Hum. Genet.* **2015**, *134*, 405–421. [CrossRef] [PubMed]
35. Powers, A.D.; Palecek, S.P. Protein analytical assays for diagnosing, monitoring, and choosing treatment for cancer patients. *J. Healthc. Eng.* **2012**, *3*, 503–534. [CrossRef]
36. Masrour Roudsari, J.; Mahjoub, S. Quantification and comparison of bone-specific alkaline phosphatase with two methods in normal and paget's specimens. *Casp. J. Intern. Med.* **2012**, *3*, 478–483.
37. Thio, Q.C.B.S.; Karhade, A.V.; Notman, E.; Raskin, K.A.; Lozano-Calderón, S.A.; Ferrone, M.L.; Bramer, J.A.M.; Schwab, J.H. Serum alkaline phosphatase is a prognostic marker in bone metastatic disease of the extremity. *J. Orthop.* **2020**, *22*, 346–351. [CrossRef] [PubMed]
38. Huang, C.W.; Wu, T.H.; Hsu, H.Y.; Pan, K.T.; Lee, C.W.; Chong, S.W.; Huang, S.F.; Lin, S.E.; Yu, M.C.; Chen, S.M. Reappraisal of the Role of Alkaline Phosphatase in Hepatocellular Carcinoma. *J. Pers. Med.* **2022**, *12*, 518. [CrossRef] [PubMed]
39. Riancho, J.A. Diagnostic Approach to Patients with Low Serum Alkaline Phosphatase. *Calcif. Tissue Int.* **2023**, *112*, 289–296. [CrossRef] [PubMed]

40. Cao, R.; Wang, L.P. Serological diagnosis of liver metastasis in patients with breast cancer. *Cancer Biol. Med.* **2012**, *9*, 57–62.
41. Urso, C.; Brucculeri, S.; Caimi, G. Marked elevation of transaminases and pancreatic enzymes in severe malnourished male with eating disorder. *Clin Ter.* **2013**, *164*, e387–e391.
42. Checa, J.; Aran, J.M. Reactive Oxygen Species: Drivers of Physiological and Pathological Processes. *J. Inflamm. Res.* **2020**, *13*, 1057–1073. [CrossRef]
43. Ściskalska, M.; Ołdakowska, M.; Marek, G.; Milnerowicz, H. Changes in the Activity and Concentration of Superoxide Dismutase Isoenzymes (Cu/Zn SOD, MnSOD) in the Blood of Healthy Subjects and Patients with Acute Pancreatitis. *Antioxidants* **2020**, *9*, 948. [CrossRef] [PubMed]
44. Nandi, A.; Yan, L.J.; Jana, C.K.; Das, N. Role of Catalase in Oxidative Stress- and Age-Associated Degenerative Diseases. *Oxidative Med. Cell. Longev.* **2019**, *2019*, 9613090. [CrossRef] [PubMed]
45. Luos, E.; Loscalzo, J.; Handy, D.E. Glutathione peroxidase-1 in health and disease: From molecular mechanisms to therapeutic opportunities. *Antioxid. Redox Signal.* **2011**, *15*, 1957–1997.
46. Ou, R.; Aodeng, G.; Ai, J. Advancements in the Application of the Fenton Reaction in the Cancer Microenvironment. *Pharmaceutics* **2023**, *15*, 2337. [CrossRef] [PubMed]
47. Handy, D.E.; Loscalzo, J. The role of glutathione peroxidase-1 in health and disease. *Free Radic. Biol. Med.* **2022**, *188*, 146–161. [CrossRef] [PubMed]
48. Eason, R. *Pulsed Laser Deposition of Thin Films: Applications-Led Growth of Functional Materials*; Wiley-Interscience, John Wiley & Sons, Inc.: Hoboken, NJ, USA, 2007; pp. 424–476.
49. Rabe, H. Referenzwerte blutchemischer Parameter bei Meerschweinchen bestimmt mit dem Vettest® 8008 [Reference ranges for biochemical parameters in guinea pigs for the Vettest®8008 blood analyzer]. *Tierarztl Prax Ausg K Kleintiere Heimtiere* **2011**, *39*, 170–175. [PubMed]
50. Islas, J.F.; Acosta, E.; G-Buentello, Z.; Delgado-Gallegos, J.L.; Moreno-Treviño, M.G.; Escalante, B.; Moreno-Cuevas, J.E. An overview of Neem (*Azadirachta indica*) and its potential impact on health. *J. Funct. Foods* **2020**, *74*, 104171. [CrossRef]
51. Shen, M.; Men, R.; Fan, X.; Wang, T.; Huang, C.; Wang, H.; Ye, T.; Luo, X.; Yang, L. Total glucosides of paeony decreases apoptosis of hepatocytes and inhibits maturation of dendritic cells in autoimmune hepatitis. *Biomed. Pharmacother.* **2020**, *124*, 109911. [CrossRef]
52. Adhikari, J.; Saha, P.; Sinha, A. Surface modification of metallic bone implants—Polymer and polymer-assisted coating for bone in-growth. In *Fundamental Bio-Materials: Metals*; Balakrishnan, P., Sreekala, M.S., Thomas, S., Eds.; Woodhead Publishing Series in Biomaterials; Woodhead Publishing: Cambridge, UK, 2018; pp. 299–321.
53. Rondanelli, M.; Faliva, M.A.; Tartara, A.; Gasparri, C.; Perna, S.; Infantino, V.; Riva, A.; Petrangolini, G.; Peroni, G. An update on magnesium and bone health. *Biometals* **2021**, *34*, 715–736. [CrossRef]
54. Vishnu, J.; Kesavan, P.; Shankar, B.; Dembińska, K.; Swiontek Brzezinska, M.; Kaczmarek-Szczepańska, B. Engineering Antioxidant Surfaces for Titanium-Based Metallic Biomaterials. *J. Funct. Biomater.* **2023**, *14*, 344. [CrossRef] [PubMed]
55. ISO 5832-1:2024; Implants for Surgery—Metallic Materials—Part 1: Wrought Stainless Steel. Available online: https://www.iso.org/standard/83775.html (accessed on 14 February 2024).
56. Liguori, F.; Amadio, S.; Volonté, C. Where and Why Modeling Amyotrophic Lateral Sclerosis. *Int. J. Mol. Sci.* **2021**, *22*, 3977. [CrossRef]
57. LAW No. 149 of 24 July 2019 for the Amendment of Law No. 43/2014 on the Protection of Animals Used for Scientific Purposes. Available online: https://legislatie.just.ro/Public/DetaliiDocumentAfis/216591 (accessed on 8 October 2019).
58. European Animal Research Association. EU Regulations on Animal Research. Available online: https://www.eara.eu/animal-research-law (accessed on 14 February 2018).
59. Jackson, N.; Assad, M.; Vollmer, D.; Stanley, J.; Chagnon, M. Histopathological Evaluation of Orthopedic Medical Devices: The State-of-the-art in Animal Models, Imaging, and Histomorphometry Techniques. *Toxicol. Pathol.* **2019**, *47*, 280–296. [CrossRef] [PubMed]
60. Shuster, A.; Frenkel, G.; Kleinman, S.; Peleg, O.; Ianculovici, C.; Mijiritsky, E.; Kaplan, I. Retrospective Clinicopathological Analysis of 65 Peri-Implant Lesions. *Medicina* **2021**, *57*, 1069. [CrossRef] [PubMed]
61. Milinkovic, I.; Krasavcevic, A.D.; Jankovic, S. Immunohistochemical analysis of soft tissue response to polyetheretherketone (PEEK) and titanium healing abutments on dental implants: A randomized pilot clinical study. *BMC Oral Health* **2022**, *22*, 484–492. [CrossRef] [PubMed]
62. Anderson, J.M.; Rodriguez, A.; Chang, D.T. Foreign body reaction to biomaterials. *Semin. Immunol.* **2008**, *20*, 86–100. [CrossRef] [PubMed]
63. Mateescu, M.C.; Grigorescu, S.; Socea, B.; Bloanca, V.; Grigorescu, O.D. Contribution to the Personalized Management of the Nosocomial Infections: A New Paradigm Regarding the Influence of the Community Microbial Environment on the Incidence of the Healthcare-Associated Infections (HAI) in Emergency Hospital Surgical Departments. *J. Pers. Med.* **2023**, *13*, 210. [CrossRef] [PubMed]

Disclaimer/Publisher's Note: The statements, opinions and data contained in all publications are solely those of the individual author(s) and contributor(s) and not of MDPI and/or the editor(s). MDPI and/or the editor(s) disclaim responsibility for any injury to people or property resulting from any ideas, methods, instructions or products referred to in the content.